Farewell to the God of Plague

Farewell to the God of Plague

CHAIRMAN MAO'S CAMPAIGN TO
DEWORM CHINA

Miriam Gross

UNIVERSITY OF CALIFORNIA PRESS

University of California Press, one of the most distinguished university presses in the United States, enriches lives around the world by advancing scholarship in the humanities, social sciences, and natural sciences. Its activities are supported by the UC Press Foundation and by philanthropic contributions from individuals and institutions. For more information, visit www.ucpress.edu.

University of California Press
Oakland, California

Library of Congress Cataloging-in-Publication Data

Gross, Miriam, 1969- author.
    Farewell to the god of plague : Chairman Mao's campaign to deworm China / Miriam Gross.
        pages cm
    Includes bibliographical references and index.
    ISBN 978–0-520–28883–6 (cloth : alk. paper)) —
    ISBN 978–0-520–96364–1 (e-edition)
    1.   Schistosomiasis—China—Prevention—History—20th century.
    2.   Schistosomiasis—Treatment—China—History—20th century.
    3.   Medical policy—China—History—20th century. 4.   Medical care—China—History—20th century.   I. Title.
    RA644.S3G76 2015
    362.1969′6300951—dc23   2015025634

Manufactured in the United States of America

24   23   22   21   20   19   18   17   16   15
10   9   8   7   6   5   4   3   2   1

In keeping with a commitment to support environmentally responsible and sustainable printing practices, UC Press has printed this book on Natures Natural, a fiber that contains 30% post-consumer waste and meets the minimum requirements of ANSI/NISO Z39.48–1992 (R 1997) (*Permanence of Paper*).

This book is dedicated to the many doctors, activists, and Party members who fought against great odds to make the snail fever campaign succeed.

It is also dedicated to my grandparents:

To my grandma Clara, whose wonderful stories of her childhood helped turn me into a historian.

To my grandpa Sam, whose clarity of vision and strategic mind set a benchmark for wending my way through difficulty.

To my grandma Mollie, whose combination of grit and caring showed me the best way to get through life.

FAREWELL TO THE GOD OF PLAGUE

Mao Zedong

When reading the *People's Daily* on June 30, 1958, I saw that Yujiang County had wiped out schistosomiasis. My mind churned with so many thoughts, I could not sleep. A gentle breeze blew warmly as the rising sun overlooked my window. Looking afar at the southern sky, I was inspired to write.

I.

Crystal-clear water
Emerald mountains,
Gorgeous to no avail.
Even Hua Tuo,
[The god of medicine],
Was helpless
Before this little worm.

In thousands of villages
Overrun with weeds,
Men are wasting away, shitting.
Thousands of homes
Are deserted.
Ghosts sing there.

Sitting here every day
We travel eighty thousand *li*.
Surveying from afar
I see a thousand Milky Ways.

Should the Cowherd inquire of the God of Plague,
The God would reply:
The same joys and grief
Pass away with the tides.

II.

Poplars and willows
Gust in the spring wind,
Swelling to a million.
The six hundred million
Of this sacred land,
All as great as the gods Shun and Yao.

At our whim,
Red rain turns into waves,
With our effort,
Emerald mountains turn
Into bridges.

With lustrous hoes,
We can flatten,
Linking the Five Peaks.
With arms like iron,
We can move the earth,
Shaking the Three Rivers.

May I ask, God of Plague,
Where can you go?
Paper boats burn,
Candles ignite scorching the skies,
[Sending you home].

Translation by Miriam Gross and Bo Kong

CONTENTS

ILLUSTRATIONS

TABLES

FIGURES

MAP

ACKNOWLEDGMENTS

This book could not have been written without the help, support, and insight of a wide community of scholars, scientists, archivists, administrators, campaign participants, friends, and family. I was very lucky to have Peter Gillette as my earliest professional mentor. He reshaped my writing along more realistic lines and introduced me to the world of hospitals, medicine, and underserved communities. I have no doubt that my decision to study the history of public health was directly related to my experiences with Peter, and his example of combining humanitarian outreach with medical expertise influenced how I researched this campaign. During my Columbia master's program, I gained my earliest graduate mentoring from Madeleine Zelin and Thomas Bernstein, both of whom combined breadth of scholarship with inspirational teaching.

My greatest debt goes to Joseph Esherick and Paul Pickowicz, who created a spectacular modern Chinese history program at University of California, San Diego (UCSD). Joe's critical inquiry and extensive knowledge shaped me as a scholar; Paul helped me to be a better writer and effectively argue my point; together they created a fantastic, multigenerational academic community of fellow students and faculty that will stand me in good stead throughout my academic career. I am particularly grateful to Ye Wa, a bosom buddy, who not only labored under the burden of helping me conquer my first academic Chinese, but also was the first person who told me about Mao's snail fever campaign and worked with me at the beginning of my research. After the UCSD program, Joe and Ye Wa became colleagues and friends. My UCSD network was also critical to my success. Marta Hanson, now at Johns Hopkins, introduced me to the history of Chinese medicine; Andrew Scull widened my inquiry to public health, colonial medicine, politics, and society;

and Martha Lampland familiarized me with the history of science and provided depth through her work on science in Hungarian Communist systems. All three have gone above and beyond as long-term mentors and inspirations. Marta Hanson, Suzanne Cahill, Lu Weijing, and Sarah Schneewind provided me with a grounding in earlier Chinese history and encouraged me to think beyond the modern period. Dick Madsen became both an academic mentor and personal friend. He helped me think about how moral and spiritual issues intertwine with politics. Finally, Gail Hershatter, my outside committee member from University of California, Santa Cruz, has been an unfailing mentor. Her incisive comments and knowledge about gender studies have served as an inspiration.

A series of fellowships enabled both my graduate experience and my work in China. I am very grateful for the UCSD Chinese History Fellowship; the University of California Pacific Rim Award; the Fulbright Institute of International Education Fellowship; the Social Science Research Council International Dissertation Fellowship; and two University of Oklahoma Junior Faculty Research Fellowships. Financial support was also provided by the Office of the Vice President for Research, University of Oklahoma. Thank-you all.

My work in China would not have been possible without my affiliation with Fudan University and the help of Gao Xi, my faculty mentor, a historian of Chinese medicine.Professor Gao shared her house, expertise, and connections, providing a true example of hospitality and mentoring. I cannot thank her enough. I also owe great thanks to the institutions, librarians, archivists, scientists, and museum directors who not only made this work possible but also helped me accomplish it. I extend special thanks to the Second Historical Archive, the Shanghai Municipal Archive, the Qingpu District Archive, the Jiangxi and Jiangsu Provincial Archives, the Beijing National Library, the Beijing Chinese Academy of Sciences Library, the Shanghai Municipal Library and its off-site book depository, Fudan Library, the Shanghai Institute of Parasitic Diseases, the Qingpu Department of Health, the Rentun Schistosomiasis Control Exhibition, the Yujiang County Songwenshen Memorial Hall and archive, the UC Berkeley East Asian Library, and the UC Berkeley Center for Chinese Studies. All of you made a special effort to work with the sometimes difficult requests of this foreign researcher.

My two departments at the University of Oklahoma, Norman—the Department of History and the Department of International and Area

Studies—were each very supportive in different ways. The women faculty in the History Department provided me with political and academic advice; Garret Olberding and Elyssa Faison, my closest peers studying East Asian history, have been particularly helpful and encouraging. I owe special thanks to my department chairs—Mark Frazier, Rob Griswold, Jamie Hart, and Mitchell Smith—for your guidance and belief in me.

University of California Press has done spectacular work on the book. Reed Malcolm shepherded the manuscript through every difficulty. My anonymous reviewers provided many wise and helpful suggestions. Ann Burgess supplied a scientist's feedback on the whole work. Julie Van Pelt did a fantastic copyediting job. Finally, Carol Benedict at Georgetown University started with the prospectus and read to the very end. She had a crucial role in shaping the work's arguments. Any remaining mistakes, however, are completely my own.

This book could not have been written without my family. My father Jerrold Gross was excited and interested in this project every step of the way, but did not live to see it published. My Chinese sister, Shiao Chin Zhu, stimulated my fascination with China as a teenager by telling me one crazy Cultural Revolution tale after another. My brother Steve, sister-in-law Cordelia, and nephew Samuel rooted for me, helped me with technological issues, and in Samuel's case, generously offered to do a last-minute edit and read of the book. Finally, my mother Carol has been the anchor of the entire project, encouraging me, commenting on the science and logic, and reading and editing multiple drafts. She has also provided an example of putting people first even while maintaining academic integrity and pursuing new knowledge with tenacity and joy. Without my family's unstinting encouragement, this work would never have seen the light.

Introduction

WORMS HAVE PLAGUED HUMANITY SINCE the beginning of time. Chairman Mao's crusade against schistosomiasis, a devastating parasitic disease, immortalized in his 1958 poem "Farewell to the God of Plague," stands as one of the most famous public health campaigns in the history of the People's Republic of China (PRC). The story of how and why it succeeded is fixed in both Western and Chinese scholarship, and its reputation is so compelling that its methods are still used in China, most recently in the campaign against SARS. When I first started research, Chinese people were dumbfounded. They always told me: "What is there to find out? It was a hugely popular campaign that totally eliminated the disease!" I pointed out that close to a million people in China have the disease now. Further, few people love anything for thirty years, particularly when it involves chasing after miniscule snails, the disease's vector. Most people shook their heads at my ignorance, reiterated that everyone loved the campaign, and promptly changed the topic.

The more I examined archival and memoir accounts, the more this campaign and the equally famous Maoist primary health medical model were called into question. These campaigns were touted for their popular support and patriotic participation in disease prevention activities, such as altering personal hygiene. However, personal accounts make it clear that there was widespread dismay at the intrusive socialist state, particularly when it got involved in telling people how to defecate. Effective local resistance and concurrent efforts at decentralization should have made it easy for local leaders to ignore such campaigns. How then did the government make people do this work? Even more surprising was the finding that many villagers and rural cadres disliked health campaigns. Why, then, did these campaigns actually succeed?

Assessments of Maoist-era grassroots science and public health efforts have changed over time. Spurred by Joshua Horn's 1969 book on Chinese public health, *Away With All Pests,* North American and European scholars became enthralled by the affordable and cooperative Chinese primary health care model, which helped inspire one of the most important milestones of global public health, the World Health Organization Declaration on Primary Health Care in 1978 at Alma-Ata. Scholarship on the campaign to eradicate schistosomiasis, hereafter called snail fever, which peaked in the 1970s, describes the effort as a unitary process of state control that was exceedingly popular among the masses, demonstrating the ability of the Chinese government to carry out its mandates at the grassroots level. Both scholars and the Chinese government ascribe campaign success to patriotic mass mobilization efforts directed primarily at disease prevention. These replaced complex biomedical solutions with simple, labor-intensive methods, like suffocating the snails, successfully bringing the disease under control in 1958.[1] Enthusiasm about both the snail fever campaign and Maoist grassroots science and public health waned in the 1980s when exaggerated government statistics about grassroots accomplishments came to light. At the same time, hyperbolic accounts of "red and expert" semiliterate rural cadres who were supposedly able to replace professional scientists, lead scientific institutes, and perform surgery after only a month of training were discredited. As scholars and policy makers learned more about the destruction of the professional scientific and medical establishments during the Cultural Revolution (1966–76), they began to doubt all Maoist claims of scientific endeavors. It seemed inconceivable that popular science could flourish even as professional science was being destroyed, a view many scholars still hold today. As a result, since the late 1970s there has been no book-length scholarly monograph assessing the Maoist primary health care model.[2] This is particularly problematic because early accounts were perforce based on government propaganda and visits to model communes, rather than on the campaign report archives now available that divulge how this model actually worked.

Farewell to the God of Plague presents the first detailed exploration of the human, technical, and organizational challenges faced by grassroots health campaigns during the Maoist era—and how the state successfully overcame them to make its will manifest at the local level. Using newly available archival evidence, my analysis shows that the campaign succeeded because of its treatment activities rather than its prevention efforts, thus revising existing scholarship in public health, history, and political science. By uncovering the

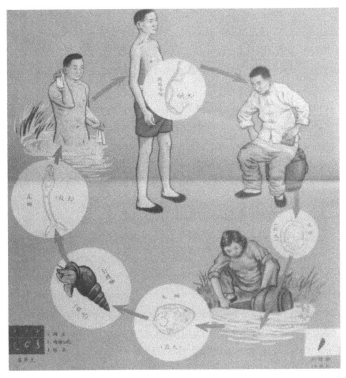

FIGURE 1. Snail fever campaign poster teaching the disease life cycle. Zhejiang kexue jishu puji xiehui and Zhejiang weisheng shiyanyuan, *Xiaomie xuexichongbing guatu* (Beijing: Renmin weisheng chubanshe, 1956), poster no. 2.

complex role of grassroots science in legitimating the regime during the antiscientific Maoist era, *Farewell to the God of Plague* also proposes a new mechanism of state power, "scientific consolidation," which facilitated Chinese Communist Party (CCP) control in rural areas without the need for an intact bureaucracy or the use of overwhelming force.

SNAIL FEVER, A SERIOUS PUBLIC HEALTH HAZARD

Snail fever, also known as bilharzia, schistosomiasis, and big belly disease, is a devastating waterborne disease caused by a parasitic worm that leads to a decades-long descent to disability and eventual death. Over 243 million people are infected with snail fever in seventy-eight countries (90 percent of them in Africa), resulting in over 200,000 deaths annually. An additional 700 million are at risk from the disease. According to the World Health Organization and the Centers for Disease Control and Prevention, snail fever is second only to malaria as the most prevalent tropical disease and "the most devastating parasitic disease."[3]

The parasitic species in China, *Schistosoma japonicum,* lays thousands of eggs daily in the intestines of its mammalian host. Eggs leave the body in the host's feces, hatch in water into first-stage microscopic larvae, called miracidia, and then find their next host, the tiny six- to eight-millimeter *Oncomelania hupensis* freshwater snail. Once in the snails, only a few miracidia mature into sporocysts (usually 1–2 percent). However, the few snails with sporocysts release as many as a thousand cercariae, the microscopic second-stage larvae, every day. Cercariae left behind in the snail's slime trail burrow through the skin of a mammalian host and then travel to the host's intestines, beginning the infectious cycle anew (figure 1).[4] Although many mammals, including humans, can be infected, oxen and water buffalo are the major reservoirs of the disease because they produce a lot of manure, often deposited close to water where the eggs can hatch.[5] Prevention activities focused on keeping the egg-laden manure from reaching water sources by instituting better sanitation and on eliminating the snails.

Snail fever has three stages: acute, chronic, and late. *Acute disease* (Katayama syndrome) is caused by an immune reaction to the invading worm and its eggs in a naïve host (one lacking worms). Often mistaken for malaria, it results in a dangerously high fever that can cause rapid death. The vast majority of people have *chronic disease,* which lasts for many years and is either asymptomatic or exhibits mild symptoms such as fatigue and diarrhea. The long period of chronic infection with few symptoms makes this disease an especially dangerous public health hazard. A few people have *late-stage disease,* whose most notable symptom is massive fluid retention in the stomach. Additional possible symptoms are fever, chronic abdominal pain, diarrhea that is sometimes bloody, malnutrition, anorexia, enervation, enlarged spleen and liver, cerebral lesions, infertility in both sexes, loss of physical and sexual development (i.e., dwarfism), diminished cognitive function in children, and eventual death.[6]

In 1949, snail fever was endemic in eleven provinces in China and in Taiwan. The disease-carrying snail covered approximately 14.5 billion square meters of territory, much of it in canals, rivers, and lakes in south and central China (map 1); 10.6 million people were infected and another 100 million were at risk for

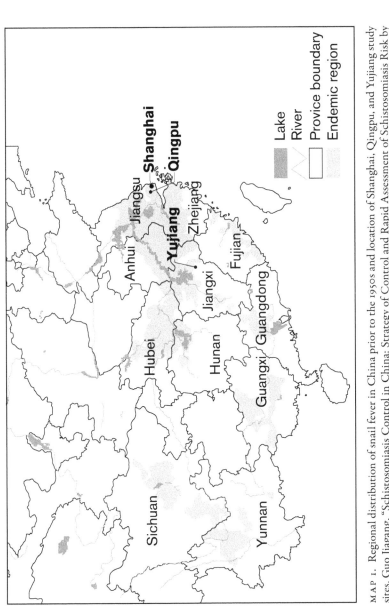

MAP 1.   Regional distribution of snail fever in China prior to the 1950s and location of Shanghai, Qingpu, and Yujiang study sites. Guo Jiagang, "Schistosomiasis Control in China: Strategy of Control and Rapid Assessment of Schistosomiasis Risk by Remote Sensing (RS) and Geographic Information System (GIS)" (Ph.D. dissertation, University of Basel, 2003), 15–16, http://edoc.unibas.ch/245/1/DissB_7169.pdf (accessed July 26, 2015). Map modified by Miriam Gross.

the disease. Prior to treatment and prevention work, snail fever killed about 400,000 people per year in China (about a 4 percent mortality rate).[7]

HISTORY OF SNAIL FEVER IN CHINA THROUGH THE REPUBLICAN PERIOD, 1911–1949

Snail fever likely started parasitizing humans in prehistory, but the first definitive cases found in China were in corpses unearthed in Hunan Province's Mawangdui tombs and Hubei's Fenghuang Mountains, which date from the Han dynasty two thousand years ago.[8] Ancient Chinese medical classics, such as the *Zhu Bing Yuan Hou Lun* (Treatise on causes and symptoms of diseases) by Chao Yuanfang from the Sui dynasty (581–618), recorded diseases that appear similar to snail fever, such as *gubing,* a disease caused by worms in the stomach acquired through contact with water.[9] In 1851, Theodor Maximilian Bilharz identified the parasite causing snail fever in Cairo. In 1905, O. T. Logan, an American doctor, was the first to recognize snail fever in China. Japanese scientists identified the East Asian disease species, *Schistosoma japonicum,* in 1903. They became world experts in the disease, mapping out its life cycle and clinical symptoms, and contributed their expertise to China in both the Republican period (1911–49) and during the early Maoist campaign in the 1950s.[10]

Early efforts to treat the disease in China (1900–1920) were scattered and unsystematic, carried out by medical missionaries and Chinese students of Western medicine. In 1920, Americans Henry Meleney and Ernest Faust joined the faculty of Peking Union Medical College, the premier Western medical school in China, established in 1915. They founded parasitology in China and laid much of the groundwork on snail fever, including determining life cycle, treatment, and initial disease distribution. In 1928, after wresting control of most of the country from warlords, the Nationalists established the country's first national Ministry of Public Health. The ministry launched a field site in south-central China. The field site's Department of Parasitology set up a rural anti–snail fever unit in Zhejiang Province that developed methods of treatment and prevention applicable to rural areas from 1932 to 1949.[11]

Additional work on snail fever was conducted by newly established provincial health departments, the British and Chinese health departments in Shanghai, and private medical research institutions, one of which, the Shanghai Institute of Natural Science, was run by the Japanese. The National

Medical College of Shanghai, renamed the Shanghai First Medical College after 1949, started test sites around Shanghai in the 1930s. Dr. Su Delong, who would later become the leading national expert in the post-1949 snail fever campaign, led one of them.[12]

Communist campaign propaganda during the Maoist era (1949–76) castigated inadequate Nationalist efforts against the disease, suggesting that this proved the Nationalists did not care for the people. However, the Nationalists had limited control over most of their territory, frequent war and budget crises, and few trained Western doctors, making wide-scale treatment and prevention work impossible. Nonetheless, the combined efforts of medical missionaries, foreign researchers, private institutions, and the Nationalists left a key legacy for the People's Republic. Early scholars identified many of China's principal infectious areas, studied the parasite and intermediate host life cycles, and investigated treatment methods. Mao Shou-Pai, director of the Shanghai Institute of Parasitic Diseases said, "The few parasitologists trained during that period [i.e., the Republican era] became the nucleus of parasitological activities after Liberation, both in educational institutions and in research institutions."[13] The People's Republic started with more professional researchers focused on snail fever than almost any other parasitic disease. Nationalist test sites also investigated how to reach out to rural populations and provided the initial strategies used by the CCP in its campaigns.

EXPLORING CAMPAIGN DIVERSITY IN THE PRC: THE CASE STUDIES

The PRC national snail fever campaign began in 1949, with peaks in 1957–58, during the Great Leap Forward; in 1966–71, during the Cultural Revolution; and most recently in 1992–2001, during a joint venture between the Chinese government and the World Bank. It was conducted in all eleven provinces with snail fever, each varying in environmental, political, and socioeconomic conditions and in reaction to the eras' complex politics. To encompass this diversity, I chose three case studies: urban Shanghai, neighboring suburban Qingpu County in Jiangsu Province (incorporated into Shanghai as Qingpu District in 1958), and rural Yujiang County in Jiangxi Province (see map 1). Information from my case studies of these sites, all of which were models qualifying for extra government resources, is supplemented with data from nonmodel areas in Jiangsu and Jiangxi Provinces.

Shanghai was the national headquarters for the snail fever campaign. With more and better Western trained medical personnel than elsewhere, Shanghai became the national center of snail fever research, as well as the location of China's pharmaceutical and chemical industries that supplied drugs and molluscicides. Because of better education, the population could assimilate more of the scientific ideas underlying the campaign and contribute more to campaign work. Finally, the city had a large tax base to provide funding. As a result, Shanghai not only ran the best campaign but often pioneered campaign practices one to two decades before other sites.[14]

Qingpu, an almost entirely rural county of 240,000 people, had the advantage of close proximity to Shanghai. Qingpu was the national test site for the campaign, developing many of the practices disseminated to the rest of China. Although inferior to those of Shanghai, Qingpu's economics, educational achievements, and medical system and personnel were far superior to those of most rural counties. By 1949, Qingpu had 17,000 elementary and 1,000 middle-school students. By 1955, every village in the county had an elementary school, thirty-four with attached middle schools, and the county even had outreach schools for children of fishermen.[15] By 1949, Qingpu had four hospitals with forty-nine in-patient beds, two health service centers, about 250 Chinese medicine doctors engaged in private practice, and forty medical workers. By 1951, all county private practitioners of Western and Chinese medicine were organized in thirty-six united clinics that eventually became the backbone for the commune hospital system. This primary care system was augmented with specialty institutions addressing leprosy, tuberculosis, mental health, and Chinese medicine.[16]

In contrast, the national model site, Yujiang County, had an entirely rural population of 137,831, with few educational facilities and medical personnel. Yujiang had only three primary schools in 1949 and only eight in 1953, producing about 147 graduates per year. More primary schools were not built until 1960. When the first middle school was built in 1967, the county still had only nineteen elementary schools.[17] Yujiang had only a single crumbling "hospital" with four personnel in 1949. By 1958, Yujiang still had only fifty-three health personnel, mostly cursorily trained Chinese medicine doctors.[18]

The study sites also differed in snail fever distribution and prevalence. Qingpu, the Shanghai suburb, was the most severely affected, with drainage both from Lake Tai, a reservoir for snails, and from the Yangtze River. Its sluggish, muddy water channels, covering 20.5 percent of the county, were a snail's paradise. With the area's constant flooding (more than once every five years in low-lying areas), snails covered most of the land (fifty-two out of fifty-eight townships), and almost all residents lived in highly infectious areas.[19] On average, 40–60 percent of the population had snail fever, rising to over 90 percent in some places, making Qingpu one of the worst snail fever sites in China.[20] Shanghai, its next-door neighbor, received snails from both Qingpu and the ring of counties encircling its noninfected core (the disease was endemic in nine of these ten counties). Shanghai also had a very large infected population, mostly in the northern and western areas of the city.

Jiangxi Province, where Yujiang County is located, was well suited for snail fever, with a northern border along the Yangtze River, which carries snails throughout central China, and China's largest freshwater lake, Poyang, a reservoir for snails, whose annual flood cycle disseminates them broadly.[21] However, Yujiang County was not among the most severely affected areas. It is one step away from the counties surrounding the lake and received snails indirectly through one of the lake's major feeder rivers, the Xinjiang, and one of its large tributaries, the Baita River. Yujiang had low to intermediate snail fever, concentrated in four townships, two state-run farms, and one town (Dengfu) that abutted the rivers. Only 12.1 percent of the county's land, about 237 acres (0.96 km2), was actually snail infested.[22] This infectious zone had a total population of 8,100 in 1949 and 13,450 in 1957, and infection rates of 17.5 percent. By way of comparison, almost twenty times as many people were infected in the Shanghai suburb, Qingpu (157,232), as in Yujiang, and snails covered an area seventy-seven times greater in Qingpu (74.3 km^2) than in Yujiang. Thus, Yujiang's snail fever problem was limited to a few very bad spots surrounded by lightly hit areas.[23]

These preexisting differences in geography, disease epidemiology and dissemination, knowledge and education levels of the population, available medical expertise, and numbers of medical personnel would all play a crucial role in what snail fever campaign personnel could accomplish and in their possible routes to success.

REEXAMINING THE MAOIST PRIMARY HEALTH MODEL AND THE ROLE OF GRASSROOTS SCIENCE

Using archival evidence from urban Shanghai, suburban Qingpu District, rural Yujiang County, and Jiangsu and Jiangxi Provinces, I revise the earlier prevailing narrative of the snail fever campaign, while refuting more recent skepticism by demonstrating how and why this globally renowned public health model actually worked. Rather than exhibiting a unitary trajectory, campaign performance depended on the resources, connections, and interest level at each site and did not succeed completely until the early 1980s. Despite the predominant story line, villagers and local cadres did not support the campaign, and educational efforts had minimal impact on fostering understanding or participation in prevention. Indeed, every aspect of the famous prevention campaign failed, including efforts to eradicate the disease vector and alter hygiene and sanitation patterns. Rather than establishing effective disease control, the Great Leap Forward campaign actually made the disease worse.

Nevertheless, the snail fever campaign succeeded, not because of prevention efforts, but because of the heretofore unacknowledged work of the campaign's treatment arm along with increased support by local leadership. Treatment was only somewhat successful during the Great Leap (1957–58), since it was hindered by limited treatment subsidies and personnel, but was extremely effective during the Cultural Revolution (1966–71). Financial subsidies, increasingly engaged local leadership, newly educated youth working as barefoot doctors starting in 1970, and, ironically, the professional physicians sent to the countryside who then mentored these new doctors all led to success of the treatment program. By 1981, almost 95 percent of the infected population had been treated successfully (only 704,982 of 11.3 million remained infected).[24] Like most endemic diseases, snail fever is almost impossible to eliminate. Despite Chairman Mao's dream of total eradication, the more realistic public health goal was to bring it under control and then maintain low infection rates. By the end of the Maoist period and shortly after (1949–80), the disease was controlled in most places. However, the Reform-era government (1976–present) paid less attention to snail fever. Today over 800,000 people have the disease, and it is rapidly escalating, reflecting the limited focus on rural health.

My conclusions about the role of science in the campaign open the door for a reassessment of the relationship between science and political control during the Maoist era. Most current scholars view Chairman Mao as antiscience and are therefore dismissive of Maoist revolutionary organizational structures, suggesting that modern, technically oriented (Weberian) bureaucracy reappeared only during the Reform era, coincident with renewed appreciation for professional science by the Party.[25] I demonstrate that although Mao's understanding of science, which I call "grassroots science," is distinct from normative science, it is tightly coupled to regime legitimacy and political consolidation and played a key role in achieving Party control in rural areas. Maoist grassroots science encouraged rural leaders to conduct field investigations and process their data to find solutions for pragmatic problems. Although grassroots science initially often lacked standard scientific criteria, such as reproducibility or control groups, it did teach educated youth the tools for scientific planning. I argue that many rural educated youth became both "red" and "expert" by participating in scientifically oriented campaigns where they learned scientific tools, as well as basic technical and medical skills, and assimilated a more scientific worldview that encouraged them to experiment and reorganize the status quo.

As Chairman Mao pushed his revolutionary agenda of decentralizing and attacking Party bureaucracy, grassroots cadres and educated youth were increasingly responsible for carrying out complicated socialist construction goals with little oversight. Local cadres found that their newly acquired scientific tools—statistics, mapping, modeling, and standardization—were absolutely essential to planning these complex mass campaigns. Notably, these are the same tools that underpin an effective technical bureaucracy. Although rural educated youth gained basic scientific expertise, their limited education precluded them from assimilating scientific skills at a professional level. Professional scientists, physicians, and engineers sent for reeducation in the countryside were also critical to campaign success, not only for their own work, but even more importantly as preceptors for educated youth. Thus, the success of these scientifically oriented campaigns derives from two previously unrecognized factors: the increasingly technical orientation of grassroots rural cadres and their integration with the sophisticated scientific work of urban, highly educated professionals.

Yet, the same scientific tools that empowered rural cadres also helped to control them, revealing a heretofore unstudied method of scientifically based political consolidation. Grassroots cadres presented a special challenge because they often put the needs of their local communities above the Party. The societal chaos and attacks on authority characteristic of revolutionary moments made it even harder for the upper Party to make its will manifest on the ground. However, when local cadres collected statistics and then gave reports in front of peers and superiors, the combination of transparency and statistical benchmarks channeled them to enact the Party's goals and mandated campaign procedures, a process I call "scientific consolidation."

In summary, my archival-based investigation of the celebrated Maoist primary health care model substantially revises the commonly accepted snail fever campaign narrative and reveals the key role of grassroots science in both the success of the campaign and in establishing Party control. I show that simple grassroots prevention activities failed due to popular resistance and that campaign success rested on technically sophisticated treatment jointly conducted by rural educated youth and urban professionals. The state used the science conveyed by these grassroots health campaigns to legitimate itself and to facilitate unpopular, but nonetheless effective, non-health-related rural socialist construction activities. Thus, even as the professional science and bureaucratic establishments were under siege, grassroots science and the consequent dissemination of bureaucratically oriented, scientific tools to rural cadres facilitated the scientific consolidation that helped establish Party control over rural communities.

The book is divided into four sections. The first (chapter 1) is an overview of the snail fever campaign from the perspective of top leadership (1949–1976). The second (chapters 2 and 3) frames campaign resistance by examining structural and economic barriers to the work during the 1950s. The third (chapters 4–6) explores the three arms of the campaign: education (chapter 4), prevention (chapter 5), and treatment (chapter 6). The final section (chapters 7 and 8), examines the many nonhealth benefits of health campaigns for the state.

PART I

From the Eyes at the Top: Overview of the Campaign

————————

CHAPTER ONE

Chairman Mao Weighs In

THE HIGH POLITICS OF THE CAMPAIGN

IT WAS THE END OF May 1949, and the People's Liberation Army had just liberated Shanghai from the Nationalists. Looking ahead, the CCP was focused on completing Communist control of China by taking Taiwan. There was only one impediment. The thirty-seven thousand crack troops from Northern China had no idea how to engage in water-based skirmishes. On August 1, the troops were sent to Shanghai's suburban counties of Songjiang and Qingpu to gain aquatic invasion skills.[1] A couple of weeks later, the swimming soldiers came down with skin rashes. Some were sick enough to be hospitalized. Since the source of the problem was unclear, doctors slowly gathered data and did experimental treatment and education. Two months later, the troops were ordered to stop swimming, but it was too late. Troops were heavily infected with worms. Over fourteen thousand troops, or 38 percent of the top soldiers in China, were incapacitated due to snail fever. Additionally, about 50 percent of the troops had hookworm, 50 percent had roundworm, and 27 percent had whipworm. Treatment by the twelve hundred medical personnel, organized in part by the snail fever expert, Dr. Su Delong, and requisitioned from medical institutions in Shanghai, Hangzhou, and Nanjing, took four months, lasting until April 30, 1950. It is unknown whether this affected the decision to delay attacking Taiwan. However, by June 1950, only two months after the last treatment of the decimated soldiers, the window of opportunity had been lost.[2] China's involvement in the Korean War prompted the United States to move from an unaligned position to protecting Taiwan with its Seventh Fleet.

When Mao Zedong and the Communist Party took over China in 1949, epidemic and endemic diseases were rampant, life expectancy low, infant mortality high, and most people outside cities had never seen a physician or been vaccinated. The military emergency resulting from troops infected with snail fever may have contributed to the decision to dedicate capital and resources toward fighting the disease. However, it is still baffling, given the multitude of problems facing the regime, that the CCP chose to expend enormous resources fighting snail fever, an unknown rural disease that generally took decades to kill its victims. This chapter examines why the national government and Mao Zedong made snail fever a priority and then provides an overview of the campaign's wider political context from 1949 to 1976.

SNAIL FEVER: A PRIORITY?

Initially identified as a threat to military and economic security, and then as an ideological issue, snail fever was a Party health priority from the CCP's very earliest days in power, garnering the personal interest of several top Party members. Except for SARS, this is the only disease campaign labeled as a political rather than a health campaign.

The top Party leadership realized that this disease was a significant impediment to military fitness after the aquatic training debacle. Reinforcing this perception, the disease devastated early recruitment efforts throughout south and central China. Due to the disease, in Jiangsu's hard-hit Songjiang Prefecture (where Taiwan-intended troops learned aquatic skills), 73.6 percent were unfit for duty in 1953; in Greater Shanghai, 33 percent of enlistees could not fight for the same reason in 1954, and Jiangxi Province had similar problems.[3] In the early 1950s, CCP concerns over military fitness and procuring healthy recruits were at an all-time high, as the Party was simultaneously trying to take control of the countryside and participate in the Korean War, where an estimated 700,000–900,000 troops died.[4]

The disease also had a large impact on agricultural productivity. After fifteen years of war, with few remaining factories, agricultural production was the major source of government income and key to obtaining the capital required for the Soviet model of heavy industrial development. Snail fever was endemic in rice-growing regions, negatively influencing the productive capacity of land, labor, and even capital (in the form of oxen and water buffalo). Land with high disease intensity became known as death traps, causing locals to flee. The most frequently abandoned land was also extremely productive prime farmland, generally with a growing season of more than three hundred days, making it amenable to multicropping. According to campaign propaganda, forty-six thousand hectares of deserted, snail-laden land in Hubei, Fujian, and Guangdong Provinces were reclaimed by August 1958, leading to large provincial surpluses.[5] In addition to killing 400,000 people per year (4 percent of an estimated 10 million sick), snail fever decreased productivity of those with mid- to late-stage disease by up to 40 percent. One report estimated that curing 3.5 million people added the equivalent of a million men's labor power to the labor force by 1959.[6] Finally, cattle studies in Jiangxi's Yujiang County found that oxen and water buffalo with snail fever plowed only half as much as healthy animals and had higher miscarriage rates.[7] Given a skyrocketing population and very slim agricultural margins for building heavy industry, the Party felt that ridding the country of this disease was a matter of economic security.

The new Chinese government was not alone in enacting health campaigns for reasons that were advantageous to its agenda. According to Ralph Croizier, particularly for new nations with limited resources, there is often a tension in government-supplied health care. Is public health enacted for humanitarian reasons to relieve individual suffering, or is it a mechanism to increase national strength economically and militarily?[8] There seems little doubt that most health work in China was done to strengthen the country. At an important meeting in Yujiang in January 1956 to launch major campaign work, the government listed four ways that snail fever had an impact, including production, population growth, energetic participation in political activities, and army recruitment. Nowhere mentioned were the human costs of the disease or improving people's well-being. Instead, the government emphasized the military, economic, and political ways the campaign would help the government.[9] This focus was incorporated into assessment of campaign success. When communities demonstrated rising production rates and grain surpluses, and when enlistment numbers and population climbed post-treatment, then the campaign must be achieving its goals. Even Chinese medicine was evaluated based on how much labor power it rescued.[10] This tendency was also true of colonial public health efforts, which were almost entirely focused on improving subjects' working potential. This emphasis became even more pronounced after World War II, when international public health was envisioned primarily as a handmaiden to economic development.[11]

Similar to other health campaigns, the initial ideological rationale for counteracting snail fever was to refute late nineteenth-century descriptions of China as the sick man of Asia. Possibly influenced by ideas stemming from social Darwinism that connected racial fitness, physical prowess, and victory on the world stage, the CCP incorporated rural health and sanitation as a core platform even before taking power in 1949. As early as April 1917, the future Chairman Mao wrote "A Study of Physical Education," where he connected national strength and military spirit to physical education. Upon joining the CCP's Public Health Commission in the 1930s, he identified hygiene as a core Party responsibility in the Jiangxi Soviet in 1934. Mao insisted on medical care and hygiene instruction for all regular and guerrilla military units.[12] Mao also established and directed a committee on public health in Yan'an, the Shaanxi-Gansu-Ningxia Border Region, and held both individual and group-level public health contests among Red Army groups. At Yan'an, the CCP allocated an impressive 6 percent of the budget to health care.[13]

Once in power, the CCP rhetoric made public health a yardstick for measuring progress toward modernity. Curing age-old endemic diseases validated Party leadership and ensured that advantages of the new society were experienced in people's healthy new bodies. Likewise, creating a cleaner living space would make villagers conscious of the new society and empowered to control nature, their age-old enemy. As Chairman Mao explained in his August 30, 1956, speech for the preparatory meeting for the Eighth National Congress: "China used to be stigmatized as a 'decrepit empire,' 'the sick man of East Asia,' a country with a backward economy and a backward culture, with no hygiene, poor at ball games and swimming, where the women had bound feet, the men wore pigtails and eunuchs could still be found. . . . But after six years' work of transformation we have changed the face of China. No one can deny our achievements."[14]

Upon realizing that snail fever helped trigger poverty and infertility, the Party made the campaign a symbol of fighting everything that was holding society back. A 1956 Jiangxi Province report explained: "Socialism will bring a happy new society—how can we have big belly disease in it? If people are lying flat on their backs in bed, how can they be happy?"[15] Newspaper articles repeatedly reported on the campaign and an entire generation memorized Chairman Mao's famous 1958 commemorative poem. In popular memory, eradication of snail fever was seated as a foundational campaign of the era, a symbol of Party success at stamping out intractable ills, and a patriotic demonstration of the power of the people.

The great success of the campaign made it an ideal ideological platform for asserting China's scientific expertise globally. Although possibly a questionable strategy internationally, it was used domestically to legitimate Party rule.

Campaign leaders explained that developed nations, including "American scientists," "up till now had no way of dealing with it [snail fever] and could only shake their heads and heave a sigh."[16] In contrast, CCP success demonstrated that the Party could wield science competitively and proved that socialism could provide benefits unavailable in a capitalist system. The Party asserted that China was the "the first place in the world to eliminate snail fever," a historic achievement with "huge international significance," a sort of medical *Sputnik* symbolizing China's triumphs on the world stage.[17] This also bolstered China's claim to leadership of developing countries. As a 1955 Shanghai report explained: "Egypt has already been treating and preventing snail fever for fifty years without any result. We have experience. We can do a cultural exchange which is of great use to politics."[18]

The personal attention of Premier Zhou Enlai, Vice Premier Chen Yun, and Chairman Mao help account for the success, prominence, and longevity of this campaign. These leaders represented a wide spectrum of political opinion, which helped the campaign to weather the tempestuous politics of the Maoist era. In March 1952, Zhou Enlai became chair of a new central epidemic prevention committee that established the CCP's initial policy toward public health and started China's Patriotic Public Health Campaigns in response to the 1952 germ warfare affair, discussed below.[19] Zhou's specific interest in snail fever is not easy to determine, but it is clear he was actively engaged. When Japanese physicians came to China in November 1955 to convey information available through the World Health Organization (which had yet to accept China as a member), Sasa Manabu, professor at the Institute for Infectious Disease at Tokyo University, met personally with Zhou. Zhou knew enough about the campaign to detail the snail fever situation in south and central China and facilitate the Japanese doctors' visit to the field.[20] When Yujiang's Party secretary came to a Beijing conference on rice production in 1966, Zhou personally rewrote his talk to highlight snail fever and link it to Yujiang's increased productivity.[21] Zhou's precise role needs further research, but he kept actively informed about campaign progress.

Vice Premier Chen Yun was born in Qingpu County, Jiangsu Province, which had some of the highest rates of disease in the country. He grew up surrounded by people suffering from snail fever. In 1957, he paid a special visit to Qingpu to investigate its campaign work and offer his support. Information he learned in Qingpu was conveyed to the State Council and reportedly influenced its decisions about the campaign.[22]

Chairman Mao spent his childhood in Shaoshan Village, Hunan Province, fifty miles from Dongting Lake, a center of regional economic interchange (fishing, cattle raising, and green reed fertilizer collection) and a reservoir for snail fever. The lake disseminates the disease during its annual flooding cycle, when its borders expand greatly. It is very likely that growing up, Mao encountered people with the disease or heard stories about hard-hit areas. Mao also passed through highly infectious areas in Jiangxi in the 1920s and 1930s when fighting against the Nationalists. According to Su Delong, a top snail fever expert and Mao's campaign advisor, Mao had dealt with so many ill villagers and soldiers that when the crack troops were discovered to have the disease in 1949, he became particularly interested in it.[23] After deciding that the Ministry of Public Health (MPH) was doing an inadequate job in 1955, Mao created a dedicated nine-person leadership small group (LSG), directly under the Central Committee, to run future campaign activities (discussed below). Mao was also personally involved in early national snail fever conferences. In Mao's December 1955 "Circular Requesting Opinions on 17 Articles on Agricultural Work," a key document for determining agricultural priorities, snail fever topped the list of diseases slated for elimination in Article 12. In "Second Preface to *Upsurge of Socialism in China's Countryside*," written at the same time, Mao repeated injunctions to wipe out diseases, with snail fever as his only specific example.[24] While in Shanghai in 1957 and the 1960s, Mao consulted with Su Delong about the campaign, and in 1958 while in Anhui, Mao visited a provincial museum exhibit about snail fever (see figure 2). Finally, upon hearing that Yujiang County, Jiangxi Province, was the first to eliminate the disease, Mao was reportedly so excited that he stayed up all night and wrote his famous poem, "Farewell to the God of Plague" (see this book's epigraph).[25] Chairman Mao's decades-long attention elevated the campaign until it was politically impossible for it to fail.

Perhaps because of linkages to military security, economic development, and Chairman Mao, the snail fever campaign was designated as a political campaign. As Wei Wenbo, deputy director of the nine-person LSG put it, "Elimination of snail fever impacts on whether our people survive or perish; it is related to the existence of our nation; to thrive or wither depends on it."[26] The campaign's unprecedented place in the political arena would have a crucial effect on grassroots work, organizational independence, and resource acquisition. These advantages made the campaign one of the most important models in the health field.

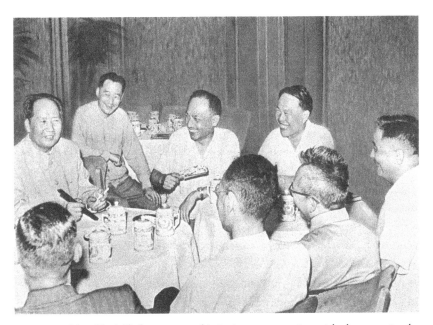

FIGURE 2. Mao (far left) demonstrates his intimate connection with the campaign by consulting with the Shanghai medical community on snail fever, June 1957. Zhonggong zhongyang nanfang shisan sheng, shi, qu xuefang lingdao xiaozu bangongshi, *Song wenshen: Huace* (Beijing: Zhonggong zhongyang nanfang shisan sheng, shi, qu xuefang lingdao xiaozu bangongshi, 1978), 11.

Beginning in 1949 and continuing, albeit intermittently, to the present, the snail fever campaign is one of the longest health campaigns in the history of the People's Republic of China. The campaign had two peaks of activity coinciding with the Great Leap Forward (1958) and the Cultural Revolution (1966–71) and a third in places participating in the 1990s World Bank project. The remainder of this chapter provides an overview of the campaign.

THE MINISTRY OF PUBLIC HEALTH UMBRELLA, 1949–1955

The Ministry of Public Health listed snail fever as a key target as early as 1952.[27] However, acknowledging the disease's significance did not mean MPH could actually accomplish this or most other grassroots work in the vast hinterland. The First National Health Conference in 1950 defined

MPH's portfolio as "1. Attention to the health of workers, peasants, and soldiers; 2. Emphasis on preventative medicine; and 3. Cooperation among doctors practicing in Chinese and Western medicine."[28] A fourth goal of "enlisting the broad masses of the people and actively participating in the health campaign with them" was added at the Second National Health Conference in 1952.[29] Although given the mandate to fight diseases, MPH lacked resources to do so and faced formidable obstacles. In addition to shortages in funding, MPH lacked personnel, materials, infrastructure, and medication. With only cursory disease surveying during the Republican era (1911–49), disease location was also unknown. Following fifteen years of war, local people had many diseases but little understanding of public health, making a focus on preventative medicine and popular participation difficult to achieve.[30] Finally, the Party encouraged reliance on Soviet rather than Western European and American medical experts. A Chinese medical delegation duly presented a paper on snail fever at a September 1954 conference in Tashkent. However, because snail fever is a southern disease, Soviet experts had no experience with the illness. Russian prescriptions were vague and depended on resources, both material and professional, that China lacked.[31]

Faced with these challenges, MPH focused its education, research, surveying, and treatment efforts in the cities where it had a hospital system connected to research and training institutions. Since research and surveys were among the Russians' nebulous advice, MPH could claim it was following Soviet injunctions.[32] Utilizing researchers trained during the Republican era, MPH established the Shanghai Institute of Parasitic Diseases in 1950, with 220 staff divided into divisions studying snail fever, malaria, filariasis, hookworm, and kala-azar. While the other parasitic diseases mainly had a single working group, snail fever had four, dedicated to prevention and control, diagnosis, clinical medicine, and pharmacology.[33] Next, MPH organized fifteen subinstitutes of parasitology or snail fever, one in each province that had endemic parasitic diseases. Provincial institutes and local health departments conducted mass surveys from 1950 to 1955. Most provincial institutes also started their own test sites, under the technical guidance of the Shanghai institute.[34]

In most areas, local health bureaus were stymied because they lacked personnel at the grassroots level. MPH continued the Republican-era effort of building a hospital in every county, but grave shortages of Western-trained personnel (China had only fifty-one thousand doctors in 1950) and funding for infrastructure made this task difficult.[35] Most rural places did have local herbalists, midwives, and Chinese medicine practitioners whose skills ranged from competence to quackery. Training programs slowly tried to improve preexisting providers' expertise. Chinese medicine practitioners in private practice were also pushed into forming united clinics, cooperative medical centers that pooled resources, including salaries. United clinics would eventually form the basis of a commune-level hospital system. However, in the early 1950s, health bureaus lacked the grassroots personnel to conduct a treatment campaign, a mechanism to convey new ideas about sanitation and public health, and the power to mandate altered behavior.

These problems were mitigated somewhat when the Party established a central epidemic prevention committee in March 1952 and launched Patriotic Public Health Campaigns (PPHCs) in response to Party accusations that America was carrying out germ warfare in China during the Korean War. Whether this was so is unknown. However, information about this attack, complete with images of dying wildlife, was broadcast all over China. Initially, all of China's disease and pest problems were presented as congruent with American germ warfare, requiring total war by patriotic citizen soldiers to eradicate the invading bugs.[36]

The government also developed a network of county-level epidemic disease prevention stations responsible for mass immunizations, maternal-child health work, PPHCs (mainly sanitation), campaigns against STDs, and site-specific disease campaigns. PPHCs often signaled health work in general, such that other health campaigns were subsumed under their umbrella.[37] Establishing epidemic disease prevention stations and PPHCs, and initiating propaganda promoting health work as a patriotic duty, were huge boons to MPH. Suddenly, the ministry had a network of personnel in the countryside and workable methods to reach out to the people. Snail fever work, however, often got lost in the shuffle and rarely gained an identity as an independent campaign.

These positive developments were hindered by the late 1951–52 Three-Anti Campaign against corruption, waste, and bureaucracy. According to an early 1950s Qingpu report, leaders of epidemic disease prevention stations in some areas came under attack. After receiving societal condemnation, leaders became cautious and were loath to fix problems lest they cause conflict. At the same time, underlings formed factions in preparation for replacing their besieged leaders. After the campaign, when leaders resumed uneasy control, many factions were less willing to follow their direction and spent time relaxing at public expense. Medical workers unhappy at being posted in the countryside took advantage of the chaos to return home. In some places, the Three-Anti Campaign affected both the quality and the quantity of public health work for up to a year afterward.[38]

The work of MPH from 1949 to 1955, later castigated as insufficient, provided a crucial foundation for the national snail fever campaign. MPH's research establishment and field test sites provided technical guidance for most of the campaign's history; the epidemic disease prevention stations developed a network of county-level personnel, some of whom would later be transferred to the snail fever campaign; personnel running PPHCs began the long process of public health education and improvements to rural sanitation; and extensive surveying for snails and sick people defined the scope of the snail fever problem. Although these were essential accomplishments, some top military and Party leaders, including Chairman Mao, were dissatisfied with the limited treatment and prevention work occurring in rural areas.

One source of complaints was from the East China Military District, one of six regional districts under military control that existed in China from 1949 to 1954. After snail fever had incapacitated its crack troops, the military district began a wider investigation in the Shanghai periphery in May 1950, probably the earliest snail fever work in the PRC. Military surveys soon revealed that many potential rural recruits were too ill for duty. It was unclear to east China's military leaders how MPH's careful research and treatment in the cities would help the countryside. Military leaders took three actions to counteract the disease. First, they started a snail fever prophylaxis committee and named Dr. Su Delong the deputy secretary of the group. Second, they instructed counties in Shanghai's vicinity to start snail fever treatment and prevention stations. These stations, including Qingpu's in June 1951, were some of the earliest disease-specific, county-level stations in China. The military government also commanded the county head or deputy of each area to concurrently assume leadership of the station, sending a clear message that the disease was an important military, political, and economic priority. Local health departments were instructed to survey the area and dispatched medical teams for initial prevention, treatment, and education work. Third, military leaders insisted that Shanghai doctors leave urban hospitals to care for rural people during Spring Festival, a monthlong holiday usually celebrated exclusively with one's family. From 1950 to 1953, doctors and medical students made the trek annually.[39] Multiple newspaper accounts, including those from leaders of the district's public health department, announced the start of a broader prevention campaign, although there is no evidence it actually occurred.[40] Chairman Mao soon echoed the military district's dissatisfaction and many of its ideas.

CHAIRMAN MAO TAKES THE HELM, LATE 1955–1958

By 1955, snail fever, an illness with devastating effects but low mortality rates, seemed doomed to be a neglected rural disease. Then, in November 1955, Chairman Mao wrested control of snail fever work from MPH; established a special nine-person leadership small group directly under the Central Committee; mandated that the group run an independent, national-level campaign; and signaled that the disease was a top priority by placing it first among the most harmful diseases in his "17 Articles on Agricultural Work."[41] Discovering exactly what stimulated this change awaits the opening of national-level archives.

Ka wai Fan and Honkei Lai address this increased focus on snail fever in their 2008 article on the campaign. They pinpoint a November 1955 meeting in Hangzhou as the "turning point," stating that at this meeting "provincial party secretaries told Mao that snail fever was a serious obstacle to the development of agriculture."[42] They further state that on November 16, 1955, after Mao met with the new deputy of MPH, Xu Yunbei, he "grew determined to eliminate the disease. Three months later, he initiated the mass campaign."[43] With the help of archived meeting reports, the present book discovers caveats to their conclusion. First, rather than promoting the campaign, most provincial leaders at the key November 1955 meeting thought the disease was unimportant. As Zhejiang delegates stated: "Prior to this meeting even the group of attendees felt this work was basically the health department's responsibility, so why do we have to attend? There are many who don't think snail fever is really that big an issue."[44] Second, Chairman Mao attacked MPH and removed Deputy Minister He Cheng in November 1955, partly because he felt MPH was following its own agenda, rather than the Party's.[45] Xu Yunbei, the nonmedical political appointee who replaced He Cheng, was unlikely to have invented a major new campaign immediately upon appointment. Finally, the campaign was announced at a special meeting on November 21, 1955, not three months later as reported by Fan and Lai.[46] Using the correct dates, Xu would have had to decide on the campaign, organize a national-level meeting in Shanghai, and gather together over ninety leaders from Shanghai, Jiangsu, Zhejiang, Jiangxi, Anhui, Hunan, and Hubei only five days after meeting with Mao.[47] Given the difficulty of travel and scheduling so many top leaders, Fan and Lai's time line seems unlikely.

This book speculates on the most likely trends and events motivating this transformation using information in newly opened municipal and provincial-level archives. It finds that three factors triggered snail fever's changed status: Chairman Mao's rapid transition to advanced producers' cooperatives as part of alterations to the first Five Year Plan; his long-standing disagreements with MPH, including those about snail fever; and his response to the Japanese snail fever delegation visiting at the same time, November 1955.

The snail fever campaign is intimately connected to concurrent developments in collectivization. When the CCP launched the first Five Year Plan in 1953, it hoped to follow the Soviet model of using the surplus produced from agriculture to drive the development of heavy industry. By 1955, it was clear that the rural surplus was increasing too slowly to capitalize industry.[48] Moreover, the rural-urban divide produced by these policies concerned Mao because he consistently valued rural people while distrusting urbanites. Furthermore, the 1956 Hungarian Revolution and the de-Stalinization process in the Soviet Union suggested that it was crucial to shore up the CCP's traditional rural support base and reaffirm that socialist policies were beneficial to the people.[49]

Chairman Mao felt that speeding up rural collectivization would solve many of the intractable problems in the countryside by creating economies of scale while increasing efficiency through shared labor, equipment, and animals. The imagined robust rural surplus would equally benefit rural and urban development, especially since it would be more directly under government control. As Mao explained as early as January 10, 1945, in a speech to model workers, once people are organized into mutual-aid groups, "not only will output increase and all kinds of innovations emerge, but there will also be political progress, a higher educational level, progress in hygiene, a remoulding of loafers and a change in social customs, and it will not take long before the implements of production will be improved, too. With all this happening, our rural society will gradually be rebuilt on new foundations."[50] By December 27, 1955, a month after launching the snail fever campaign, Chairman Mao put forward another encomium for the cooperativization process in his second preface to the book *Upsurge of Socialism in China's Countryside,* saying that eliminating illiteracy would rid rural people of ignorance, fatalism, and superstition—deficits of the mind; and eliminating snail fever would rid people of disease, weariness, and indolence—deficits of the body.[51]

Agricultural collectivization went through a number of stages in China, but the most important from the public health perspective was the move from lower-level cooperatives to advanced producers' cooperatives (APCs). This shift was completed in most places by late 1956, concurrent with alterations to the snail fever campaign.[52] APCs and communes (1958 and after) were critical for four reasons. First, pooling money created a small surplus to pay for basic health care, loans for people who could not afford treatment, and health infrastructure. Second, because APCs allocated work, they were able to assign people to incomprehensible jobs related to health campaigns, such as eradicating snails. Third, APCs appropriated people's free time for government propaganda education and forced treatment. Finally, APCs facilitated organizing mass campaigns. A retrospective report from Yujiang explained that prior to cooperatives it was difficult to implement an "overall program of prevention and treatment because there was no unified way of assigning the labor force or planning the use of the land."[53] Thus, the move to APCs made it possible to carry out mass health campaigns, especially those against endemic diseases that required massive labor power and large alterations to the environment. Additionally, as discussed in chapter 7, the promise of medical care was also an easy way to legitimate collectivization and validate CCP benevolence to villagers, key concerns of Mao.

Chairman Mao's generally contentious history with the medical establishment and with MPH in particular undoubtedly contributed to his decision to take over the snail fever campaign. As early as 1953, Mao was accusing both government and army medical establishments of being bureaucrats who sat around eating at public expense and acted like "lords and masters" toward regular people.[54] He felt their unbending rules and slow processes epitomized bureaucracy and would keep China's development forever behind its Western competitors. He suggested replacing existing bureaucracies with new organizations but apparently lacked the wherewithal to accomplish this goal at that time. By the mid-1950s, Mao's frustrations with MPH had crystallized into two major concerns: MPH was disregarding two of the national medical priorities set in 1950—cooperation between Chinese and Western medicine doctors, and strong rural outreach. MPH was dominated by doctors trained in Western medicine, who generally believed that Chinese medicine was superstitious nonsense. The ministry rarely hired Chinese medicine practitioners and often sidelined or excluded them from medical work.[55]

Additionally, given its focus on intensive Western scientific medicine, MPH used a model of treatment radiating out from urban centers, rather than focusing efforts in the countryside.

Chairman Mao thought that including Chinese medicine and its practitioners was essential to the success of health campaigns for practical, patriotic, and pedagogical reasons. With only 51,000 Western doctors, using Chinese medicine and its practitioners was the only practical way to extend medical care to the countryside. As Mao explained in an October 30, 1944, speech while in the Shaanxi-Gansu-Ningxia Border Region, "To rely solely on modern doctors is no solution."[56] The few Western medicine doctors required expensive, slow training and costly drugs and equipment mainly manufactured outside China; and these doctors focused on providing high-quality care in the cities. Yet, in 1957, China already had about 360,000 Chinese medicine practitioners working with the rural population. They needed only cheap, locally grown herbs and a set of needles.[57]

Chairman Mao also saw Chinese medicine as a unique cultural heritage that could be contributed to the world. For this reason, Mao wanted to transform and legitimate Chinese medicine. As he put it, "Based on the theories of modern science, ... we must ... organize the principles of traditional Chinese medical science and summarize its clinical experience by scientific methods... to gradually... turn it into a major component of modern medical science."[58] Mao also wanted to institute certificates for those who completed Chinese medical training, thus creating unified norms and professionalizing the group.[59] Potentially, Chinese medicine allowed China to be internationally competitive in science. If Chinese medicine was accepted as scientific and successfully addressed areas of medicine unreachable by Western medicine, then China had an advantage stemming from its own cultural heritage.[60]

Finally, while this is speculative, Mao likely appreciated Chinese medicine because it epitomized his idea that knowledge should primarily be acquired through practical experience. While Chinese medicine doctors had a few key written volumes, students learned mostly through hands-on apprenticeship programs. Thus, Chinese medicine was living proof of a theory of experiential learning that was increasingly important to Mao's revolutionary thinking.[61]

In the Maoist period, Chinese medicine and its practitioners played a key role in the snail fever campaign both practically and rhetorically. This campaign was one of the first and most prominent attempts to unify Chinese and

Western medicine in practice and to forge direct linkages between private practitioners of Chinese medicine and the Chinese government. In national and international propaganda, pride in campaign successes was often directly linked to accomplishments of Chinese medicine. Indeed, the most famous campaign movie prominently featured a Chinese medicine doctor serving the people as the face of the campaign. Notably, this emphasis on Chinese medicine was absent in grassroots propaganda.

Chairman Mao's second problem with MPH, its urban rather than rural focus, pointed to a broader difference in policy orientation: scientific versus state (social) medicine.[62] Practitioners of scientific medicine, influenced by the germ theory of disease, believed that treatment should focus on discovering and then eradicating pathogens. This paradigm relied on sophisticated urban-based scientific institutes, top-flight hospitals, and lengthy training programs that emphasized quality over quantity and resulted in medical care that was unaffordable and inaccessible for most of the population. In contrast, state or social medicine policy analysts posited that diseases originated in a social context, were linked to poverty, and could lead to the entire social unit becoming sick. Therefore, state medical efforts should focus on community-wide prevention and basic medical care for all, and be linked to comprehensive social reconstruction. To accomplish this, states should focus on low-cost rural prevention work and simple treatment by a multitude of grassroots and midlevel providers, such as retrained Chinese medicine practitioners. Not surprisingly, the highly trained, urban-oriented MPH physicians were unlikely to address Mao's state medicine–oriented concern of caring for the rural masses.

This schism was brought to Mao's attention in an especially pointed way. While the East China Military District was in existence, it mandated that the Shanghai medical establishment send doctors to the countryside to conduct an annual Spring Festival snail fever campaign. Upon dissolution of the military district, the city health department announced in December 29, 1954, that it "supported doing the treatment, but was not willing to send out any more people to do it!"[63] Following a second query, the health department replied in March 1955 that it did not have enough doctors with knowledge about how to treat the disease, saying, "We already had sent them out there for you before."[64]

The Shanghai medical establishment actually had a valid reason for refusal—Shanghai itself was having a snail fever epidemic. Every fall, impoverished Shanghai citizens, particularly pedicab drivers who were able to reach the suburbs, trawled for crabs and crayfish, a Shanghai specialty, as a source of both food and income. Thousands were infected with acute snail fever while wading in muddy canals and had to be immediately hospitalized—4,576 in 1954 and 4,131 by mid-September 1955. This caused panic in the city and created a shortage of hospital beds. Sending the few competent personnel to the countryside would have been a grave disservice to Shanghai doctors' first responsibility, their own urban residents.[65] However, from Mao's perspective, MPH's doctors were callously ignoring the needs of the people and the mandates of the Party while sitting on their backsides in the comfort of the city.

MPH's refusal to reorient its methods and goals to suit the Party challenged CCP leadership, both over medical objectives for the new society and more broadly over who would dominate science in the public sphere. Unlike most ministries that were packed with political appointees, most of MPH's top personnel had medical backgrounds, and they were unwilling to capitulate to ideological decisions that contravened scientific truths or professional norms.[66] MPH's continued resistance to Chinese medicine and its refusal to treat rural people gave Chairman Mao fodder for attack. In March 1953, Mao criticized the deputy minister of MPH for opposing the unification of Chinese and Western medicine. In November 1955, He Cheng, the deputy minister of MPH who had handled the Party's health work since the early 1930s, was forced to resign after publishing a self-criticism castigating himself for opposing Chinese medicine. That November, Mao took the snail fever campaign away from MPH and launched a campaign directly under Party control.[67] At the November 21, 1955, national meeting inaugurating the campaign, Shanghai's health department leaders were forced to criticize themselves publicly because they "had not energetically received the reactions and regulations of the government and Party authority and . . . had neither cared enough for the people . . . allowing their power to come forth, nor had they made use of the potential of Chinese medicine in treatment."[68] Speculatively, Mao's decision may have been his opening gambit in achieving his wider goals of using the campaign to model the new era's health methods and targets while asserting Party control over how medical science should be enacted.

A final impetus shaping the campaign came from interaction with Japanese researchers. In November 1955, Dr. Sasa Manabu from the Institute for Infectious Disease at Tokyo University, part of the first Japanese medical delegation to visit China, suggested that Chinese leaders bring over Dr. Komiya and other experts to communicate new strategies for addressing snail fever. On November 7, 1955, just a couple of weeks prior to Mao's takeover of the snail fever campaign, this delegation also signed an "Agreement of Friendship between the Chinese Medical Association and the Japanese Medical Mission" that facilitated an ongoing relationship between the two medical establishments.[69]

In 1956, the renowned Japanese scholar Yoshitaka Komiya, from the Japanese Society of Parasitology, brought a delegation to China for two months. Importantly, Komiya had a long relationship with China and with the Chinese medical establishment. After getting his medical degree, Komiya established the Association for Social Medicine, which focused on workers' health, joined the Communist Party in 1929, and was arrested and dismissed from the university one year later. After his release, he worked at the newly opened Shanghai Institute for Natural Science under the auspices of an old mentor, the institute's deputy director, Yokote Chiyonosuke. Komiya's research turned to parasitology, particularly malaria and snail fever. He returned to Japan only after World War II, as head of the newly established National Institute for Preventative Hygiene, where he developed methods to control Japan's snail fever problem.[70]

Komiya's delegation conducted its own research by doing surveying and clinical and preventative care in Jiangsu and other provinces. The delegation also presented a series of lectures about the most advanced treatment regimens and provided suggestions for the most effective prevention tactics in China's countryside. Binational consultations about the disease continued. In 1957, top Chinese parasitologists went to Japan as part of their own medical delegation. In light of China's complicated relationship with Japan, the willingness to follow the delegation's advice is interesting but was likely aided by Komiya's Communist affiliation and long-term connection to China. As researcher Iijima Wataru notes, Komiya's suggestions transformed the early snail fever campaign and continued to influence it long after the binational delegations ended. Although never acknowledged by the Chinese, Japan's contributions were observed by the 1975 American snail fever delegation, who reported that Komiya had mapped out "a blueprint for each phase of the control measures" that had then been carefully "followed and implemented" by the Chinese.[71] Komiya's blueprint would have been impossible to carry out under MPH. Speculatively, some of Mao's campaign restructuring, early involvement in national conferences, and expansion of the research establishment may have been a response to Komiya's suggestions.

As a result of Chairman Mao's intervention and Komiya's proposals, the snail fever campaign changed its goals, timing, structure, actors, and activities. The MPH goal was to control, not eliminate, this endemic disease, in line with the global consensus. For this reason, MPH had never established an endpoint for campaign work. In contrast, Chairman Mao's target was to permanently eliminate this and most other diseases affecting people, animals, and crops. The notion that snail fever could be eliminated was just as revolutionary as his projects in other arenas. At the first nationwide conference on snail fever, in November 1955, Mao announced that he wanted the disease completely eliminated in only seven years, a time frame reached in a discussion with Su Delong, the top Shanghai-based snail fever expert involved in the early East China Military District work. In Mao's plan, communicated through the new campaign deputy director Wei Wenbo, two years would be spent on preparation (i.e., surveying, propaganda education, establishing test sites, etc.); three years on treatment and completely eliminating the disease from the environment; and two years on mop-up.[72] Jiangxi's leaders attending the meeting tried to provide a reality check. According to their best estimate, their province had over 300,000 patients and could treat 2,000 a year, implying that the campaign would take 150 years to finish.[73] Instead, this already implausible schedule was made worse when provincial leaders, whether because of socialist fervor or political acumen, competed to claim they could finish even sooner than seven years. Rural provinces with limited resources were soon pushed into plans they knew were not viable. As the head of Jiangxi Province's department of health plaintively explained when reporting on the national meeting in January 1956: "The Central Committee came up with a seven-year plan, but Zhejiang and Anhui, etc., all said they'd eliminate in five years. Our original plan was for seven years. The result is that it's backward, and the provincial committee also criticized us for being conservative and backward, so we have no choice but to . . . also do it in five years."[74] Over time the campaign time line would shrink repeatedly, until Shanghai announced that it could complete elimination in just two years.[75]

Chairman Mao also created a new research organization and campaign structure, with Dr. Su Delong as the deputy head of the new National Schistosomiasis Research Committee, from 1956 to 1985, where he directed research protocols for the duration of the campaign.[76] This new campaign structure reinforced party control down to the township level. This change helped the snail fever campaign become one of China's most famous and successful health campaigns. The concurrent launching of advanced producers' cooperatives made social and political pressure difficult to avoid and greatly expanded mass mobilization campaigns. These changes ensured that villagers, rather than MPH personnel, carried out the health campaigns. The snail fever campaign joined other health and kill campaigns, which focused on eradicating human, animal, and plant pests, reaching a high point during the Great Leap Forward, when improving rural public health was a core part of Mao's revolutionary agenda. Since health campaigns were supposed to teach people about science, they were also associated with a larger concurrent campaign against superstition.

Under Mao's leadership, the snail fever campaign expanded the MPH focus on research, surveying, educating new personnel, and establishing test sites to develop appropriate methods. The fifteen original provincial-level parasitic institutes grew to forty-two research organizations and thirty-eight hospitals. Some medical colleges dedicated units to clinical research on snail fever. Additionally, over two hundred new hospitals were created to specifically treat the disease.[77] However, the bulk of the Maoist campaign concentrated on two new activities: prevention and treatment, directions greatly influenced by the Japanese scholar Dr. Komiya.

In contrast to Mao's focus on prevention, the MPH campaign followed the advice of American Republican-era (1911–49) experts Ernest Faust and Henry Meleney to concentrate on treatment, mostly at model sites, to garner local support. It limited prevention work to feces management, because eliminating a vast number of snails, without local support from villages with individually managed irrigation systems, seemed impossible.[78] Dr. Komiya, however, advised leaders to focus on prevention, rather than treatment, and to switch from feces management to snail killing. Japan had identified four environmental control methods: burying snails, constructing stone walls, making concrete enclosures, and draining marshes. While Japan used the last three, Dr. Komiya felt that snail burial was China's best option because it was cheaper and required less technical sophistication.[79] This approach was possible because advanced producers' cooperatives and communes were able to mount unified efforts aimed at snail killing. Eventually, snail killing became the participants' most memorable campaign activity.

At the same time, a number of developments made mass treatment feasible. Advanced producers' cooperatives provided monetary and logistical support for treatment. Party control over the pharmaceutical industry and top-level endorsement increased supplies of the drug to treat snail fever. Most importantly, the 1957 Anti-Rightist Campaign gave Mao increased control over doctors. During the preceding Hundred Flowers Campaign, leaders such as the head of the Peking Union Medical College wrote critiques of

Party medical management. In the ensuing Anti-Rightist Campaign, scientists and medical professionals were scapegoated as those who caused problems, rather than those who helped solve them. Mao explained to his physician that "power over personnel, finance, and administration were the concrete manifestation of party authority," a judgment that left little space for the nonpolitical professional agendas of the scientific and medical establishments.[80] During the Great Leap Forward that followed, doctors were dispatched in disgrace to the countryside to learn from the masses. Such attacks devastated professional science but were extremely helpful for grassroots campaigns. Some big municipalities, such as Shanghai, had done limited mobile medical outreach to near suburbs and more consistent work in model test sites. However, the snail fever campaign peaks during the Great Leap (1958), and to an even greater extent during the Cultural Revolution (1966–71), were the only times that the urban medical establishment was emptied out and dispatched to the far hinterland, staying long enough to really make a difference. In the countryside they disseminated scientific knowledge, trained local personnel, and treated massive numbers of people, albeit some by protocols of short duration.[81]

Chairman Mao's late 1955 takeover that, speculatively, was linked to the rapid shift to advanced producers' cooperatives, fundamental disagreements with MPH, and Komiya's medical delegation, made the snail fever campaign viable while entirely transforming it. Mao decided to totally eliminate the disease in seven years and established a new campaign structure, making the campaign a responsibility of political cadres rather than MPH. The newly ascendant campaign made prevention activities primary, particularly snail elimination, and also made treatment a major focus. Exaggerated statistics and the focus on quantity over quality make it hard to judge this period's achievements. However, Mao's changes established the basic contours of the campaign for the rest of its history.

THE COLLAPSE OF THE CAMPAIGN, 1959–1965

From 1959 through 1961, as part of the Great Leap Forward, China endured one of the worst famines in history, leaving people more interested in hunting food than chasing snails. Neither individuals nor localities had economic resources for treatment, and people's bodies were so malnourished that few could endure it. Despite continued exaggerated plans and statistics, during the famine the campaign ground to a halt, allowing the snails to recover. At the same time, earlier successful treatment from 1957 to 1958 created a group of snail fever–free individuals, susceptible to acute disease. The result was that the disease rebounded in epidemic proportions in the early 1960s, particularly dangerous acute cases.[82] Even Jiangxi's Yujiang County, the place Chairman Mao had just lauded in his July 1, 1958, poem "Farewell to the God of Plague" as the first to completely eliminate the disease, had many new cases.[83] It was a political nightmare that the campaign kept quiet. To this day many Chinese people think the disease was eliminated in 1958.

The years from about 1961 to 1965 have often been called the recovery period, when Mao's revolutionary methods were discredited and Liu Shaoqi and Deng Xiaoping tried to rebuild society by reinstituting economic techniques from the early 1950s, reasserting centralized control, moving away from self-reliance to greater economic inputs from national and provincial governments, and allowing scientific expertise rather than politics to determine the Party's processes and goals. However, this was less true in the health arena, due to the terrible legacy of the famine and the dual loss of most of the few experienced personnel and local funding sources. Additionally, lack of pressure from Mao made it easier for local cadres to neglect prevention.[84] The limited health funding for snail fever and other health campaigns was expended on a few test site areas, and health work was carried out by small groups of trained educated youth rather than by mass campaigns.[85]

In contrast, research institutions and tests sites became more rigorous. On July 19, 1961, the government issued the "Fourteen Articles on Science," emphasizing that research needed to be conducted in "relative stability," according to the "five fixes" (fixed direction, duties, personnel, equipment, and system), and most importantly with five days out of six dedicated to research (rather than political concerns).[86] This directive provided a national-level mandate to revamp research establishments and reorient them toward science. Most of the excellent parasitic disease research complex had been seriously affected by both the 1957 Anti-Rightist Campaign and the politicization of science during the Great Leap. This new focus on research allowed the Shanghai Institute of Parasitic Diseases to adjust its personnel and add the word "research" to its name, signifying a focus on science, not politics. It established a new prevention research unit headed by foreign-trained leaders in July 1963, impossible only a few years before.[87] Many medical and parasitic research institutes started doing lab work, halted during the Great Leap, and some test sites engaged in more stringent research, asking sophisticated questions and employing control groups for the first time. Due to the devastation from the famine, these changes were mainly not incorporated at the grassroots level.[88]

CAMPAIGN REVIVED: MAO TAKES CHARGE AGAIN, 1966–1971

Health care, health care, it benefits high officials,
Peasants, peasants, their life and death are nobody's business.

MAO ON MPH, *circa 1965*

In 1966, at the start of the Cultural Revolution, Chairman Mao regained power and revitalized the snail fever campaign.[89] Campaign activities during the second campaign peak (1966–71) were similar to the first, but often more extreme. Mao once again signaled that he he was taking back control from MPH, which guided work during the recovery period (1961–65), by attacking the ministry for its politics and priorities. Mao seems to have been concerned that despite a decade and a half of compliant rhetoric from MPH, resources remained entirely skewed toward the cities. Indeed, of the 1.5 million Western medicine professionals working in China in 1965, 70 percent were in cities, 20 percent in county seats, and only 10 percent in rural areas. Rural areas received only 25 percent of national medical expenditure; the other 75 percent went to the cities.[90] On June 26, 1965, MPH was accused of serving only "the lords in the national government," a mere 15 percent of the population, all of whom were located in cities, and not taking care of the masses in the countryside. Mao suggested changing the agency's name to Ministry of Urban Lord's Health.[91] While themes and word choices were similar to earlier attacks, there were some differences. First, Mao now had the power to demand fundamental shifts in MPH's financing, resource utilization, training, and personnel distribution. MPH was one of the most criticized organizations during the Cultural Revolution. By June 1967, the minister and all six vice ministers had been removed from office.[92] Second, Mao's views on self-reliance had crystallized further. He insisted that the material and professional resources for rural health work should be entirely supplied by the locality, a position that Liu Shaoqi, president of the PRC, argued was unrealistic. Third, many of Mao's critiques of MPH seem linked to disagreements in high politics with Liu Shaoqi, rather than responses to MPH actions.[93] Early criticism of MPH for building limited centers of competence (i.e., scientific medicine), rather than dispersing meagerly trained personnel throughout the countryside (i.e., social medicine), became a wider condemnation, analogous to those against Liu Shaoqi of overreliance on professionals and scientific criterion, rather than on the power of the people backed by ideology (such as Mao Zedong Thought).[94]

Mao's criticism caused large changes in the revitalized snail fever campaign and prompted a greatly expanded effort to bring health care to rural areas. Since the snail fever campaign was so closely associated with Mao, campaign participation was framed as repudiating Liu Shaoqi and espousing Mao Zedong Thought by showing support for the peasant masses.[95] Supporting the campaign became a political necessity, unrelated to cadres' interest in this particular disease. Renewed attacks on the scientific and medical establishment caused professional science to plummet while, once again, rural communities benefited from urban doctors dispatched long-term to the countryside. Mao's rekindled focus on social medicine and his belief in experiential, rather than book-based learning, led to an unstinting assault on the medical profession's training program. As he put it, "The more books one reads the more stupid one gets."[96] He felt that a few years of training for graduates of higher primary school should be enough, since their learning would mainly come from practical experience in the countryside. He explained that "even if they haven't much talent, they would be better than quacks and witch doctors and the villages would be better able to afford them."[97] Through these words Mao shaped the "barefoot doctor" program, started in 1968, which transformed rural health care by incorporating educated youth as midlevel health providers and allowed the system to expand access down to villages.[98] Although this basic idea had existed since the 1930s in the Dingxian Mass Education Movement and was tried in the 1950s, it was now possible for the first time. Educated youth, trained in the new rural school system, became barefoot doctors who worked with sent-down doctors to make rural health campaigns function. In 1969 the government encouraged communes to establish cooperative medical services, where fees paid by commune members and brigades supposedly supported the entire system. Chairman Mao also removed the economic barriers to snail fever treatment, thereby vastly increasing the numbers receiving treatment. Finally, starting in 1970, the government started a massive national herbal medical campaign to encourage collecting, growing, and processing local herbs to make affordable medicines. Together these changes transformed rural medical care and the snail fever campaign along with it.[99]

The campaign continued after 1971, but most of its motive force was lost. The realignment of top power relations was a major contributor to this decline. Lin Biao, Chairman Mao's well-publicized designated successor, allegedly attempted a coup in 1971; he then fled on a plane toward the Soviet Union, crashed due to insufficient fuel, and burnt to death. For many people across China, this was the last blow to the Cultural Revolution that "transformed [it] from a crusade for ideological rectitude that would give birth to an egalitarian and collective society into a power struggle."[100] As sent-down youth in Chen Village put it, "We came to see that the leaders up there could say today that something is round; tomorrow, it's flat. We lost faith in the system."[101] As the Gang of Four increasingly dominated politics, this problem was made worse because they seemed less dedicated to the campaign than Chairman Mao. For example, Zhang Chunqiao, a member of the Gang, reportedly remarked that Party committees engaged in snail fever work were "busying themselves about tiny flukes while neglecting major affairs."[102] Faith in the Party and in Mao Zedong Thought (or the appearance of it) that had been a primary catalyst for this campaign was now lost.

In addition to this general change in revolutionary ambiance, the snail fever campaign's scientific and political leadership structures were attacked. The Shanghai Institute of Parasitic Diseases, the institution responsible for scientifically guiding the campaign and for maintaining its statistics, was closed from 1972 to 1978 and all its records were burned.[103] Chairman Mao abolished the national nine-person leadership small group responsible for overall coordination of the campaign in 1971. He categorized Wei Wenbo, its deputy director and chief spokesperson, and Fang Zhichun, Jiangxi's Party secretary, both of whom had strongly supported a scientific approach, as "political gods of plague" (along with Liu Shaoqi) and removed them from office. Without these structures to hold local leaders responsible, push for the campaign to continue, and check on it results, campaign work tended to degrade significantly.[104]

A final factor in the demise of the campaign was that in the wake of the Lin Biao Incident, Chairman Mao felt the need to rebuild trust and support by rehabilitating many senior cadres and professionals who had been sent to the countryside. As a result, by late 1972, more than 80 percent of senior professors and physicians had returned to cities, greatly diminishing medical expertise at the grassroots level.[105] The upshot was that the campaign's most extensive and effective Cultural Revolution work occurred from 1966 to 1971. The campaign briefly resumed after the Cultural Revolution, from 1977 to the early 1980s, before drifting into malaise for much of the Reform era (1976–present).[106] However, the Maoist-era campaign and its short-lived post–Cultural Revolution aftermath successfully treated 95 percent of the sick people by 1981, eliminating the disease in many places and controlling it in most.[107]

CONCLUSION

Chairman Mao's interest in the snail fever campaign left a complicated legacy. Without his engagement and sustained sponsorship, it is doubtful the campaign would have existed. MPH, working alone, lacked the resources and the power to make the campaign succeed. Mao's sponsorship, the new campaign structure, the designation of the campaign as political, the incorporation of political cadres in campaign work, and the decision to run the campaign through mass mobilization, rather than small, specialized prevention groups, transformed the campaign and led to considerable popular engagement. Mao's commitment also contributed to the development of the parasitic disease research establishment, which functions effectively to this day. His focus on practical solutions helped sustain and cultivate an extensive system of model test sites whose pragmatic, affordable, and localized tactics were the benchmarks of the campaign. Mao's focus on rehabilitating Chinese medicine and his demand that it be incorporated in this campaign helped ensure Chinese medicine's integration and acceptance into the current Chinese medical scene. Mao's continued interest during the Cultural Revolution revitalized the campaign, leading to treatment and prevention work on an unprecedented scale. Finally, Mao's close association with the campaign and the widely disseminated propaganda trumpeting its successes meant that in the Reform era, when most rural health work was neglected, snail fever remained both a priority and a political necessity. Due to sustained effort throughout the Maoist period, the disease was either eliminated or brought under control in most of China. China was one of the very few developing countries to accomplish this impressive feat.

At the same time, Mao's involvement with the snail fever campaign also had important deleterious effects. Mao used this campaign, along with his support of Chinese medicine, to attack professional expertise within the

Ministry of Public Health and, in more revolutionary moments, within the parasitic disease research institutes. This made it extremely difficult for MPH to fight for the resources and cross-departmental support it needed and made it impossible for it to criticize politically based policies that were detrimental to public health. Mao's growing desire to undercut scientific and technical expertise filtered to the grassroots-level campaign, where it negatively affected treatment and prevention activities. However, the unintended consequence of banishing doctors was a dissemination of urban medical knowledge to the countryside. Finally, because Mao claimed that snail fever had been eliminated in 1958, many Chinese naturally assume the disease is no longer a problem. According to the Shanghai Institute of Parasitic Diseases, this makes is extremely difficult to develop an effective prevention strategy today.[108] The remainder of this book presents Chairman Mao's campaign from the grassroots perspective. In the face of the complex dynamics of rural resistance, the Party's attempts to keep the campaign running and use it to consolidate power without an intact bureaucracy or the use of force make for a fascinating story.

PART II

The Campaign Nobody Wanted

STRUCTURAL AND ECONOMIC UNDERPINNINGS TO RURAL RESISTANCE

CHAPTER TWO

_____

Dodging Leadership in an Era of Decentralization

STRUCTURAL PROBLEMS OF THE 1950S

IT WAS THE LATE 1950S, at the height of Chairman Mao's campaign. Upon hearing that the quality of snail suffocation work by a Shanghai brigade had dropped precipitously, Shanghai Party Secretary Zhou Jianbang gathered all heads of production brigades and any cadres above them and dragged them straight to the erring brigade. He insisted they redo the manual labor on the spot, a strategy that immediately solved the quality control problem.[1] Support by local leadership was the most important prerequisite throughout the snail fever campaign. Even in resource-strapped Yujiang County, where most lacked understanding of the campaign's purpose, simply having one prominent figure energetically promoting the campaign propelled it forward. As one Yujiang villager put it when asked about his interest in the campaign, "Cadres understand things better than me. If they go do it, I will too!"[2]

Grassroots leadership was an enormous challenge for the early CCP government. As it took power from the Nationalists, territory under Party control rapidly expanded in 1949, spreading government very thinly. The new rural cadres, who were mainly peasants and demobilized soldiers, had limited knowledge of Communist ideology, values, and norms and very low literacy levels, making it difficult for the Party to disseminate complicated information. It also made gathering statistics and keeping records, the essentials of state building, almost impossible.[3] Moreover, although enthusiastic about the new government, cadres were bound by family, friend, and client networks whose needs often came first.[4] When goals of the Party and local cadres aligned, as in the push for increased agricultural production, education about new techniques and proof of their efficacy were often sufficient for participation. However, when goals were discordant, as in grassroots health campaigns, it was very difficult to promote participation.

The decades-long decentralization push by Chairman Mao to rid China of bureaucracy enhanced the difficulty of conducting campaigns. Decentralization eliminated supervisory and accountability systems and attacked bureaucracy, making it hard to ensure local compliance and almost impossible to guarantee unitary standards and quality control. Decentralization also placed semiliterate rural cadres in charge of complex campaigns outside their experience, discouraging them from willingly assuming leadership. The snail fever campaign is an excellent example of Party efforts to manage these problems. Many local cadres did not understand why the campaign was necessary and found campaign activities, like attacking miniscule snails, bizarre. The increasingly detailed strategies for snail eradication also seemed overly complicated and out of touch with rural realities. Top-level Party officials had to figure out how to persuade these cadres to not only participate but also perform activities correctly. A primary mechanism was to institute political structures that encouraged local cadres to become campaign leaders, whether or not they were interested.

This chapter examines leadership in the campaign. It first explores the benefits of good local leaders. It then describes leadership small groups, a new leadership structure started around 1956, and explores how LSGs both helped and hindered medical and political leadership of the campaign. The chapter concludes by considering the impact of efforts to decentralize on both LSGs and health campaigns.

THE MANY ADVANTAGES OF GOOD LEADERS

Engaged local cadres made an extraordinary difference to campaign work. Based on archival evidence (and critiques) of grassroots and provincial-level campaign reports, most examples of excellent leaders were at model test sites, a finding explored in chapter 3. Aside from championing snail fever personnel and helping them gain limited local resources, excellent leaders could mobilize their villagers, underlings, and other cadres to participate. They were particularly good at forcing compliance and neutralizing attempts to undermine the campaign. For example, in 1956 the head of a Jiangxi production team allowed only three of his ten workers to receive the monthlong treatment, fearing damage to his production numbers. The Party secretary assessed the situation, using scientific tools such as statistics to calculate the amount of labor needed for the various agricultural tasks. The secretary then organized the stream of patients to minimally disturb production. Without his intervention, the treatment arm of this local campaign would have ground to a halt.[5]

Leaders also modeled good behavior to overcome barriers to testing and treatment. Campaign personnel consistently had trouble collecting stool samples. Good leaders demonstrated compliance by publicly brandishing their own stool samples. After a Party secretary from a Qingpu commune solicited people's stool samples and personally brought them to be tested, he was able to mobilize all those who needed treatment with only an hour's work.[6] Leaders could also pressure recalcitrant sick people into getting treated. "Often the cadre had to do extra work to get people into the clinic. There was one cadre . . . [who] for the sake of one patient took a trip to this village seven–eight times."[7] Perhaps the most effective encouragement was for cadres to get treated first. Deng Shilin, a local Yujiang leader, noted, "After leadership went first, other people wanted to be treated."[8] Once on the wards, some patients tended to run away midprocess. Good leaders paid consolatory visits, helped solve people's problems in paying for living expenses, and even supplied money for food gifts, especially welcome when people were missing holidays. After Jiangxi's Wanfeng County Party secretary brought special food, "the patients were very moved and those who had thought to leave decided to stay."[9] His county's government also gave five hundred yuan to subsidize sick patients. Impressed with this outpouring of support, villagers decided that the treatment teams were worthy of respect and brought them eggs and zongzi (a traditional holiday food) for the Dragon Boat Festival. A positive leadership presence could alter the entire dynamics around treatment.

Engaged leadership also profoundly influenced prevention activities by effectively organizing and supervising work. Leaders had the interest and technical ability to plan large campaigns that went off like clockwork, they solicited community-wide support, and they led by example. In Yujiang, Party Secretary Li Junjiu doffed his outer clothing and started silently digging, which "spurred them all on" (figure 3).[10] In contrast, snail elimination teams without leaders sometimes did not "even wait for the machines to start up before taking off. This is a big waste!"[11] Lack of organization also wasted labor power. In 1961, when urban health personnel rallied several thousand students for rural snail elimination work, they discovered that local cadres had made no preparations for them, wasting the day's effort.[12]

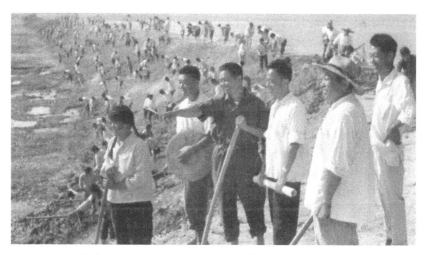

FIGURE 3. Leadership involvement spurs on the snail fever campaign. *Qianjunwanma song wenshen* (Guangzhou: Zhongguo chukou shangpin jiaoyihui, 1973), 4.

Leadership involvement also raised the morale of treatment and prevention personnel. When campaign workers encountered problems or had suggestions, they could rarely talk to upper-level leaders directly. When Party secretaries helped solve problems and gain resources, personnel tended to feel empowered and were inspired to take a more activist approach themselves.[13] In contrast, local leaders intent on impeding the campaign made sure that requests stopped with them. With no mechanisms for solving problems, many personnel decided that apathy was the best way to weather their current situation.

Committed cadres also promoted the campaign to their dubious and disengaged peers. Li Junjiu, who started out as Yujiang's deputy county secretary, spent half a year trying to convince fellow snail fever committee members that, despite their not understanding the concept of prevention, prevention activities kept them from getting reinfected. He tried to explain that successful agricultural production and the people's health were intertwined, making campaign participation a necessity.[14] Luckily, the then county secretary, Li's boss, backed him up, agreeing that his ideas were the "correct way to lead the cadres and the masses."[15] Since the disease was thought to cause both physical and spiritual enervation, the campaign was framed as curing two big problems of local cadres: the inability to reach acceptable grain quotas and the difficulty of persuading people to throw themselves into the societal transformations demanded by the Party. As

Jiangsu's Jiangdu County leaders explained, the disease "leads to no energy for production and then [the people] can't afford to pay the grain tax."[16] Consequently, supporting the snail fever campaign would mitigate both problems.

Dedicated cadres clearly made a big difference to the campaign. Unfortunately, most grassroots leaders seemed happy to remain uninvolved indefinitely. Therefore, Chairman Mao and the upper echelons of the Party initiated a structure of leadership small groups to implant a sense of responsibility, even if it could not instill enthusiasm.

LEADERSHIP SMALL GROUPS: THE NEW CAMPAIGN STRUCTURE

The PRC government is organized in a *tiao/kuai* system (vertical and horizontal lines of authority) that Kenneth Lieberthal describes as a "matrix muddle" run by a "bureaucratic leviathan" that leads to "fragmented authoritarianism."[17] While fairly good at funneling information down the ranks of a single ministry, this system has difficulty connecting horizontally even within a ministry, let alone across ministries. Because "units (and officials) of the same bureaucratic rank cannot issue binding orders to each other," when cross-ministerial problems arise, it is rarely clear who has administrative authority over whom.[18] This impedes unified ministerial work at the national level and cross-departmental work at lower levels.

The snail fever campaign had to be coordinated across health, science, propaganda, education, production, and water conservancy departments. Cadres from each department were accountable to higher-level cadres within their ministry, with some reference to the local CCP committee and county government. At the county level, departments protected their turf from incursions by other departments, viewing each other as potential rivals competing for the limited pot of local resources.[19] Forcing departments to waste assets on a health campaign was particularly egregious when they lacked sufficient resources to accomplish their primary mission. Thus, from 1949 to 1955, the campaign was relegated to the health department.

The CCP developed a governmental structure superimposed over the *tiao/kuai* system, called a *kou,* or gateway, system, to solve the problem of projects that needed groupings of functionally related bureaucracies. This second system was headed by a top cadre, to ensure cross-departmental compliance and signal the importance of the proposed activity. This leader directed a hierarchy of LSGs whose members often held key positions in the lower-level groupings of relevant bureaus and departments. Upon joining the LSG, they served as middlemen between their own department and the LSG, and they were held responsible for guiding the joint project to completion.[20]

The cross-departmental nature of snail fever work made it a perfect match for the LSG structure. The national nine-person LSG directing the campaign was immediately under the CCP's Central Committee. Beneath the national LSG were seven-person provincial LSGs, five-person county LSGs, and three-person district/township LSGs. As of 1956, the first Party secretary or his deputy at each level was mandated to run the LSGs. Other LSG members were drawn from health, agriculture, irrigation, culture and education, and the Woman's Federation. LSGs directed the campaign, disseminated information, and encouraged coordination and buy-in from the various nonhealth departments.[21] Nominally underneath the LSGs, but mainly directed by the provincial health department, were a network of snail fever stations doing the actual work, most covering at least one county. Stations had on-site treatment wards and departments responsible for propaganda education, surveying and testing, prevention, and research. Most also had mobile treatment and prevention groups to conduct on-site surveying and testing and to establish makeshift rural wards.[22]

IMPACT OF THE NEW CAMPAIGN STRUCTURE ON MEDICAL LEADERSHIP

When Chairman Mao established the new campaign structure, he signaled his dissatisfaction with the Ministry of Public Health's campaign by taking leadership away from the ministry and forcing it upon Party secretaries at all levels via the LSG structure. This created a quandary. MPH was the obvious leader for a health campaign, while cadres supposedly running the campaign lacked the knowledge and the interest to do so. An early assessment of the snail fever campaign's high politics by David Lampton in the 1970s, when archival sources were unavailable, concluded that the new structure successfully marginalized MPH. Based on archival evidence, Lampton's assessment was only true at the national level.[23] Instead, the new structure simultaneously confirmed provincial health department leadership of the campaign and helped the campaign gain maximal resources, while causing serious chain-of-command problems and contributing to the leadership vacuum of both medical personnel and political cadres.

Lacking medical expertise, lower-level cadres perforce depended on local health personnel to provide training and medical materials and to do most treatment work and some prevention work. Provincial health departments supplied some funding for campaign activities and salaries for nonlocal campaign personnel. Indeed, Great Leap Forward campaign plans in Jiangsu gave its health department full responsibility for treatment, surveying, and technical guidance. The head of different levels of health departments or his deputy was a member of almost all LSGs, often as the second-in-command. This was made explicit in Shanghai in 1956 by deciding that its health department and the LSG would share the same seal—the seal of Shanghai's health department.[24] Retention of real power by the health department made the campaign possible, but contributed to a gap in leadership by justifying the belief of rural cadres that health campaigns were not their responsibility, thereby providing convenient justification for taking a lesser role in the campaign.

At the county level and below, heads of the snail fever stations directed by provincial health departments and the medical personnel serving as their local representatives were the logical campaign leaders. They had the joint advantage of medical knowledge and dedicated job responsibilities, allowing them to devote themselves to the campaign. They were also held accountable for the number of patients they treated, ensuring that they were active in carrying out their duties.[25] Yet few doctors were successful at mobilizing people because they lacked sociopolitical credentials. Doctors needed the active support of local cadres, which was rarely forthcoming. Doctors were often posted in unfamiliar areas, making it challenging to find every little hamlet to drag people in for treatment. Few locals trusted these unknown outsiders, especially when they requested stool samples for disease testing and a major portion of the family budget for treatment fees. When advanced producers' cooperatives were formed (late 1956) and accorded the power to apportion labor, doctors' situation became even more tenuous. They could neither gather people for prevention activities nor guide prospective patients through the mass of red tape that a month's loss of labor entailed.

Few doctors viewed mobilization and outreach as part of their job, or received training in how to do it. Doctors were few, their responsibilities heavy, and treatment drugs were dangerous, requiring constant monitoring on the ward. Physicians felt their skills would best be used to cure people, rather than enticing them onto the wards. These challenges would have been mitigated if local cadres had taken a leading role in the campaign. However, most cadres responded that "this year our focus is on work. We don't have time. Maybe next year."[26] The cadres generally "depended on the specialized snail fever personnel to fight the battle themselves."[27] Meanwhile, the treatment personnel "waited for patients to appear and for cadres to mobilize them and don't go get them themselves."[28]

Ironically, while compounding issues with assigning responsibility and leadership, the new structure made the campaign possible. Because health care was chronically underfunded, provincial and lower-level campaigns that were funded took money from other campaigns. When it was part of the health department disease prevention system, snail fever work competed for funding with diseases that caused higher and more immediate mortality rates. Slow-acting snail fever generally did not receive enough resources for a viable campaign.

Once snail fever received Mao's personal imprimatur and MPH management was critiqued, provincial health departments were assigned direct control and told to develop a system of dedicated county-level snail fever prevention stations. This placed the snail fever campaign on par with the entire disease prevention system. In 1956, the Jiangxi Province snail fever campaign garnered 3.5 times as many personnel as the entire disease prevention apparatus (2,010 personnel versus 559).[29] Since Jiangxi had limited capacity to train health providers in the early 1950s, most medically trained personnel seem to have been transferred to the politically supported snail fever campaign, leaving a tiny remnant to address all other problems. Being directly under health department control meant more resources for administration and field-level supervision; more funding and professional medical personnel; and direct funneling of special government resources designated for snail fever work, which might otherwise have been consumed by the starved disease prevention system. The snail fever campaign became successful only when it was removed from disease prevention system management.[30] Thus, the key administrative issue for campaign functionality was how the campaign was positioned within the health department hierarchy, rather than whether MPH or the LSGs had control.

This structural shift muddied provincial health departments' chain of command. Previously, health departments provided funding, informed people about national mandates, and supplied general guidance for the work; hospitals and clinics offered medical care; and the disease prevention station, the activist arm of the apparatus, reached out to the rural population, providing everything from vaccinations to STD campaigns. Now, an independent structure for snail fever stations was created, focused on sanitation-oriented prevention activities, a core mission of disease prevention stations. These snail fever stations were guided by county-level LSGs and by provincial level snail fever bureaus that directed effort and resources under the immediate supervision of the provincial health department. This organization removed county-level health departments and their disease prevention stations from the chain of command. Moreover, as health department personnel had just been transferred into snail fever stations from disease prevention centers, they were unsure whether to follow their old leaders or the new ones.[31]

The result was that MPH national leaders and provincial health departments were supportive of the campaign, but local health departments often were not. If the whole purpose of snail fever stations was to conduct this campaign, why should local health departments be responsible? Indeed, many local departments had insufficient personnel, as many had just been transferred to the snail fever campaign. A 1952 Shanghai report commented, "The treatment brigades and the local health department tried to mutually shift the responsibility on each other."[32] Many local political cadres concluded that snail fever was not "really that big an issue" because "even in the health department it's only the cadres in the snail fever stations who are dealing with it."[33]

Chairman Mao's institution of the LSG system had a profound, if unintended, impact on medical leadership. The LSGs did not succeed in removing health department influence at the grassroots level because no one else had the expertise to replace it. However, LSGs, along with the earlier attack on MPH, forced provincial health departments to elevate the campaign so high in their hierarchies that it finally gained enough human and material resources to be viable.

HOW POLITICAL CADRES EXPLOITED THE NEW SYSTEM TO EVADE THE CAMPAIGN

LSGs had a structural flaw. The LSG structure was supposed to facilitate cross-departmental work and signal the centrality of the snail fever campaign to political cadres. However, LSG leaders retained their primary jobs while assuming responsibility for the campaign. Thus, time or resources spent on the campaign came at the expense of their own work—yet it was their own work where they were judged and that determined their political futures. Local cadres noted that "upper leadership only look at production and look little at snail fever work."[34] As one Yujiang leader put it in 1956, "This thing is a central activity, that thing is also a central activity; no matter what, we'll get blamed for it. At meetings we let the snail fever work become the priority, and the result is my own work is put on the back burner."[35] Moreover, campaign work originated outside the chain of command, so local leaders felt that "those above them haven't assigned them to this work and they are afraid it will impact on production and get them criticized."[36] Long-term, local cadres had to focus on their primary job of maximizing production to retain power.

The early campaign was often a net loss both economically and in terms of political capital, except in model areas examined in the next chapter. As few villagers understood the campaign, leaders did not gain popular appreciation by forcing it upon them. Cadres from Qingpu's national test site explained, "Not only is the task so big it appears unsolvable; it's also a task that will be very hard to mobilize people to do."[37] Cadres from Jiangxi "feared that villagers would have many objections" and that they would "receive criticism" from the community.[38] Similarly, in a broader exploration of statecraft by Vivienne Shue, when asked whether he paid attention to upper cadres or villagers, a commune cadre from Guangdong told her that "the first thing we thought about was whether or not the peasants would accept it. . . . If it was something that the peasants might not accept, . . . then it would be a lot of trouble for us. We'd have to find a way to take this policy and change it a little. . . . Or we might even not carry it out at all."[39] In the wake of the Three-Anti Campaign (1951–52), where popular criticism successfully toppled leaders, popular dissent was not something to dismiss lightly. Cadres had to mobilize people for many socialist construction activities and address complaints coming from villagers forced to work together in collectives. Given limited political capital, it was best to expend it on the most critical campaigns and those with the best chance of success.

With the advent of the LSG structure in 1955, the snail fever campaign no longer had medical leaders solely responsible for its function. Medical leaders could not succeed without the backing of political leaders; and political leaders had every reason to disregard the campaign in light of other duties, creating a power vacuum. By trying to mitigate one structural problem, the new organization created another.

The increasingly complicated scope of work compounded avoidance of the campaign. As Harry Harding notes, "Collectivization and communization broadened the range of activities for which local cadres were responsible to include not only agricultural production, but also capital construction, social services, militia work, and local industry."[40] As decentralization progressed, campaigns devolved lower in the hierarchy to less educated cadres, who were unable to manage the increasingly large numbers of participants or provide the sophisticated documentation required. As A. Doak Barnett put it, "While many of these cadres were experts in farming, very few had had special training to prepare them for new responsibilities such as keeping accounts, maintaining statistics, and reporting to higher authorities."[41] For example, by 1957 Jiangxi cadres were instructed to prepare for a snail elimination campaign by

> surveying to determine snail distribution, density, relationship to river systems, and key areas. [Find out disease] death rates, numbers of sick people, and means of infection. . . . Draft a plan for snail elimination, and after meticulous survey, calculate the amount of engineering, labor, funds, equipment, and technical personnel needed, and then [assess the] engineering efficacy, collect good data, prepare engineering drawings, tabulate, do statistics, do registration, and put forward a snail elimination plan . . . for the second half of the year. Discuss it with the local people and determine the . . . work time, engineering specs, and the operating procedures.[42]

Semiliterate cadres took one look at this work scope and decided that ignoring the campaign was a good pathway to sanity.

Qingpu's Chengbei Township, the national test site, which received technical guidance from Shanghai, had the best chance of any rural site to determine how to run the campaign. Yet, in January 1956, they reported, "We also have no idea how to provide guidance to get the job done."[43] In rural places without this help, the problem was worse. Halfway through the purportedly three-year campaign, a May 14, 1957, letter from Jiangxi's five-person LSG to the national nine-person LSG reported, "In terms of preventing areas' people from getting sick and snail elimination, it's still a case of having no idea what to do and being unable to put forward concrete measures for dealing with things. The Party committee can do nothing about organizing the snail elimination work."[44] Since Party legitimacy depended on leadership based on "scientific" plans, admitting that they could not devise an initial work plan was shocking. If provincial LSGs had no idea how to run the campaign, one can imagine the confusion at the county level and below.

To avoid being held accountable, many cadres tried to avoid participating in the LSG system. Initially, many rural counties palmed LSG leadership off on relatively powerless personnel. The national campaign mandate in 1956 that Party secretaries or their deputies lead these groups was circumvented by taking as long as possible to start LSGs. Jiangxi was still sending out notices from the national LSG in April 1957, stating, "Anyone who hasn't established a snail fever LSG should do it soon and have it run by a secretary. . . . Each party committee should do a survey, have a discussion, and formulate a 1957 treatment and prevention work plan."[45] Clearly, even the most basic work, such as surveying and planning, would not happen until LSGs were formed. Jiangsu sent out similar memos demanding the start of LSGs as late as October 1957.[46]

Unfortunately, LSG formation did not guarantee active campaign engagement. The next tactic was transferring LSG members without refilling slots, justified as necessary to meet production goals. In 1957, the LSG of Jiangxi's highly infectious Shangrao County had six different heads in one year. Transient leadership made it almost impossible to get anything done. This avoidance strategy became so widespread that Fang Zhichun, the head of Jiangxi's government, announced in late 1957 that rosters of LSG members had to be sent to the provincial office for ratification and that "after this . . . it is forbidden to arbitrarily swap them."[47] Unfortunately, having a named roster did not solve these problems. A 1957 report from Jiangxi noted that though some places did have a full complement of snail fever personnel, "in reality nobody is doing [the work]."[48]

Part of the problem in Jiangxi was the inability of leadership to decide who had the authority to determine staffing. An August 15, 1957, report from Nanchang Prefecture mentions "maintaining personnel in the LSG offices" as a big problem, "since in terms of staffing the province is very changeable."[49] Apparently, the prefecture had drawn up a plan for personnel distribution that was later revoked by the provincial human affairs bureau. As a result, said the report, staffing "up till now still hasn't definitely been established or strengthened."[50]

Many county LSGs compounded these problems by having few to no group meetings. A February 1956 report from Jiangsu found that many places had "duly established snail fever LSGs," but "some haven't met or established themselves directly before [an upper-level] meeting occurred."[51] Eight years later, Jiangsu's highly infectious Kunshan County still found that many LSGs "have not put into play the potential usefulness of the group. . . . In more than a year they haven't met once."[52] Additionally, members of grass-roots LSGs often refused to attend higher-level snail fever campaign meetings. When Jiangxi's De'an County tried to hold a meeting of top-level cadres in May 1957, only thirty-six of the over one hundred mandated participants appeared. Even personal phone calls from the County Committee did not result in a single additional participant. Similarly, Fang Zhichun, head of Jiangxi Province, noted in 1957 that "cadres don't view this work as important enough. We've asked them many times to come to meetings and they never come. Since they don't come to meetings, of course they can't understand the Central and Provincial Committee's intentions and naturally can't do the work well."[53] The result was that the places least interested in the campaign did not have their work monitored by superiors, failed to learn the newest government campaign mandates, did not absorb how neighboring areas had done successful campaign planning, and evaded the peer pressure that was an important component of these meetings' dynamics. As discussed in chapter 8, it took until the 1960s for enough youth to receive a basic education and to work in special teams, assimilating scientific tools before acquiring the mass planning skills that would help make the snail fever campaign a success during the Cultural Revolution.

THE STRUCTURAL EFFECTS OF DECENTRALIZATION—AND WAYS TO COUNTERACT IT

With wider attacks on bureaucracy during decentralization drives, starting in 1957 and peaking during the Cultural Revolution (1966–76), the minimally effective LSG system became even more problematic. Decentralization gutted most supervisory structures. When the bureaucracy was functional, upper-level cadres were responsible for oversight and prodded local leaders to respond to national directives. This critical intermediate level of supervision disintegrated when Chairman Mao attacked the old system, leaving no one to insist that the snail fever campaign be done according to national mandates—or done at all. This same problem haunted medical work. Lack of medical supervision led to a high malpractice rate and increased fatalities. In Shanghai and Qingpu, experienced doctors supplemented by top-notch Shanghai specialists, comprised a midlevel, county-based supervisory structure during the early and mid-1950s.[54] This structure was dismantled during the Great Leap and famine. Jiangxi had only two technical guidance groups totaling fourteen people for the entire province. Originally, the Jiangxi government planned to abolish these groups in 1957, but it soon realized they had to be continued because the quality of personnel was so low.[55] Without medical guidance, inexperienced medical personnel were left to flounder, leading to devastating results. Similarly, without systems ensuring compliance, local cadres were empowered to make their own decisions about the campaign.

Many cadres used their power over health campaigns and the health department to adjust staffing to reflect their own priorities, which rarely included public health. When there was a natural disaster, such as a flood, all medical personnel would be transferred to flood control; at moments of peak production, personnel were transferred to the fields; and when literate people were needed, medical personnel were reassigned. As the head of Jiangxi's Guangfeng County health department put it, "I've been the head of the department for five to six years. I'm frequently sent out to the countryside to do production. I've nearly become an agricultural specialist."[56] In one September 1957 report from Jiangsu Province, work included road construction, repairing rivers, surveying and exploration (prospecting), and constructing national defense engineering projects. Up until 1957, the originating organization often paid for the salary and expenses of health workers. This added a further incentive for transferring medical personnel to other tasks, since they were free help.[57]

The results for the snail fever campaign could be devastating. In 1957, when thirteen million mu of land in Jiangxi were experiencing drought conditions, concerned campaign reports stated, "In some places the whole campaign has ground to a halt; all the labor is collected together to counteract the drought."[58] Since transfer decisions were effective immediately, personnel rarely had time to transfer knowledge or impart skills to new campaign workers. One September 1961 Qingpu report explained, "The people who are managing medicine and treatment change frequently. They don't often communicate the state of affairs to the next incoming person, making for a very chaotic situation."[59] Similar problems hindered prevention work. A December 1963 report from Yujiang commented that "too much transferring of personnel meant that the snail situation was not passed on. So things got dropped."[60] Once original personnel were reassigned, they were not always transferred back, and with scarce personnel, often no replacements were available.

The impact of transferring personnel differed by both place and time. Relatively well-endowed Qingpu had difficulties with transfers in the early 1950s but had fewer problems during the first campaign peak, 1957–58.

However, after the famine in the early 1960s, Qingpu and Jiangsu's health personnel and health systems fell apart, causing the snail fever campaign to go dormant. The campaign did not revive until its peak in the early Cultural Revolution (1966–71) prompted the government to reassign personnel. In impoverished Jiangxi, even at the peak of the Great Leap, campaign personnel were transferred away, but during the Cultural Revolution, increased numbers of educated youth provided partial compensation.[61]

There was one incongruous result of devaluing health work and transferring medical personnel. From the perspective of political cadres, the only individual of unquestioned value was the accountant, leaving many local health departments staffed solely by this individual. Realizing their value, accountants gained more power than merited. One report noted, "The station head's office doesn't have a desk lamp, but the accountant has everything down to an ashtray. [The accountant] emphasizes that accountant work is special."[62] Many treatment personnel were not paid enough to survive, necessitating borrowing money. Such disbursements were supposed to be decided by the head of the snail fever station, but in fact the accountant usually made the decision. This individual's power over the communal pocketbook could result in a subordinate position for treatment personnel. A May 1957 report from Jiangxi's five-person LSG reported that when the station head reprimanded the accountant for getting into a fight with personnel, he replied, "These are my snail fever station personnel! There is no need for other people to manage them."[63]

Continuous transfers also made it difficult for remnant personnel to become competent. Prior to the campaign, few had experience treating or preventing snail fever. A March 1956 report from Qingpu's Chengbei Township test site complained, "It's very common that those who understand the work are dispatched to do other things, leaving those who don't understand it to do the work. These new people are then quickly transferred to other things as well, making it difficult to do the work well."[64] Transfers were frequent for treatment personnel and even worse for prevention personnel, as it was unclear to most cadres what prevention was accomplishing. Together, these factors made it very challenging to develop experienced personnel and competent medical leadership or to conduct a coherent, long-term campaign.[65]

These dynamics caused big problems for provincial leaders. The snail fever campaign was a priority for Chairman Mao. Provincial authorities knew there would be repercussions if their campaigns were not successful. Jiangxi leadership rapidly initiated the mandated LSG campaign structure in late 1955, established a snail fever bureau and provincial test site, and held meetings to motivate lower-level leaders' participation. Fang Zhichun, Jiangxi's Party secretary, took an energetic role, exhorting his underlings to give the campaign their best support. Yet by the end of 1956, some areas had only achieved 32.9 percent of their treatment goals.[66] Originally planning to treat 100,000 people in 1957, Jiangxi dropped the annual target to 60,000 but still only managed to treat 13,151 in the first half of the year.[67] The prevention front was equally lamentable. A May 30, 1957, report from the Jiangxi LSG to the national LSG reported, "In the whole province 68,683 people in thirty-two counties were mobilized to eliminate snails."[68] Importantly, 20,000 of these were mobilized just in the limited infectious area in Yujiang, and many of the rest were in places trying to become models. These data provide a benchmark for the numbers required for an effective campaign and indicate how little work occurred in most counties. Jiangxi's minimal campaign work was particularly problematic because the campaign was on a tight time line. Most places, prompted by Shanghai, announced in late 1955 that they would eliminate the disease in three years.[69] By 1957, halfway through the campaign, Jiangxi provincial leadership realized that their campaign was faltering badly, in good part due to local obstructionism.

To counter the problems of decentralization, in 1957 the Jiangxi government made structural modifications to the campaign. It was politically impossible to alter the LSG structure, but the province could change the snail fever stations that did the work. Jiangxi leadership transferred 40 percent of snail fever station personnel to mobile teams and reduced the number of stations from forty-four to twenty-six. They also decreased the number of station administrators and increased medical and professional personnel. County-level, circulating guidance and monitoring groups were added to improve quality control.[70] This countered two problems of the station-based system and would ideally increase treatment numbers.[71] Because stations were fixed in place, local cadres had to mobilize people for treatment, but the statistics indicate that cadres were unwilling or ineffective at doing so. Mobile units solved this problem. Second, a distant station-based system extracted a much greater economic burden than a local ward, where a patient's family could provide food, firewood, and sometimes nursing care. Accessibility also enabled locals, particularly women with caretaking duties, to get treatment.

The Jiangxi government also realized in 1957 that it lacked sufficient resources to address the disease everywhere. Thus, while all reorganized stations were kept running, the government designated ten of the thirty-five infectious counties, including Yujiang, and one city as focus sites. Three monitoring groups were dispatched to assess the work and suggest improvements. The result was working meetings at the county level and below to determine work process and to ensure that all LSGs were, in fact, led by county secretaries or their deputies and had a full complement of personnel. Such high-level political notice also resulted in some county departments and communes providing extra resources to the campaign.[72]

Jiangxi's snail fever system was restructured again in mid-1958 to counteract the extreme decentralization during the Great Leap that cut provincial government out of the process by making LSGs responsible to local government. In 1958, all snail fever units were placed directly under provincial government leadership, though they were still supposed to inform local governments of their activities. All their expenses were included in the province-level budget, paid by the provincial finance department, and managed by the provincial health department. These changes were made "to facilitate the goal of mainly eliminating snail fever in a three-year period," something that was unlikely to happen if local cadres were left to their own devices.[73]

The Great Leap restructuring transferred leadership and funding to the province, with counties responsible for performing the work. After the famine, even this was not enough, as villagers and local cadres were unwilling to participate. Thus, in 1962, provincial health departments assumed responsibility for all the work too. These organizational shifts transferred responsibility from counties to the province and reversed the trend toward decentralization. These changes quietly acknowledged local resistance by cadres and made clear the inability of the LSG structure to make up the difference.[74]

CONCLUSION

China experienced two countervailing political trends during the Maoist era. New national leaders were forming a government and extending Party power down to the grassroots, where effective local government had been missing for at least a generation. Simultaneously, Chairman Mao was decentralizing government and deconstructing China's bureaucracy. The CCP developed a number of novel structures to cope with these competing imperatives. LSGs tried to engender cross-departmental work and mandate that local leaders take responsibility for the Party's agenda, even without oversight. When local and national interests coincided and local cadres felt competent to do the work, such methods were often successful. However, when interests were not coincident, as in the snail fever campaign, local political leaders gained little by promoting the national agenda. They could not figure out how to run the campaign and, especially in areas with limited disease, it was not apparent why cadres should exhaust resources and political capital on a project that seemed clearly designated for the health department.

The new LSG organization had a profound, if unintended, impact. Attention from Mao, and earlier attacks on MPH, prompted provincial health departments to create a network of snail fever stations that moved campaign work directly under their control while leaving leadership nominally under the LSG system. This allowed the campaign to maximize the human and economic resources it gleaned within provincial health departments. Thus, instead of removing health departments' involvement from the snail fever campaign and constraining their activities, the new structure actually reinforced provincial health departments' core relationship to and leadership role in this campaign. At the same time, the new structure contributed to a lack of grassroots leadership, one of the largest impediments to effective campaign work during the 1950s and early 1960s. Local leaders proved perfectly capable of sabotaging the new system, while sociopolitical and structural realities made it impossible for the medical establishment to take sole responsibility for the work. As the trend toward decentralization continued, local leaders' lack of buy-in and power over health department staffing contributed to the paucity of campaign coherence and continuity and undermined medical leadership. Unfortunately, the fact that the campaign was an unfunded mandate, discussed in the next chapter, probably constituted an even bigger barrier to campaign success.

CHAPTER THREE

Denying Economic Responsibility While Brandishing an Empty Purse

FANG ZHICHUN, JIANGXI'S PROVINCIAL LEADER, arrived at the national snail fever conference in Shanghai intent on learning the best way to address his province's massive snail fever problem. Molluscicides were being used around the world and in China's own top test sites to eliminate snails. Fang was seriously considering investing the province's limited budget when he learned that these imported chemicals cost five hundred yuan for every mu of ground. Fang noted that 300 million mu in Jiangxi were affected by snails. As he put it, "They want how much money?! We can't afford it!"[1] These economic realities set the parameters of the campaign until the Cultural Revolution. From whole provinces down to the individual villager, campaign work was determined not by what was most effective but rather by what was affordable.

Health campaigns were unfunded mandates. This chapter examines the reactions of local cadres, villagers, and medical personnel to the imperatives of such a campaign. Rural cadres had unprecedented control over budgets because decentralization and its concomitant emphasis on self-reliance placed funding squarely in their hands. At the same time, collectivization changed the resource base from an individual to a group basis, providing cadres with a larger pool of funding. The chapter begins by exploring the reasons why grassroots cadres concluded that the conflict between production activities and campaign work was unsolvable, and it then moves on to document how cadres undermined the prevention portion of the campaign by withholding resources. Next it considers how pushing villagers to receive expensive treatment without providing sufficient subsidies affected their lives, their relationship to doctors, and the medical personnel themselves. The chapter concludes by considering the model test site in Yujiang County, famous because it inspired Chairman Mao's poems about snail fever. It explores how and why Yujiang County chose to become a model site and what resources it garnered as a result.

THE ECONOMIC RATIONALE FOR LOCAL CADRES TO SABOTAGE THE CAMPAIGN

In the early 1950s, agricultural productivity had been demolished by fifteen years of war, a problem compounded by hyperinflation. Understandably, food production was the top concern of the CCP, which was intent on not just rebuilding agriculture but increasing it beyond prior levels. This goal pushed cadres to focus on production at the expense of all other activities. This mandate was laid out in Chairman Mao's March 1953 speech "Resolving the Problem of the 'Five Excesses,'" among others, where he stated, "Agricultural production is the predominant work in the countryside. . . . All other types of work revolve around . . . [it] and serve its interests. All so-called work assignments and work methods that may hinder the peasants from carrying out production must be avoided."[2] In a country where much of the population lived close to subsistence, this was a proposition that both local leaders and villagers could wholeheartedly support.

The fact that most health campaigns were unfunded had a devastating impact on the engagement of local leaders with these campaigns. When local cadres became responsible for health work in late 1955, they had to decide how many assets to allocate for this work. Campaign propaganda education argued that health campaigns increased production because healthy people have more labor power and would produce more in the future. For most grassroots cadres this logic was not obvious. As one 1954 report from Qingpu lamented, "They don't see a relationship between health and economics and as a result neglect health."[3]

Prevention-oriented health campaigns were hard to sell, because possible future benefits came at the expense of diminished chances for a successful harvest now. With limited material or human capital (tools, animals, pesticides, fertilizer, or technical knowledge), increasing the amount and intensity of labor was the best route for improving production. However, prevention activities needed massive amounts of labor, and treatment required sick people to lose production time while being cured. A 1956 Shanghai report noted that snail fever treatment took forty days per person, including recuperation.

In Shanghai's western district, with 28,737 sick people, treatment would cost 562,928 days of labor. Furthermore, cutting snail-infested grass, spraying molluscicides, and redoing irrigation would take a minimum of 40,000 work days.[4] Labor costs were even higher in grassroots areas, where lack of resources meant that snail removal was mostly by hand and shovel. People from Yujiang noted, "We already have a lot of land with few people to work it. How do you expect us to put more labor into preventing the disease and killing the snails? You are increasing the amount of labor without increasing production. What are we going to eat, the northeastern wind?"[5] Liu Fu, head of Yujiang's agriculture and industry bureau, commented, "It's right to do this work, but a huge area needs prevention work. There's a total population of thirteen thousand and over half have the disease. We have to work on agriculture and on irrigation. How do you think we can mobilize the labor to eliminate the snails?"[6]

In addition to an immediate impact on production, the campaign could have longer-lasting negative effects. Many people treated were asymptomatic, but the aftereffects of treatment could be severe, especially in rural places lacking access to decent doctors, palliative drugs to cushion side effects, or clean wards. Some patients died on the ward or were left with lingering problems from treatment, diminishing available labor. Moreover, those sent for treatment or to do prevention work might be permanently transferred, making it impossible to complete production goals. Local cadres could be blamed for not safeguarding their most precious resource if there was an enduring loss of labor power.[7] More than a decade into the campaign, the benefits were still not evident. Even in Qingpu, where very high rates of disease should have motivated popular participation, locals concluded by 1962 that "too much time expended on health work before impacted negatively on production."[8]

Salary and additional monetary considerations also strongly influenced local cadres. The state payroll supported commune and higher-level leaders, but team and brigade leaders' salaries stemmed entirely from the crops they grew. If work on health campaigns decreased grain production, then salaries of local leaders dropped. Moreover, only county-level leaders got "regular state budgetary allocations for their operations," so to finance prevention work, communes and local cadres had to deplete the miniscule funds designated for local projects that built political capital and client networks.[9] Because departments at each level of government had to negotiate for a share of limited local money, support for the snail fever campaign could preclude support for pet projects later. The length of the campaign also created special problems. Cadres noted that "it's hard to keep fighting for money for snail fever for such an extended period."[10] Thus, choosing to promote this campaign tended to diminish what little leverage cadres had over the local budget. As increasing decentralization made rural health-care financing dependent on commune resources, campaigns became contingent on annual fluctuations in local assets. Only an excellent harvest made it possible for the commune to support an extravagance like a health campaign.[11]

The snail fever campaign also negatively affected crop production by making improvements to the irrigation system more difficult. Suffocating snails while reconstructing the irrigation system, described in chapter 5, was a major method of eliminating snails, but it altered the work process. A 1956 report on Jiangsu's Nanhui County irrigation system said, "The whole county's engineering had already been more than half completed when the snail fever leadership small group realized it should put forth its requirements and said that the [irrigation department] must put snail elimination in their specifications as the first and most important thing. The engineers and the people all wouldn't agree to it."[12] Compounding irritation, at least in Shanghai, and likely elsewhere, the irrigation department was instructed to use its limited budget to pay for this work: "At the time when [it] formulates its plan, all the costs for the labor and expenses needed to eliminate snails should be united in the same plan."[13] Realizing that this problem was systemic, at the third national snail fever meeting in December 1956 a person from the irrigation bureau was added to the national nine-person LSG and a member of the agricultural bureau was designated as the group's deputy secretary. Their purpose was "to get active engagement and support from nonhealth bureaus, particularly agriculture and irrigation."[14] This strategy, replicated down the hierarchy of LSGs, seems to have had negligible impact. Prior to this change, a January 1955 Yujiang report complained about an "arrogant" doctor who "gave directions for the burial process that came out of his own head and had no reference to the needs of the irrigation work."[15] Almost a decade later, in December 1963, Yujiang still found that "prevention and regular work are not united well together.... When fixing irrigation channels, they don't pay attention to snail elimination and vice versa."[16]

There were few repercussions for neglecting health campaigns, as cadres at the county level and above often shared local cadres' viewpoint. According to a 1956 report from Jiangsu that evaluated campaign problems, "All the leading comrades from the county committee, upon encountering the comrades who do the basic work, yell that there's little money and economic difficulties."[17] Similarly, in Jiangxi, a 1956 report from Shangrao Prefecture explained, "Only Yujiang and Yushan County leadership [the two models] view [health campaign] work as important; the rest only attend meetings and use slogans. Especially the township- and district-level cadres think that if they don't do production well they'll receive a swat in the rear, but if they don't do health work well no such swat will be forthcoming."[18] Without effective penalties, most cadres, knowing that they would not receive governmental support and observing the scarcity under which they labored, determined that it was unrealistic to do both production and health work. Thirty years of propaganda claiming there was no inherent contradiction between prevention and production failed to change this basic stance.

Finally, cadres who were active proponents of treatment discovered that their main recompense was endless inconvenience and irritation. When Jiangxi villagers went to receive treatment in the city, they expected the government to subsidize their medical fees, food, traveling expenses, and, if they died, a coffin. Thus, before committing to treatment, villagers wanted cadres to find them a loan, to address subsistence costs, and even to help them locate extra bedding. Jiangxi cadres concluded that these complex demands made it too much trouble to organize treatment. As Zhang Fuliang from Yujiang's Magang Township put it in a February 1957 report, "Here they don't have a quilt, there they don't have firewood, whatever the thing is they look for a cadre."[19] These problems filtered up to the highest levels of provincial government. In a February 20, 1957, report from Lü Liang, a member of Jiangxi's five-person LSG, he complained that "some people think treatment is the government's business. Due to this, whatever the problem, they want the government to help. They purely overdepend on the government."[20]

Because the campaign was evaluated almost entirely on economic criteria, local leaders did a cost-benefit analysis. During the Maoist era, performance assessments were based on short-term production statistics. Annual cycles of hunger during the winter and spring encouraged cadres to maximize production within each year. Moreover, fluctuating national mandates generated an unstable work environment that favored short-term planning. Finally, local leaders' salaries were dependent on boosting current food supplies. When a short-term gradient was employed, the snail fever campaign's economic benefits were doomed. It was clear that production trumped prevention.

Assessing these realities, many cadres exploited their control of economic and human resources to actively undermine the snail fever campaign, particularly prevention activities, which took more labor power and netted fewer obvious results. Economic sabotage was the easiest mechanism to undercut the campaign, because the campaign ground to a halt when food, material resources, salaries, and labor power were withheld.

Limiting access to food and material resources deterred campaign participation. To discourage treatment, cadres withheld food for patients and made treatment difficult to obtain. A 1957 Jiangxi report remarked, "Some of the township cadres are afraid that campaign work will impact preparations for plowing and don't let sick people get treated. They consciously do not solve sick people's difficulties and push people to withdraw."[21] To discourage prevention, cadres withheld essential work implements. Since most tools or boats (necessary to hunt down snails) were in short supply, it was easy to claim they were needed elsewhere. In the rare instances when the government provided money for the campaign, cadres sometimes decided to spend it on more valuable activities. For example, in 1963 a Yujiang production brigade given five thousand yuan to build public toilets, promptly invested it in production activities instead.[22] Both prevention and treatment personnel were discouraged from visiting by denying them food or only offering them rice without vegetables.[23]

Cadres also manipulated village labor and monetary resources, removing patients from wards, and refused funding for village treatment support personnel. In Jiangxi's Fengcheng County, people had "already entered the hospital to receive treatment when the commune asked them to leave to go fix dikes."[24] A September 1953 report from Jiangxi's snail fever bureau indicated that outside expert treatment personnel were used to cook food and wash quilts because local cadres were unwilling to reimburse village helpers.[25] Agreeing to provide money from campaign funds often did not help because, as a July 1956 report from the Yujiang health department indicated, such money came from the limited funding for prevention work.[26] They were simply robbing Peter to pay Paul.

The most blatant manipulation of labor and money was reserved for the prevention campaign. For snail elimination teams, in addition to withholding labor or calling people back after only a couple of days' work, cadres often selected people with half labor power, such as the elderly; teenagers with a poor work record; and landlords, intellectuals, and others deemed bad or from reactionary political categories by Chairman Mao. Leaders chose these people, not only to maximize production, but also because workers received the same mediocre number of work points, no matter how much effort was expended. As a 1965 Qingpu report remarked, "If that's the case, why not send children to do it?"[27] In relatively prosperous Qingpu, villagers did receive some recompense, but in many places leaders refused to give work points for snail elimination or surveying.[28] Not surprisingly, villagers remarked in a 1957 Jiangsu report, "We'll only eliminate snails if we receive work points for it."[29] There was no easier way to stymie prevention activities than to stop reimbursing workers for them.

Lack of reimbursement had an even greater impact on feces management, the other prevention activity. Almost all feces management personnel were elderly and semi-incapacitated people who communes had to support, the *wubaohu* (the five welfare guarantees). Even the low salary paid in places like Qingpu collapsed in hard times like the great famine and its aftermath (1959–66), when the work reverted to the villagers, to do in their spare time. Impoverished Jiangxi Province repeatedly tried to establish feces management systems with stable personnel but failed even in model sites like Yujiang. One description of Yujiang's campaign remarked, "Whether these people were useful was mainly dependent on whether we could solve the problem of decent compensation."[30] Even elderly women with few job opportunities were unwilling to do the work in Jiangxi. At the height of the campaign, a January 1958 Yujiang report lamented, "Some production brigades have nobody specially managing the feces. The result is that when the toilet is broken nobody fixes it; nobody watches that covers are put on; nobody takes care that it is brewed for the correct amount of time; and nobody washes the extremely dirty toilets!"[31]

Control over the communal pocketbook and labor power provided cadres with great scope to hinder the snail fever campaign. As soon as it became apparent that the campaign came at the expense of immediate production targets, leaders effectively utilized the powers they had gained through government decentralization to hinder campaign work by withholding food, funding, supplies, salaries, and adequate labor power.

VILLAGERS' PROBLEMS WITH THE UNFUNDED
TREATMENT MANDATE

Economic constraints strongly influenced villagers' reception of the campaign. Although lack of reimbursement affected people's participation in prevention activities, it had a far greater impact on treatment. Until July 7, 1966, when the government made all snail fever treatment free, villagers were required to pay their own treatment and board fees. Treatment was a double burden because they also lost a full month's salary and, later, work points. In addition, all fees were supposed to be paid up front in one lump sum.[32]

For most rural people, receiving treatment was a fiscal impossibility, costing the major wage earner 25–50 percent of his average annual salary. Agricultural salaries were low: 60 yuan (1957) in Shanghai; 37 yuan (1949) and 63 yuan (1965) in Jiangxi's Yujiang County; and 28 yuan (1957) and 42 yuan (1965) in Jiangsu, which probably had the most accurate statistics. Meanwhile, treatment cost at least 16 yuan (medicine: 5; board: 6; lost salary: 5).[33] Even though the government was making a good-faith effort (treatment cost eight times as much in Shanghai), receiving treatment was basically impossible for most rural people.[34] A 1952 summary of treatment work in Qingpu noted that "up till now, most of the people who have received treatment are those who were paid for at public expense. If people have to self-pay, most don't receive treatment."[35] A 1956 report summarizing work in Jiangsu concurred: "People want treatment but have no money to pay for it. This causes the phenomenon that there are many sick people and many empty beds."[36]

Late-stage patients faced even heavier economic burdens due to more expensive drugs, extended hospital stays, and possible surgery. Since these patients were almost entirely bedridden, their families also tended to be the most destitute.[37] In the early campaign, the government capped drug fees at five yuan for all patients, providing a large hidden subsidy to the few late-stage patients treated. After the government shifted to less expensive short-course treatment for early-stage patients (three to seven days rather than twenty), it still charged the same amount. With these excess fees, these patients' were unknowingly subsidizing late-stage patients. Later the government realized the true costs of acute and late-stage patients and switched to charging late-stage patients more, usually around fifty yuan.[38]

As the campaign progressed, the government tried to mitigate payment difficulties without much success. The subsidies available for the truly indigent required complicated procedures in order to obtain a government verification letter.[39] In addition, subsidies covered only drug fees, which were already capped to keep costs down, but did not address board fees, which could be twice as much. This problem was made worse because leaders' often did not pay local treatment support staff enough, so the latter sometimes demand bloated board fees. A July 1954 Qingpu account noted that cooks, frustrated with their salaries, "gathered in extra money by way of supplement."[40] When Jiangxi's Shangrao Prefecture tried to treat forty-five hundred patients in 1957 mostly for free, two-thirds were still unwilling to enter the hospital because they could not pay for board.[41] Indeed, a Jiangsu report noted, "As the amount of fees owed slowly increases, they start not paying drug fees. By now they're not even paying money for their food!"[42]

The inability of patients to pay for treatment, combined with the national treatment push, affected villagers' view of both the government and medical personnel. As Qingpu villagers observed in 1953, "You [the government] say you are concerned about our health, yet you are still trying to make money off our drug fees. If you are going to be that way, it's worse than not giving us treatment at all."[43] In an effort to meet treatment quotas, entice patients, and avoid the anger of ill patients pressed to get unaffordable treatment, many doctors obfuscated about payment, addressing the issue only when giving villagers their bill, or they initially underestimated the cost, only to present people with a seemingly bloated bill later. However, these misrepresentations made villagers distrust medical personnel and resist treatment. One early Shanghai report warned, "The content of propaganda education should avoid vague generalizations and irresponsibly or casually catering to people's needs. If you cheat people by saying they won't need to pay for treatment . . ., it makes people have a negative reaction and feel unsatisfied as well as influencing the government's prestige."[44]

The disconnect between the propaganda, which emphasized complete disease eradication, and the reality of treatment, with only a 60 percent cure rate, or lower for the short-course regimen, also caused problems for doctors. Patients expected that if they bankrupted themselves for treatment, then their disease would be cured. Instead, many were asked to pay repeatedly, leaving them feeling cheated or that the medical teams were quacks. It was not until 1957 that Shanghai decreased fees for those treated multiple times. There is no mention of similar adjustments in rural places.[45]

Doctors sometimes gave up on collecting fees, palming the problem off on the government. As one report complained: "The problem of collecting fees was not closely attended to. Instead, they carelessly asked patients what they could give and then accepted whatever was given to them. Some places entirely ignored undertaking this work. They were afraid of the trouble it would cause. The treatment brigades and the local health department tried to mutually shift the responsibility off on each other. At base this aspect of the work was a total loss."[46] This created a downward spiral in terms of fee collection, since "many people looked to see what others were doing and only paid if they did."[47] Although wreaking havoc with campaign financing, this tactic explains how some precooperative treatment occurred.

Once advanced producers' cooperatives helped support fee payments and provide loans, views of treatment improved. A 1956 Yujiang report remarked, "Before, even if you sold off your house and land, you might not get treated; now you only have to pay eight to nine yuan and no matter what the problem, you can think up a way to overcome it."[48] When communes were established in 1958, loans were offered through their public welfare fund, and workers sometimes received excess hours pre- and post-treatment to make up the difference.[49] In addition, short-course treatments used during revolutionary periods, while retaining drug fees, diminished board fees. However, the fact that most treatment occurred only after 1966 when it was made free, suggests that insufficient subsidies were still an important barrier.

THE UNFUNDED TREATMENT MANDATE AND THE SALARY DYNAMICS OF MEDICAL PERSONNEL

The terrible shortfall in snail fever campaign coffers had a devastating impact on medical personnel, since their salaries were often dependent on these fees. By the end of 1956, Jiangsu had treated 110,000 patients and received only about 10 percent of their total treatment fees. A 1956 report notes that "this became a huge stumbling block to conducting the treatment work."[50] Similar shortfalls due to rural people's inability to pay were experienced by the entire rural medical system.[51] Consequently, the chronically overextended provincial health departments had difficulty providing supplements to the snail fever campaign.

Most rural physicians were private practitioners who lacked experience managing treatment in a group setting. Newly railroaded into united clinics, mobile snail fever treatment teams, and snail fever stations, doctors often mishandled their inadequate supplies of drugs, equipment, and money.[52] As an April 1953 report from Qingpu described, "Funds are completely mismanaged such that next month's funds are used this month and much money is diverted for other things."[53] There were no records or accounting systems, no receipts for drugs consumed, and no habituation to reporting what one did to the group. The result was terrible wastage and mismanagement and many opportunities to make up salary shortfalls at the expense of the group.[54]

The impact of the shortfall in fees varied depending on doctor category. Hospital and snail fever station doctors were immune, as they received fixed rates of compensation from their home institutions. Physicians at united clinics, a new medical structure staffed using previously independent Chinese medicine doctors, were paid partially by their home clinic and partly from treatment fees. Finally, Chinese medicine private practitioners who were dragooned into the campaign were entirely dependent on the nonexistent treatment fees. As a late 1956 Jiangsu report lamented, "Because of the difficulty in getting fees, [Chinese medicine doctors'] living is not guaranteed, making for very bad morale and having a huge impact on them enacting their potential. . . . In most areas these doctors have no way to support themselves while trying to do their work."[55] These structural differences created a terrible livelihood problem and reinforced preexisting fissures in the medical establishment between Western and Chinese medicine practitioners.

Government pricing regulations compounded this fracture. Whereas house calls by Western doctors had a rising scale of twenty cents for 0.6 mile and fifty cents for 1.6 miles or more, those by Chinese doctors were fixed at ten cents.[56] Snail fever station physicians had resources to cover administrative and travel fees, as well as auxiliary equipment and drugs. Salaries provided by their home institution also acted as a hidden medical subsidy to rural areas. Together, this ensured that they required fewer resources from cooperatives, making them more welcome. In contrast, treatment fees for Chinese practitioners were also supposed to magically cover these additional expenses as well as provide funds for fixing up ward spaces—a problem that should be "voluntarily solved by the doctors and the cooperatives."[57] Not surprisingly, Chinese medicine wards tended to be more decrepit and crowded than those of Western doctors.[58] Because Chinese medicine was particularly helpful for late-stage patients, bolstering their bodies so that they could endure the treatment drugs, many Chinese doctors were assigned to treat them. Unfortunately for these fee-starved doctors, late-stage patients were the least likely to pay fees and the most likely to need more care than paid for by the minimal fees collected. The government made this dynamic worse by providing a subsidy for Western medicine for late-stage patients, but none for Chinese herbal medicine. This, as a 1956 report from Jiangsu pointed out, "led to few people receiving Chinese medical treatment."[59] The disproportionality between Western and Chinese medicine was made clear in a

1956 five-year Jiangsu treatment plan, which mandated that Western medical care should charge around 7 yuan, while Chinese medical care should cost 1–1.5 yuan. Thus, the few treatment fees received for the latter covered an even smaller proportion of expenses. Together, these provincial-level structural and pricing decisions created a large disincentive to offer Chinese medical treatment and reaffirmed Chinese medicine's second-class status.[60] These choices are particularly interesting in light of Chairman Mao's concurrent attacks on the Western medical establishment for not incorporating Chinese practitioners as equals, his repeated promotion of Chinese medicine in internal directives (discussed in chapter 1), and his editorials and articles in the *People's Daily*.[61] Apparently, Mao's high-level policy goals had limited impact at the provincial-level and below.

From the local perspective, it was clear that Chinese medicine providers were charging more and providing worse care. In addition to their poor economic situation and limited access to medical herbs, Chinese doctors were forced to provide Western medical treatment, including giving shots, which few had mastered. Lack of treatment fees meant they had no money to replenish medicines aside from government-supplied tartar emetic, and they could not supply the supplementary drugs used to buffer the tartar emetic's side effects. Most Chinese doctors were also unable to treat patients' many other concurrent diseases. Given a choice, many rural people selected Western doctors.[62]

Rural Chinese medicine doctors were mostly from despised landlord families, the only group that could afford to educate their sons. The few patients who could pay felt vindicated in withholding money from this denigrated group, leading to even smaller revenue streams.[63] The doctors' families could not help either, because they had lost any resources they previously possessed. Chinese doctors tried to survive by increasing prices above the government-mandated amount, appropriating drugs or campaign materials and selling them on the side, pilfering money from the communal campaign account, or running away to resume private practice. However, due to government pressure and simultaneous efforts to eliminate private practitioners, their participation was often mandatory.[64]

The upper campaign echelons frequently discussed the structural problems making Chinese doctors poor. Some reports, ignoring that patients were not paying fees, suggested that the funding gap "encourages them: the more they treat, the more fees they will receive."[65] Other reports proposed that local governments give doctors a loan for living expenses, to be repaid later out of treatment fees. In the absence of methods compelling villagers to pay for treatment or plans to designate more money for subsidies, this strategy transferred local debt to the medical provider.[66] In relatively more prosperous Jiangsu, the provincial government provided an initial salary subsidy of 4.6 yuan per patient; this was eliminated in 1956 and revived in 1957 at a lower rate. However, a September 1957 report from Jiangsu still deemed the subsidy "very unreasonable."[67] Around the same time, patients' fees were raised to around 7 yuan. The exact amount, according to a May 1956 report, should depend on what would "support the livelihood of the [Chinese medicine doctors'] treatment groups . . . but should take into account fee standards in bordering areas."[68] Apparently, villagers were unearthing the places with the lowest treatment fees, helping drive down regional prices and decreasing Chinese medicine doctors' salaries.[69] The subsidy solution was also tried in less affluent Jiangxi in 1958, but at least in Jiangxi's Shangrao Prefecture, it was ineffective because Chinese doctors were still advised to bring their own grain when they went to the countryside, to cover basic subsistence needs.[70] Once communes started in 1958, the Jiangsu campaign mandated that doctors sign contracts making the commune responsible for members' treatment fees "in order to ensure that treatment teams get a salary."[71] Given the continued discussion of this issue into the 1960s, there is no indication that such contracts were widely used.

The nadir of all these compensation problems occurred during the famine and its immediate aftermath (1959–63), when almost all treatment stopped and most communes' dining halls closed, leaving treatment personnel no source of food. Because the provincial health bureaus also made significant cutbacks, previously secure snail fever station personnel also had difficulty.[72] At least in Jiangsu, this problem was solved in 1963: "We also took care of [doctors'] living issues and helped them solve concrete hardships associated with their jobs so that they could tranquilly go about their work."[73] After this effort, the same report notes that "previously 92 percent of the snail fever station personnel had concerns and now more than 90 percent are without them."[74]

With the Cultural Revolution, all the prior salary dynamics changed. Snail fever treatment became fully subsidized, greatly assisting Chinese doctors.[75] However, it was now politically difficult for Western doctors to continue to receive salaries from their institutions, especially because this separate funding allowed the doctors to retain some autonomy, which contradicted government goals. Thus, the economic situation of Western doctors and snail fever station personnel was equalized with their Chinese medicine peers. A 1967 report from Shanghai recorded that medical personnel in cities and towns received thirty-two yuan per month, but those working in the countryside were given only six yuan, with the rest distributed as work points by the production brigade.[76] Thus, judgments about a doctor's output and efficacy were firmly in the hands of the peasant masses. A later report noting that agricultural workers' salaries had grown beyond thirty-two yuan, but doctors' had not, asked whether doctors' pay should be adjusted upward. Shanghai's Patriotic Health Campaign Committee advised the report's authors to "keep doing the old system," a safe decision for a dangerous era.[77]

The lack of steady compensation, frequent anxieties over basic sustenance, and the inability to procure most medicines had a profound effect on the morale of treatment personnel, their ability to work together, and their capacity to carry out treatment. For both villagers and doctors, insufficient subsidies became a primary reason to avoid the campaign. However, once this structural problem was addressed by the government's comprehensive 1966 treatment subsidy, it became a major impetus to the Cultural Revolution snail fever campaign and helps explain its success.

THE MANY ADVANTAGES TO BECOMING
A MODEL TEST SITE

Given that most local cadres did not actively support the snail fever campaign, it is interesting to determine what was different about leaders of model sites. This section explores how Jiangxi Province's rural Yujiang County achieved national model status and why its leaders supported this effort. While campaign propaganda asserted that all the campaign needed was local leadership, the Yujiang test site makes clear that in addition to leadership and a rare comparative economic advantage, outside professional medical expertise was integral to the success of the campaign.

Yujiang had not been identified as an infectious county during the Republican era (1911–49), but fortuitously, in February 1951, a government irrigation team at the Baita River near Yujiang's Dengfu Town observed that 70 percent of the population had snail fever. A subsequent provincial health department survey in March 1951 made Dengfu one of the earliest sites recognized as having the disease by the new provincial government. The provincial health department's snail fever bureau, established in June 1952, was moved to Dengfu Town in April 1953, providing Yujiang early access to the province's top personnel.[78]

Upon becoming Yujiang's deputy Party secretary in 1954, Li Junjiu recognized a golden opportunity. The county had no industry, few natural resources, limited infrastructure, and almost no possibility for educational advancement, and it was unlikely that impoverished Jiangxi Province would supply Yujiang with such resources. However, the county was the center of the province's snail fever campaign, and Li used this fact to propel both the county and his career to new heights. Over the next four years, Li's campaign leadership elevated him to county Party secretary (1956) and then to national recognition, media acclaim, and invitations to provincial and even national meetings in Beijing (1958); the county experienced a similar unprecedented trajectory.[79] As Yujiang achieved prominence, leaders at the county and subcounty levels signed onto the campaign too.

Having the provincial snail fever bureau provided Yujiang with a huge organizational advantage over other potential model sites. Moreover, the provincial health department set up a treatment station in Yujiang, making it home to three traveling treatment and prevention teams and ten small groups. Yujiang's Magang Township was designated as the provincial test site and assigned the continuous use of one group to do experimental work. In August 1954, the snail fever bureau was renamed Shangrao Prefecture's number 1 snail fever station, with three groups to care for six counties, one of which was still dedicated to Magang. In April 1956, the station was assigned solely to Yujiang because of a province-wide expansion, starting with a full complement of thirty personnel and one small group. Crucially, the deputy head of the provincial snail fever bureau (who unlike the bureau head was a medical expert) was retained as the first head of the county station.[80] It is unknown how many other provincial snail fever bureau personnel Yujiang managed to keep, but assuredly they were the cream of the crop.

When Chairman Mao launched the national campaign in November 1955, Yujiang was in an exceptional position. At a time when almost none of Jiangxi's rural counties had started surveying, Yujiang had completed three years of campaign work, garnered some of the best provincial personnel, and ensured a future stream of top professionals and political attention by inaugurating the provincial test site, as documented in table 1.

With the launch of the national campaign, Yujiang immediately established a snail fever committee, appointed the head of the county as its leader, and had its five-person LSG running by the end of 1955. Many counties had

	Yujiang	Fengxin	De'an	Guangfeng
First Provincial Survey*	March 1951	1953	August 1952	August 1953
First County Survey*	Spring 1952	1956	September 1955	April 1956
First Prevention/ Treatment Station	April 1952	Unknown	1956	1956
First Mass Campaign	Winter 1955	March 1956	March 1957	Winter 1958
Number of Participants	20,000	800	1,000	1,000+

SOURCES: Yu Laixi, "Yujiang renmin fangzhi xuexichongbing de weida douzheng," Yang Daozheng, "Qumo you dang yizhi jian yin chu pikai xin tiandi (Fengxin)," Ye Songling, "Xuexichongbing fangzhi gongzuo de huigu (De'an)," and Mao Zhixiao, "Wo canjia songwenshen de licheng (Guangfeng)," all in *Song wenshen jishi*, ed. Liu and Wan, 1, 3, 16–19, 23–25, 37; Mao Zhixiao, "Xuefang Jishi," 18; Wang Jingui, "Song zou wenshen, renshou nianfeng," 113, 118.

* First the province conducted a survey of the population; then the county performed its own survey. Generally, a county-level survey indicated serious local engagement with the disease.

yet to begin this process by 1957. Yujiang leaders optimized the mandated organization to achieve the best performance. Since the Party secretary ran the county committee, lower-rung committees had to follow suit. In addition, the head of Yujiang's public health clinic was named head of the LSG office, the entity that actually implemented the work. The LSG office was moved to Dengfu Town in February 1956, the area with the highest intensity of disease, to personally oversee the work. Wu Zaocun, Yujiang's deputy Party secretary moved permanently to the affected area to oversee the campaign and to "guarantee that production and prevention [were] carried out together."[81] These appointment choices meant that those with the most political power sponsored the campaign at all levels and appeared on-site for the most important mass mobilization campaigns; and those with the best medical knowledge were the guiding force behind actual campaign practice.[82]

Yujiang had another key advantage in its fight against snail fever: the government had established state-run farms on two of the most infectious tracts of land, totaling about twenty thousand mu, which were empty because local people fled these plague spots.[83] The newly imported workers experienced very high rates of acute disease: of the two hundred workers, seventy had been admitted to the hospital by September 1955.[84] However, this single, mainly male population, some of whom were prisoners and all of whom had recently moved there, had fewer long-term habits associated with that terrain, less ability to evade spare-time work, and much less power than local villagers to resist treatment or objectionable work, like suffocating snails. Thus, Yujiang's worst areas were also those with the least amount of popular resistance to prevention activities.[85]

State farms were also advantageous because their direct link to the government granted them much more extensive funding and equipment than a normal community. When many workers got ill, Jiangxi's agricultural and forestry department allocated forty million yuan in 1954 and eighty million yuan in 1955 to reconstruct the irrigation system while eliminating the snails. By 1955, the farms had tractors and bulldozers, machinery that was unaffordable for normal communities for at least a decade. The farms also loaned this equipment to Yujiang's four infectious townships, increasing the efficacy of their campaigns. The Yujiang leadership's ability to requisition this prized machinery was likely due to top-level political attention (discussed below), which made it politically impossible for farm leaders to refuse. The fact that funding and equipment could be targeted to the areas where the snails were worst undoubtedly helped Yujiang eliminate the disease.[86]

Energetic leadership, enormous organizational and personnel advantages, and increased resources mark the limit of what could be accomplished through the authorized campaign structure. However, Yujiang lacked medical infrastructure, medical and technical personnel, educated youth who could become grassroots health workers, and medical supplies, and the county did not have the assets to buy, build, or train what it needed. Yujiang circumvented these problems with its network of connections. As documented in table 2, from 1955 to 1958 this network provided Yujiang with the province's few fully trained medical personnel and visits by political bigwigs and outside medical experts, which undoubtedly contributed to the success of the campaign.

Thus, Yujiang's success reflected an extraordinary level of outside assistance, in addition to self-reliance and grassroots know-how. Specifically, most treatment of both people and animals, a large percentage of technical guidance for prevention work, some of the county's campaign monitoring, and its ability to rapidly assimilate new campaign techniques all derived from outside sources. Multiple oversight visits by both the national and provincial LSGs and their entourage of specialists ensured that Yujiang's work happened consistently, maintained the highest quality, and did not deteriorate between major mass mobilization efforts (see figure 4). While it is unknown how much Yujiang's high-level connections facilitated access to drugs, they

TABLE 2 Outside help and attention received by Yujiang, 1955–1958

Date	Visitor	Campaign Contribution
Summer 1955	Provincial health department and hospital personnel	Help with comprehensive surveying and treatment
February 21, 1956	Members of the national government and national nine-person LSG	One-day visit gives encouragement to the early campaign and assures locals that it has attention from the highest levels of the government
February 1956	Provincial medical expert (studied in Japan, which had top snail fever experts)	Medical expertise, surveying, and treatment strategies; links to and recommendations for more provincial personnel. This person sent at the behest of the national nine-person LSG. (See 1956–58, below).
March 1956	Li Junjiu and Zhang Denglai	Li and Zhang, head of the hospital, attend national snail fever meeting in Shanghai. They gain newest protocols for the campaign and national recognition for their efforts.[1]
Spring 1956	Five national specialists (including Su Delong)	Supervision, top technical and medical expertise, recognition and promotion of model status
Fall 1956	National leaders and specialists	Central government sends another group to examine Yujiang's work.
Winter 1956	Two Yujiang people	Yujiang helps consolidate its advantages by sending two people to Qingpu to learn feces management strategies.[2]
1956–57	Two groups of medical personnel from Shangrao Prefecture	Each group conducts many full treatment cycles, staying for a half year and quarter year, respectively.
1956–58	Three groups of medical personnel from Jiangxi's best hospitals	Each group stays for three months or three full treatment cycles, doing most of Yujiang's snail fever treatment.
1956–58	Ten medical personnel from county medical organizations	Stationed long-term in the infectious area to help with treatment[3]
1957	Technical personnel	Transferred by the provincial irrigation bureau to ensure that Yujiang's channels are reconstructed correctly
Winter 1957	Three of the province's top Chinese medicine doctors	Treatment for the majority of Yujiang's challenging late-stage patients
Winter 1957	Sixty-nine new prevention staff	Staffing for Yujiang's snail fever station. Due to the 1957 provincial reorganization, Yujiang received disproportionate numbers of new top prevention personnel.[4]

May 1957	Provincial supervisory group	Extra guidance and technical assistance. Jiangxi recognizes it cannot help everybody; Yujiang is one of ten provincial sites receiving such help.
July 30–August 10, 1957	Three members each from Jiangxi's five-person LSG and the national nine-person LSG	These top provincial and national campaign leaders pay an oversight visit to Yujiang and conclude it has "basically" eliminated snail fever. They disseminate a report to the wider campaign.[5]
May 1958	Professor and twenty-five students from provincial agricultural school	Survey and treat many of Yujiang's cattle
May 1958	Thirty-seven provincial medical experts	Confirm that Yujiang is the first county to eliminate the disease
May 1958	Fang Zhichun, Jiangxi's provincial secretary	Comes to celebrate Yujiang's successes (Fang visited earlier, but dates are unknown).[6]

1. YJA: 8, 1-12/1955; Li Junjiu, "Diyi mian hongqi shi zenyang chashang de," 98; Zou Huayi, *Kuayue siwang didai*, 98–100.

2. Zhong and Jiangxi sheng jiachu xuexichongbing fangzhi zhan, *Jiangxi sheng jiachu xuefang zhi*, 173; Li Junjiu, "Diyi mian hongqi shi zenyang chashang de," 98; Zou Huayi, *Kuayue siwang didai*, 110–11.

3. Yu Laixi and Zhonggong Yujiang xianwei xuefang lingdao xiaozu bangongshi, *Jiangxi sheng Yujiang xian xuefang zhi*, 64.

4. JXA: X111-02-269, 12/1957, 13; Zou Huayi, *Kuayue siwang didai*, 145; "Jiangxi sheng xuexichongbing ji," in *Song wenshen jishi*, ed. Liu and Wan, 219.

5. JXA: X009-01-010, 1957; Li Junjiu, "Diyi mian hongqi shi zenyang chashang de," 100.

6. Yu Laixi and Zhonggong Yujiang xianwei xuefang lingdao xiaozu bangongshi, *Jiangxi sheng Yujiang xian xuefang zhi*, 78, 133; "Jiangxi sheng xuexichongbing ji," 219; Sun Yongjiu, "Gonggu chengguo ying nan er shang; ba xuefang hongqi ju de genggao," in *Song wenshen jishi*, ed. Liu and Wan, 103.

did help with snail campaigns. While most Jiangxi counties averaged 1,000 people for their first mass mobilization campaign, Yujiang mobilized 20,000 people drawn from twenty-eight townships, working 181,169 days (see table 1). Twenty-four of these townships and 11,950 (60 percent) of the people were from outside the infectious area and did 95,723 days (53 percent) of work.[87] The political wherewithal needed to push local cadres, particularly those from noninfectious areas, to contribute a large percentage of their labor force existed only in counties like Yujiang. This abundant labor power meant that the most arduous work could be done a few times, rather than endlessly. Finally, outside technical personnel and supervision meant that work was more likely to be done correctly the first time. Together these factors made it

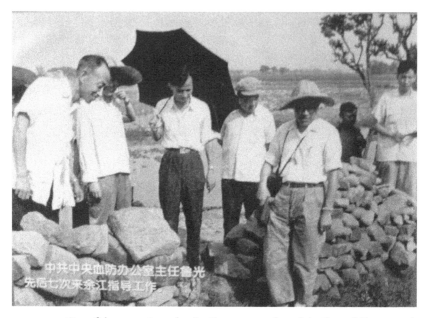

中共中央血防办公室主任鲁光
先后七次来余江指导工作

FIGURE 4. One of the seven times that Lu Guang, a member of the Central Committee's snail fever prevention office, visited Yujiang to guide and encourage their work. Top-level attention helped make Yujiang a success. Photo from the collection of Miriam Gross. Picture taken in the Yujiang County Songwenshen Memorial Museum.

possible for Yujiang villagers to do less work with fewer repetitions, making the campaign seem less intrusive and more worthwhile.

While Yujiang did not truly eliminate snail fever in 1958 as it announced, it was one of the first counties to control the disease. Because of Yujiang's huge political cachet, local leaders received national attention and enormous pressure to maintain their accomplishments after 1958. When Sun Yongjiu was appointed county secretary in 1960, he was called before the provincial head, Fang Zhichun, and told, "Yujiang is the first county to eliminate snail fever. Because of this, Chairman Mao specially wrote two poems. It's in a historic position. We've decided that the work here can only succeed and we will not allow you to fail.... If you have any problems we guarantee to support you."[88] Sun's association with this famous county led to an invitation to Beijing to meet the national minister of health in 1961, who told him that "Yujiang was the first red flag in the prevention battle field. You made us win glory. I hope you can raise the red flag higher and higher."[89] After hearing that Yujiang had snails again in eight different places in 1961, top leaders from the national and provincial LSGs rushed to Yujiang to express their concern, provide "guidance," and personally go to affected areas to monitor cleanup work.[90] In 1963 Sun was asked to talk at the national snail fever conference in Shanghai, and in 1966 he was invited to a conference on rice production in Beijing. While at the latter, Premier Zhou Enlai previewed his speech, "corrected" it to emphasize the link between campaign work and agricultural productivity, and changed the title to "After the Elimination of Snail Fever, a Great Development in Agricultural Production Occurred."[91] After these interventions, Sun realized that he had to make the campaign a success.

The copious political leaders, technical specialists, and outside visitors who came year after year to glory in Yujiang's successes likely helped it maintain long-term control of the disease. Each time a new visitor was on the horizon, Yujiang had to survey and eliminate remnant snails and treat any patients to avoid losing face. As a 1973 report explained about visitors from fifteen provinces and several foreign countries, "These visitors have a positive impact on local people, reaffirming the definiteness of their success. . . . This also encourages them to do work."[92] (See this chapter's appendix for a list of visitors and commemorative activities, 1958 and after.) Most rural counties had none of the advantages brought by high-level connections, let alone top medical personnel, leading to a much longer campaign trajectory that often led to disease control, but not elimination.[93]

CONCLUSION

Economic limitations made it impossible for the snail fever campaign to accomplish most national mandates. Rural leaders noticed that the campaign wasted labor power, one of the only resources for transforming productivity. Faced with hungry people and pressure from above, many decided that production and campaign work were mutually incompatible. Local cadres exploited the powers they gained through decentralization to quietly undermine the campaign by not supporting outside personnel, ensuring that limited local resources were unavailable, assigning insufficient and weak workers, and, as described in the prior chapter, transferring personnel to other jobs and undercutting the new LSG campaign structure. These efforts were especially effective at obstructing water and feces management, undermining a major focus of prevention work.

Villagers were rarely enthusiastic about unpaid prevention work, but they might have supported treatment. However, the government could not afford to subsidize treatment, let alone fees for board and supplementary salaries. The constant pressure from campaign personnel and some cadres to get treated, when it was fiscally impossible, undoubtedly contributed to the many exasperated comments from villagers in the archives. Advanced producers' cooperatives and short-term treatment increased access by providing loans and decreasing board fees, but it was only after the government's full subsidy in 1966 that most were able to reap the benefits of treatment that had been promised for the last fifteen years.

For Chinese medicine doctors, the drastic shortfall in treatment fees and skewed government fee regulations meant that they often had trouble surviving. The comparative prosperity of Western doctors reinforced the subordinate status of Chinese doctors, despite government propaganda valorizing them. Moreover, Chinese doctor survival strategies caused villagers to become hostile to and distrust the campaign. Government stopgap measures did little to mitigate this problem until the 1966 government subsidy.

At the same time that most cadres sidelined the campaign, leaders of model areas energetically supported it. Championing the campaign brought these leaders and their counties a network of high-level connections, political capital, media attention, national recognition as leaders, and a cascade of human and material resources. They espoused the campaign for the same reason their peers abjured it: to maximize resources in the way that best benefited both their people and their careers.

The Yujiang model test site and confirming data from the Qingpu model suggest that dedicated grassroots cadres combined with the might of the masses and local know-how were not enough for campaign success, despite the Party's assertion to the contrary. In addition to committed leadership and additional resources, such as tractors and outside labor in Yujiang (and chemicals in Qingpu), as documented in table 2, medical personnel played a large role in success. Yujiang, Qingpu, and more typical nonmodel areas relied heavily on outside professional expertise to conduct the campaign's treatment work and to ensure campaign continuity and provide quality control. Chapter 8 examines how places lacking high-level connections partially compensated during the campaign peak during the Cultural Revolution. Part 3 of the book explores the campaign's three arms—education, prevention, and treatment—to determine how they functioned despite the dearth of leadership and funding.

TABLE 3 Keeping success in mind, Yujiang 1958 and after

Date	Visitor/Activity	Campaign Contribution
May 25, 1958	Fang Zhichun and other provincial bigwigs	Big celebration held for eliminating the disease.
June 5, 1958	Telegram	MPH sends a congratulatory telegram.
June 30, 1958, and May 28, 1959	Newspaper articles in the *Jiangxi* and *People's Daily*	Articles bring Yujiang provincial and national attention.
May 25–28, 1959–66	Annual commemorative days and party	Annual focus on the campaign keeps snail fever and Yujiang's success at the forefront of people's attention.[1]
September 1959	Movie	A film company comes to Yujiang to create an education film about the campaign.
August 1961 and March 1962	Members of nine-person LSG and provincial disease elimination office	Leaders check on Yujiang's work.
April 1962	Yujiang starts planning a commemorative museum	Museum planning leads to collecting a lot of memorabilia and talking to people about the campaign.[2]
1963	Commemorative stele	Stele (4 x 2 meters) with Mao's poem is erected outside Dengfu Town train station, ensuring that all visitors know why Yujiang is famous.
May 5, 1963	Big meeting attended by members of the national and provincial LSGs	This commemorative meeting draws over five hundred people and is publicized nationally by Xinhua news.
October 21–November 9, 1963	Provincial and prefectural disease elimination team	They conduct a multiweek oversight tour and write a report on it.
January 1964	Museum opens	Yujiang's first commemorative museum opens.[3]
1967 and after	*People's Daily* articles	The newspaper publishes memorials: small ones annually and big ones every ten years.
May 17, 1967	Nine years after 1958 commemorative meeting	The whole county is required to recite Mao's poem from memory. Each level of the county government is asked to celebrate with discussions, pictures, and songs. The Xinhua bookstore is supposed to send one copy of Mao's poem to every household in the infectious area.
June 26, 1967	Thirteen members of the provincial health department and nine medical students	They conduct treatment and do propaganda education about Mao Zedong Thought.[4]
1968–71	135 health professionals	A large group of urban health professionals is sent down to Yujiang, staying at least until 1971; they help with health work in all domains[5]

(continued)

TABLE 3 *(continued)*

Date	Visitor/Activity	Campaign Contribution
1968	Over twenty stele erected	Most steles are at the county seat. All are inscribed with Mao's poem. They help ensure that the campaign is kept firmly in the leadership's mind.
October 3, 1968	Ten-year anniversary party	Fifteen thousand people, provincial bigwigs, and the provincial head attend. The event is covered by multiple newspapers, including the *People's Daily*.
October 3, 1968	Museum revamped	The museum is renamed, its contents brought in line with the Cultural Revolution, and it is enlarged from 160 to 486 square meters.
1971	Museum revamped	The museum is revised again to suit current political trends, and it is enlarged to 762 square meters.[6]
1973, August 1974, July 1977	Outside and foreign visitors	Forty-seven teams from fifteen provinces (2,761 people) and people from England, Germany, Japan, Sudan, and foreign students from twelve countries visit to learn about the campaign.
1977	Commemorative stele	Another stele is erected at the county seat.
October 1977	Movie short	A short movie is made about Yujiang's campaign.[7]
1978	Commemorative stele	The provincial committee allocates 150,000 yuan for a stele in front of the museum.
1978	Museum enlarged	The national and provincial health departments allocate 150,000 and 250,000 yuan, respectively, to build a bigger museum.
October 3, 1978	Twenty-year anniversary party	This huge party is held in front of the museum. All the provincial bigwigs and all past county Party secretaries attend.
October 3, 1978	Museum renamed	The museum is "eliminated" and renamed. An exhibition hall commemorating the campaign continues.
1979	Exhibition hall attendance	During 1979, 23,600 people visit the museum. The exhibition hall continues to the present day.[8]

1. Yu Laixi and Zhonggong Yujiang xianwei xuefang lingdao xiaozu bangongshi, *Jiangxi sheng Yujiang xian xuefang zhi,* 78, 84, 133–34, 146; Mao Huiren, Li Guifa, and Jiangxi sheng Yujiang xian xianzhi bianzuan weiyuanhui bianji, *Yujiang xianzhi,* 596, 597.

2. Yu Laixi and Zhonggong Yujiang xianwei xuefang lingdao xiaozu bangongshi, *Jiangxi sheng Yujiang xian xuefang zhi,* 135; YJA: 19, 1–12/1961; YJA: 21, 1–12/1962; YJA: 29, 1–12/1964.

3. Mao Huiren, Li Guifa, and Jiangxi sheng Yujiang xian xianzhi bianzuan weiyuanhui bianji, *Yujiang xianzhi,* 597, 598; YJA: 27, 1–12/1963.

4. Mao Huiren, Li Guifa, and Jiangxi sheng Yujiang xian xianzhi bianzuan weiyuanhui bianji, *Yujiang xianzhi,* 597; YJA: 32, 2–10/1967; YJA: 33, 1–12/1968.

5. YJA: 38, 1–12/1972.

6. Mao Huiren, Li Guifa, and Jiangxi sheng Yujiang xian xianzhi bianzuan weiyuanhui bianji, *Yujiang xianzhi,* 597, 598; YJA: 34, 1–12/1968.

7. YJA: 40, 1–12/1973; YJA: 41, 1–12/1973; Yu Laixi and Zhonggong Yujiang xian xuefang lingdao xiaozu bangongshi, *Jiangxi sheng Yujiang xian xuefang zhi,* 139, 142; Mao Huiren, Li Guifa, and Jiangxi sheng Yujiang xian xianzhi bianzuan weiyuanhui bianji, *Yujiang xianzhi,* 598.

8. Yu Laixi and Zhonggong Yujiang xianwei xuefang lingdao xiaozu bangongshi, *Jiangxi sheng Yujiang xian xuefang zhi,* 86, 142–43; Mao Huiren, Li Guifa, and Jiangxi sheng Yujiang xian xianzhi bianzuan weiyuanhui bianji, *Yujiang xianzhi,* 598; YJA: 42, 1–12/1979.

PART III

The Three Arms of the Campaign

EDUCATION, PREVENTION, AND TREATMENT

CHAPTER FOUR

Building the New Scientific Socialist Society

EDUCATING THE MASSES

> Their minds have been freed from the fetters of old ideas and traditions, and this in turn has released their latent energy and talent.
>
> WEI WENBO, *deputy director of the national campaign, 1958*

FEW PARTS OF THE SNAIL fever campaign were more important than disseminating scientific knowledge and attitudes to the masses.[1] A half century of debate in China had positioned science as the stimulus to modernization that would finally overcome China's traditional culture.[2] Building on this legacy, Chairman Mao joined other world leaders in the 1950s in believing that science could bring physical, socioeconomic, and spiritual uplift. Furthermore, Mao's populist version of Marxism, "not only looked to the peasantry as the popular basis of the revolution, but attributed to the peasants themselves those elements of revolutionary creativity and standards of political judgment that Marxist-Leninists reserve for the party."[3] From this perspective, implanting grassroots scientific endeavor and eradicating supposedly superstitious traditional practices were essential if Communism was to succeed. As a result, during the Great Leap Forward (1958–61), at the height of revolutionary fervor, Mao suggested that although earlier Party initiatives neglected science and technology in favor of social revolution, now "the party's focus of attention can be transferred to technological revolution."[4] Jiangsu's 1958 snail fever plan incorporated this new emphasis, explaining, "If we only have mass mobilization without the guidance of science and technology, then we will have blind warfare where we can't hit the enemy's strategic points; but if science and technology don't merge with the people, then they won't normally have the strength to progress."[5]

For true societal transformation that would help craft a new sort of person, Chairman Mao felt that science needed to be enacted by the masses. That way, peasants would stop seeking advice from elders and replicating their solutions. Instead, when faced with a problem, they would incorporate scientific thinking, practical experiments, and cost-benefit analyses into their problem solving. The resultant burst of practical technological development in fields and factories would greatly increase productivity, a main governmental aim of the era.[6]

Unfortunately, conveying scientific knowledge and instilling scientific patterns of thought in a mostly illiterate rural population were easier said than done. Schools were a logical place to teach people science, but establishing a comprehensive rural education system would take decades. Many Chinese leaders believed they could not wait that long. Health campaigns seemed like a good place to jump-start scientific understanding, because the science involved in counteracting diseases was concrete, pragmatic, and directly relevant to improving people's livelihood.[7]

This chapter examines how the Party tried to teach rural people scientific knowledge and states of mind. The Party used many pedagogical approaches, but most did not succeed because they used language that was incomprehensible and relied on a disease paradigm discrepant from that understood by most of the people. Education failed to convey even the fundamental idea that pathogens caused disease. Unfortunately, prevention campaigns did not make sense without this concept. The inability to convey scientific rationales for snail fever campaign activities made it difficult to mobilize rural people for prevention work, especially in view of the limited support of local cadres for prevention (see chapter 2). Although the Party was somewhat more successful in teaching scientific states of mind, these attitudes did not translate to increased campaign participation. Instead, educators embedded campaign work in organizational structures so that participation was no longer voluntary, a strategy effective for treatment and mass snail campaigns, but not for hygiene and sanitation work.

TRANSMITTING NEW KNOWLEDGE

Using scientific knowledge to construct the modern new society was a strong component of the pedagogical agenda of health campaigns. Most of them tried hard to convey the scientific underpinnings of their work. The CCP tried many different approaches, including incorporating science education into entertainment, specially produced texts and images, and lectures and using experiential learning. As discussed below, each of these approaches had shortcomings that prevented the bulk of the rural population from understanding the link between the snail and the disease, thus undermining broad acceptance of prevention work.

The CCP realized that securing an audience by making the science entertaining was a very high priority, and it used many different media to accomplish this, culminating in movies produced during the 1960s. As early as April 1950, a Central Committee directive suggested that campaign personnel use "the effective [teaching] methods employed in the northeastern campaign against plague: movies, slideshows, and modern drama/stage plays."[8] But in the 1950s few places had access to electricity, projectors, or slide sets. Instead, personnel enticed villagers using methods stemming from popular culture: opera, theater, songs, and drumming and musical instruments, creating a strong story line about the happy, disease-free new society.[9] Unfortunately, such methods were better at stirring emotion than conveying detailed scientific information (see figure 5). Even worse, the underlying principles explaining the science tended to be lost, presented vaguely, or eliminated entirely. Western forms of theater and musicals were also tried and proved equally ineffective. Furthermore, employing traditional entertainment undermined a core Party mission of eradicating superstitious popular culture in favor of a modern scientific society. By using the types of entertainment employed in religious festivals, the Party gave popular culture tacit support, helping it to find a way to persist in the new society. In the early 1950s, even the location of these theatrical productions and educational shows were often the same as religious festivals, occurring during large markets, fairs, and holidays. Although reaching many people, they turned snail fever campaign education into simply one more sideshow.[10]

In the 1960s the government made a number of entertainment-oriented movies focused on the campaign, the most famous of which is *Kumu feng chun* (Spring comes to a withered tree). This renowned feature film tells the story of star-crossed lovers unable to marry because of lives ruined equally by snail fever and the Nationalists. When they meet again in New China after 1949, all things are possible by working together to eliminate the disease. Familiar caricatures include the downtrodden, disease-ridden heroine; her future husband, an innovative tractor driver; the local leader of the snail fever station, who demonstrates that quietly sacrificing for the people can bring

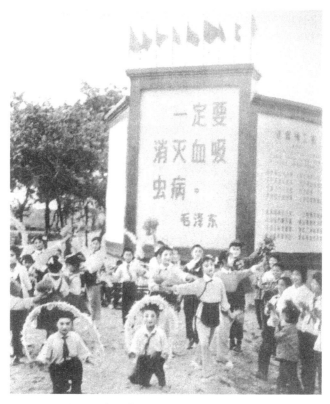

FIGURE 5. Theatrical productions were a wonderful way to popularize the snail fever campaign but were not effective at conveying scientific information. Zhonggong zhongyang nanfang shisan sheng, shi, qu xuefang lingdao xiaozu bangongshi, *Song wenshen: Huace* (Beijing: Zhonggong zhongyang nanfang shisan sheng, shi, qu xuefang lingdao xiaozu bangongshi, 1978), 55.

miracles; and the urban medical doctor who focuses on theoretical research instead of caring for the people.[11]

Unfortunately, little disease information was disseminated. The film mentions the danger of walking barefoot in contaminated water, and indicates that snails have to be eliminated and night soil managed, but does not explain why. It states that late-stage disease is a death sentence treatable only by Chinese herbs, both of which are untrue. It credits grassroots science with developing snail killing by burial, rather than acknowledging that it came from the Japanese expert Dr. Komiya. Interestingly, in urban/rural doctor clashes, the urban physician is castigated for neglecting treatment and focusing on snail elimination. Indeed, prevention receives only twelve of ninety-seven minutes of screen time, compared to endless scenes of suffering people in clinics. The motivation for contradicting the campaign's core stricture of the centrality of prevention is unclear.

As a second approach, the government developed a wide variety of written and pictorial educational materials, which were produced by an entire publishing industry dedicated to health campaigns. It churned out everything from ballads and poems to detailed treatment and prevention manuals and health comic books. Many of these efforts were stymied because most rural people in the 1950s and 1960s were illiterate. Provinces also developed teaching poster sets and blackboard newspapers. Perambulating artist groups were dispatched to draw big wall paintings, cartoon slogans, big Chinese character posters, and even luminescent paintings that could be seen at night. Pictorial and textual material shared the same problem: few could read well enough to understand the explanatory texts and the images transmitting complicated scientific ideas were alien.[12] This was particularly the case because pictorial and photographic representations of the disease almost always chose late-stage patients with a distinctively protruding stomach. The vast majority of patients did not believe they were ill because they were only lightly symptomatic and did not have the characteristic big belly. Such images reinforced villagers' perception that the campaign had nothing to do with them.

Local ballads, poems, slogans, and rural sayings were collected by the provinces at the behest of the national government and published in newspapers or books, repeated in grassroots reports, and recounted in major meetings as the voice of the masses. Some were disseminated orally as entertainment; others were distributed as another textual method. Catchy work songs and slogans that delineated work requirements and processes probably acted as a good motivator and memory tool. However, such sayings, like other entertainment, contained negligible scientific content.[13] Since few villagers in the 1950s could read and most lacked access to or funds for reading matter, this material was probably intended for a more educated urban audience. Disseminating these texts may have had unintended negative consequences for the relationship between urban and rural areas. The folksy poems and ballads likely reinforced urban stereotypes about rural people's ignorance, confirming the idea that villagers needed their guidance for campaign success. It also may have given urban residents and Party members the false impression that rural people backed the campaign.

A third educational method involved content-heavy education like didactic lectures and discussions. The use of this approach became possible starting in 1956, both because of Chairman Mao's campaign sponsorship and because the entry of rural people into advanced producers' cooperatives (end of 1956) and communes (1958) allowed the Party to enforce attendance. Personnel tried to structure education so that they had a captive audience. In addition to educating students stuck in school and patients trapped in wards, compulsory meetings for political cadres or villagers sometimes were infiltrated with a mandatory piece on snail fever. When elders spoke about the bitterness of the past at compulsory meetings, they were directed to describe how snail fever had previously ravaged society. Lunch breaks during communal work in the fields, when people were too tired to escape, were another favorite time for propaganda.[14] The coercive potential of cooperative life provided unprecedented opportunities for propaganda education and allowed campaign workers to try more content-rich forms of education.

While lectures were more accessible than books and could clearly lay out the disease's life cycle and the science behind various prevention activities, they bored people unused to classroom-based learning. Moreover, lectures (and campaign texts) used specialized terms like "cercaria" *(weiyou)* and "miracidium" *(maoyou)* that rural people found arcane, and the talks were often presented by outsiders, diminishing enthusiasm for the material. Many villagers used such lectures as an opportunity for daydreaming or a nap. As a June 1955 report from Qingpu explained, "Many are utterly uninterested in receiving training and refuse to come." Once forced, some participants "arrived late," sat glumly "not saying a word," "chatted in the middle of class," or found various ways to "purposely cause trouble. . . . Many didn't learn much or change their old habits."[15]

The fact that teachers usually knew little more than their students also diminished the effectiveness of a didactic approach. A few areas, like Shanghai, were able to use health department personnel as educators. Qingpu, with higher literacy rates than most areas, considered using grassroots cadres as educators but decided against it because of their resistance to the campaign, settling instead on elementary and middle-school teachers.[16] However, with only a short training course, the teachers were not very effective educators. Rural places like Yujiang employed a tiny pool of elementary teachers, students, and occasional health personnel, who were supplied with very cursory training. Until educated youth were trained as grassroots health workers in the 1960s, most rural places had insufficient educators with minimal training.[17]

A final strategy involved experiencing science by gazing through a microscope or attending a science exhibition. A major attraction of this approach was that it showcased Western technology, which one account noted "greatly attracts the people."[18] This seems to have been more effective than the other methods, but many people still had difficulty interpreting what they experienced. Microscopes were the method of choice for campaign leaders. According to an official account of Shanghai's campaign, "Making existing scientific skills graspable by the people has become the weapon for the war against snail fever."[19] In fact, microscopes became a key symbol of all health campaigns. They adorned almost every health propaganda book's cover, campaign pictures inevitably focused on peasants peering intently through them, and provincial newspapers ran articles guiding people how to use them.[20]

Microscopes had many advantages, both as a method to teach science and a mechanism to achieve the wider goal of creating a scientific citizenry. Microscopes were portable, already available to do testing, and did not require energy sources, making them ideal for villages. Whereas movies, slides, or phonographs were viewed as entertainment or teaching tools, microscopes were envisioned as unadulterated science. Microscopes also turned a theoretical discussion about disease life cycle into real objects that people could see and touch. Microscopes were also appealing because they had previously been used only by experts, but now, at least symbolically, their scientific power was placed in the hands of villagers, affording them an opportunity to conduct empirical research. Finally, seemingly no prior knowledge was required. Villagers simply gazed through the lens and could see with their own eyes how the disease worked, affording even illiterate villagers an experiential interaction with science. As one campaign worker put it, "After looking through a microscope they will know it is a small worm . . . that actively harms people and will [stop] treating the campaign as a big joke."[21] Personnel thought they could use the microscope experience to encourage villagers to employ the scientific method of investigating things for themselves, as advocated by Chairman Mao.[22] In this way, remarked one optimistic report, "scientific information will be disseminated and scientific knowledge will be universal."[23]

Many educators began by fingering the snails, which were so pervasive that they faded into invisibility. This got villagers' attention and turned the snail into an object of study. Then they would bring out the microscope, plopping it down in the middle of the village and waiting for a crowd to gather around this alluring alien object. Like a magician prepared to show miracles to the credulous, campaign personnel would then unveil their star exhibit, the shit sample, ideally taken from someone in the village. After villagers gazed at the eggs in the stool, the educator would dissect snails before people's eyes, revealing for all to see the cercariae embedded inside them. Each villager got the novel pleasure of handling the machine and looking through its lens.[24]

Unfortunately for the prevention personnel, "seeing is believing" works only if those participating share a similar knowledge base and an intellectual paradigm that leads to analogous interpretations. In the 1950s, few villagers' understanding of the world included microscopy, microorganisms, or the notion that a specific causal agent triggers a disease. This made the sight in front of them impossible to decode. Some villagers were horrified. Once they focused on the impenetrable visionary field, they saw what appeared to be monsters. Yet the minute they hastily leaped back, the little demons disappeared. Prevention personnel told the villagers that they were seeing larvae, but this was unconvincing, since many had never heard the term. Many villagers accused personnel of "playing tricks and demonstrating magic just to try and scare us."[25] In fact, sometimes villagers were correct. Figuring that they would never know the difference, some educators simply fixed the microscope on the first worm that appeared in front of the lens: "Actually it was not the schistosome they saw, but they had plenty of worms in the water anyway, and it helped to convince them."[26] Villagers also found it unbelievable that something so small could hurt them. As some local cadres remarked: "A red mark is left by a mosquito bite. Blood is shed as a result of bites by ants and locusts. But the larvae discharged by snails are not even visible, how can they enter the body?"[27] Another problem was that personnel were not providing all the necessary empirical evidence. Even when villagers understood the idea of microscopic creatures, they were not shown that it was the worms in their water sources that were entering their skin. It was not clear what eggs in stool samples or cercariae in snails has to do with a big belly and diminished strength.[28] In the end, villagers were being asked to take something on faith, the opposite of a data-driven scientific understanding.

It was possible for villagers to gain understanding through microscopes but it required significant investment in education. One such success, highlighted by an October 5, 1957, *Jiangxi Daily News* article, recounted the efforts of a farmer, Zou Luode, placed in charge of the Meizhuang snail fever prevention station. When Zou had trouble understanding the booklets about prevention, he asked the doctors nominally under his supervision for help in understanding how people could safely dine on river snails, while the *Oncomelania* snail was dangerous, and why one kind of snail was infected with the parasites' larvae and the other was not: "Out of curiosity he gathered two bunches of river snails and two bunches of *Oncomelania,* crushed them, and examined them both under the microscope."[29] A doctor stood by and helped him interpret what he saw and connect it to the disease's life cycle. After months of interaction with his doctors, Zou understood the ideas behind prevention and became a successful educator. Thus, people with minimal education were perfectly capable of understanding the concepts of prevention if afforded long-term, intensive science tutoring.

Scientific exhibits offered another means for mass experiential science and were reportedly one of the most well-received and effective methods for conveying new ideas about science and disease transmission. In addition to traveling exhibits, key campaign sites like Yujiang and Qingpu established exhibition halls in 1964 and 1973, respectively. Exhibitions were filled with photographs, X-rays, slides, material objects, and even three-dimensional models. Many also displayed charts, graphs, maps, and statistics proving the potency of campaign work. Some also had sick people and those who had been cured ready to talk to fellow villagers about their disease and how it could be treated. Proctors stationed at exhibits helped people interpret what they saw. Microscopes were the centerpiece of most exhibits, the culminating piece of evidence linking the information to physical reality (see figure 6). Microscopes were much more effective as part of an exhibit than when presented singly in villages. Explanatory material in the exhibit provided villagers with a context for understanding what they saw in the microscope. For some villagers, the exhibition space was like an alternative world, completely different from the village environs and very exciting as a result. When Jiangxi's Shangrao Prefecture held an exhibit in 1954, it attracted 14,500 people who swarmed in from the neighborhood, fascinated to see this new spectacle. After viewing Qingpu's exhibit in 1954, which combined heart-wrenching photographs about the ravages of the disease with scientific evidence about how to counteract it, an eighty-five-year-old women said, "It was the best I ever attended."[30] She returned home and encouraged everyone else to go. Many people reportedly attended multiple times and came from miles away. Qingpu's spring 1956 exhibition was an even greater success, visited by 80,130 people, according to campaign reports. After viewing this exhibit and gazing through the microscope, one villager remarked, "Previously I'd only heard the name of *Oncomelania* snails. Now I can see it's a tiny little thing. I know its appearance and can go find it." Another villager commented, "Previously I didn't believe snails had cercaria. Now that I can see them it's

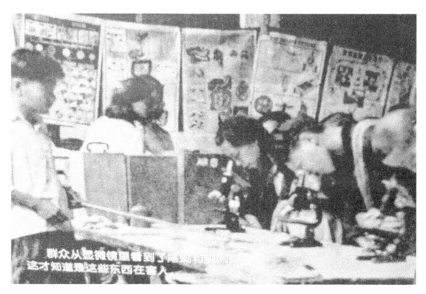

FIGURE 6. Educational exhibit about snail fever that also popularizes basic science. Photo from the collection of Miriam Gross. Picture taken in the Yujiang County Songwenshen Memorial Museum.

really frightening!"[31] Exhibits seem to have spurred interest and perhaps higher campaign participation levels. They may also have extended understanding by creating a holistic environment, employing a comprehensive approach, and likely having more knowledgeable educators.[32] Unfortunately, this approach was a very resource-intensive and complicated pedagogical strategy. For this reason exhibits did not play a major role in most rural areas.

Starting in the 1960s, Party efforts to increase literacy through conscription, adult literacy education, and vastly expanding the rural education system, which also taught basic hygiene and health information, began to pay off. Likely as a result of education, rural people, especially youth, started assimilating some of these new ideas about the origins of disease. The Party trained many of these educated youth as grassroots health workers to disseminate knowledge in the villages and act as a force for change. Due to their education and literacy, these workers were better equipped to understand and retain the knowledge they received, enabling them to provide clearer and more specific presentations. The large number of concurrent health campaigns instructing people about new pathogen-based diseases also mutually reinforced new concepts of disease causality. By 1964, after seeing a movie on the life cycle of snail fever and then looking at miracidia under a microscope, local cadres and villagers from Jiangsu's Kunshan County remarked, "Wow! It really makes my hair stand on end. It makes it all come alive [huolonghuo-xian]! Previously our thinking was too apathetic. From now on we must definitely eliminate the snails!"[33] In Yujiang, after a villager, Chen Qiguo, saw the ova in his own feces under the microscope, he went home to educate others about the disease and encourage them to get their stool tested too.[34] After years of scientifically oriented education on multiple fronts, some members of the younger generation were in a different place by the campaign's second peak during the Cultural Revolution (1966–71). The world behind the lens began to make more sense and provided a convincing rationale for previously inexplicable campaign activities.

PREVENTION: THE CONCEPT THAT NEVER GOT ACROSS

The CCP hoped that the prevention arm of the snail fever campaign would be cheap, effective, and empowering and would help to construct a scientific socialist society (see chapter 5), but lack of understanding of the concept of prevention significantly undermined this goal. As a 1952 Qingpu report explained, "Some people on the surface are doing the work—like cleaning their house nicely—but inside they totally don't understand the purpose behind it. In many cases it is a task-oriented approach—the top ordered the bottom to complete the task, and it was done, but there was no understanding of the hygiene behind it."[35] County and provincial reports consistently remarked, "There is a discrepancy between the policy, which is that prevention should be primary and treatment a supplement, and what people are doing on the ground, which is to neglect prevention in favor of treatment."[36] Grassroots personnel were unsuccessful in making prevention compelling. "If we only do prevention," noted a 1953 Shanghai report, "then the masses won't be mobilized; but if we only do treatment then we violate the principle that prevention should be the main activity."[37] Even this report writer did not see the reason for doing prevention except to uphold Party discipline.

The fact that rural people did not understand prevention is demonstrated by responses to vaccination campaigns. Shots have an easy conceptual link to prevention, since a single shot protects against one disease. Popular responses suggest that many people thought vaccines were a new type of medicine, effective only when the disease was occurring. When there was a summer upsurge of malaria in Qingpu in the 1960s, villagers were infuriated that they got preventive medicine only the next winter when they were no longer sick. As a group of Qingpu residents said when trying to resist vaccinations in 1952, "Whether we are healthy or not has nothing to do with you [the vaccine givers]. Moreover, if you don't give us shots, it's not certain that we'll die."[38] If vaccines were a medicine, it made no sense to give them to the healthy. Some people decided vaccinations were a magical cure-all that, due to government sponsorship, might actually work.[39] Whether eager or resistant, villagers consistently assessed vaccinations as a new type of treatment, rather than as a prevention mechanism.

If the prevention concept was incomprehensible when there were direct causal links between the activity and result, it is not surprising that education failed to convince people that they had to alter their water usage, work, and bathroom habits and change the whole environment by leveling hills and digging a new irrigation system to attack snails that caused a person's big belly only many years later. In snail fever, eggs found in feces are not the infectious agent. Instead, the cercariae, or second-stage worms emitted from free-living snails, infect humans. Yet in 1958, after years of education, Yujiang villagers speculated that dogs should have a higher rate of disease than cows because dogs ate human feces and the eggs got into their bodies. An equally confounded report author commented, "We can't open their stomachs so we don't know."[40] Thus, even the connection between the life cycle of the parasite and risk factors was unclear, let alone any connection with prevention activities.

Many common pedagogical strategies actually obscured the conceptual basis of prevention. The biggest reason why health campaigns were unable to convey the fundamental idea that pathogens cause disease was that they rarely directly taught this idea. Instead, the posters, comic books, and simplistic texts for the semiliterate immediately plunged into the life cycles of particular organisms without explaining the underlying principles of disease transmission. Speculatively, this may have reflected broader trends in medical education, especially in the public health arena, where material was simplified and theoretical underpinnings removed. As C. C. Chen, a distinguished medical professor explained, "Premature specialization produced graduates who were ill-prepared, especially because of their lack of clinical training and scientific background. To some teachers, too, they appeared to have failed to gain an adequate understanding of the broader meaning of public health."[41] Not surprisingly, when these students produced educational materials and most likely when they taught, they replicated their own training by producing texts and images narrowly focused on single diseases. For most villagers, it was impossible to generalize from one example, particularly one with such a byzantine life cycle as a parasite. This was especially the case because this idea challenged the preexisting paradigm that diseases were caused by environmental imbalance, past life indiscretions, dissatisfied spirits, and an excess of heat, cold, or wind—in other words, diseases were caused by forces beyond human control.

The inability of the snail fever campaign to convey that pathogens cause disease had devastating consequences. If a microorganism causes disease, then it is logical to either kill the germ or to create an environment where it cannot live, validating the logic of prevention-based campaigns. However, if disease is beyond human power to control, a prevention campaign is irrational. At an important Jiangxi 1956 prefectural meeting, cadres said that the occurrence of the disease "is a matter of bad environment [shuitu buhao] so there is nothing to do to treat or prevent it."[42] In 1973, after decades of work in Yujiang's test site area in Magang Township, a female hygiene leader had a child who got sick. Her neighbor said, "I don't do hygiene work and my child hasn't gotten sick. Sickness has to do with your fate and not with hygiene work."[43] Interestingly, African malaria campaigns faced similar challenges. Because people thought diseases' origins were beyond human power to influence, "people [were] unwilling to participate in time-consuming malaria [prevention] control activities."[44]

Educational material also unintentionally reaffirmed the idea that forces beyond human control caused disease. The earliest antidisease campaigns, the Patriotic Public Health Campaigns, were premised on attacking evil germs allegedly spread by Americans conducting germ warfare against China during the Korean War in 1952. Germs were portrayed as tiny twisted American soldiers with big noses, who would be eliminated by the Chinese populace in patriotic battles. This representation built on prior depictions in which the demons, ghosts, and gods causing disease were shown as evil twisted people with bold features. Initially, the snail fever campaign propaganda represented the disease through malicious, deformed figures, still wearing the olive drab of American soldiers. After Chairman Mao's famous poem, instead of being "germs," these figures were termed the evil "god of plague." Both visual representation and the poem's title reaffirmed that, as usual, a malevolent god caused this disease (see this book's cover and figure 7). The sense that germs and ghosts were interchangeable can be seen in people's use of realgar or red orpiment, an arsenic compound. To get rid of

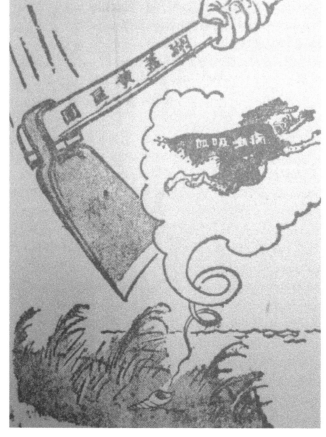

FIGURE 7. Newspaper representation of snail fever reinforces evil spirits and miasmas as the cause of the disease. Lü Qizuo, "Ganzou wenshen," *Jiankang bao*, no. 695, November 26, 1958, 2.

ghosts, realgar was sprinkled on the affected area of the body or was drunk. Even after villagers heard that diseases did not come from ghosts, a July 1955 Qingpu report noted that they "still used realgar to kill all the germs in the environment."[45] Villagers had learned that the malicious force was external, rather than internal, but did not understand that an entirely different entity caused the disease.

Confusion about disease life cycles was compounded by linking prevention with more appealing activities that helped production, citing gains in efficiency to motivate participation. Thus, people reconstructed the water system to improve irrigation, create more arable land, *and* kill snails. They managed night soil to bring manure strewn around the village into the feces management system, thereby increasing the amount of available fertilizer. They also brewed manure longer to kill a variety of parasites' eggs. However, if efficiency and speed were the goal, it was most effective to stop doing the portion of work directed against the disease, because it had no impact on production. Villagers could dump snail-laden earth in the river (spreading the snails further), while still effectively reconstructing the irrigation channels. People could collect manure around the village, usefully increasing their fertilizer stock, without brewing it, a lengthy process that brought no obvious dividends but is the crucial step for killing the schistosome eggs. Linking prevention activities and production made it easy for people to focus on production, the concept they understand and valued. It also meant that villagers were trying to parse the meaning of prevention in the context of agricultural production, rather than in relation to discussions of disease.[46]

The snail fever campaign, like the Four Harms Campaign *(sihai yundong)* and the Patriotic Public Health Campaigns, was a kill campaign focused on obliterating a specific pest from the environment. Unfortunately, kill campaigns obscured prevention rationales by using what was discernible (i.e., rats, snails, and feces) as a proxy for the invisible pathogen. After hearing campaign propaganda, a co-op member cleaned out his animals' shed because "he didn't want his oxen to come down with a disease."[47] He thought the feces itself was dangerous, rather than the pathogens it contained. Once the threat lay in a visible object or creature, it was easy to attack it for the damage one saw, rather than for the invisible disease-causing agents it carried. While rats were supposed to be killed to prevent plague, propaganda suggested eliminating them because they ate grain—the threat people could see. This strategy backfired because creatures that caused no obvious damage and were merely annoying, such as mosquitoes, flies, and bedbugs, seemed unworthy targets. Snails were the most innocuous of all. Villagers concluded that the Party had a hidden agenda for forcing rural people to kill them. As some Qingpu villagers said in 1956, "You're just afraid we'll be idle in winter time and had to find make-work for us to do."[48] When the main explanation was the harm caused by the snail vector people could see, rather than the pathogen it carried, the whole logic behind the prevention activity became unintelligible. This problem was compounded when educators again invoked the virtue of efficiency by enlarging the original Four Harms Campaign to five, six, and, then seven harms, one of which was snails.[49] As multiple campaigns became bundled, it was hard to distinguish the details of any one. Then the thing they all shared, obliterating a creature, became the preeminent component of them all.

Chairman Mao's focus on complete disease elimination, rather than control, created a final problem. Since the benchmark was elimination, positive assessments used the language "basically eliminated" or "completely eliminated." This focus undermined the long-term nature of prevention work. Additionally, when villagers heard the word "eliminated," they assumed their work was done. Since endemic diseases like snail fever are almost impossible to eradicate, a standard based on elimination established unattainable expectations. This led to great dissatisfaction at endlessly repeating work and made it difficult to link the concept of prevention to ongoing attempts at keeping diseases under control.[50]

The large disconnect between the educational messages delivered and the knowledge actually required to understand how pathogens cause disease makes it unlikely that people participated in the 1950s and early 1960s campaigns for scientific reasons. Villagers conducted prevention activities based on faith in the Party, societal pressure, and active leadership, when it existed. As a result, postfamine (1961–65), when faith was low and coercion light, almost all prevention and sanitation activities stopped. By the early Cultural Revolution, an understanding of some of the basic science, mainly among youth, joined other reasons for campaign participation and also provided a new way of understanding the world. However, the fact that the majority of villagers did not understood the concept of prevention for decades probably was the final blow to prevention work.

INCULCATING NEW STATES OF MIND

Most health campaigns tried to inculcate people with the new scientific states of mind thought to be the foundation of a modern scientific socialist society. Scientific qualities included neophilia, efficiency and rationality, and creativity and innovation, attributes counteracting characteristics ascribed to the old society during the New Culture Movement (c. 1915–30s).[51] The old society, particularly peasants, were cast as unchanging for thousands of years, leading them to absorb a backward, superstitious, apathetic, and irrational mind-set. Health and other scientific campaigns were key to reconstructing the attitudes of villagers, who through conscious participation for rational reasons were supposed to be transformed into innovative members of society.

Unlike scientific knowledge, a scientific mind-set was easy to engender, but outcomes were not what the Party expected.

One of the crucial attitudes for effective societal transformation was neophilia: embracing the new while vilifying the traditional. Neophilia was a key strategy for consolidating power, as most resistance stemmed from past experience and entrenched patterns. The CCP was represented as embracing all attributes that were new and progressive while valiantly bettering the lot of rural people by battling "our country's most harmful infectious disease," whereas the prior Nationalist government was castigated as the epitome of backwardness.[52] Unfortunately, the more that propaganda emphasized snail fever's longevity and prior government incapacity, the more impractical it seemed to eliminate the disease. As a 1955 Shanghai report explained, "[People] feel it was transmitted from the past, and therefore they have not tried to do anything and further are afraid of it."[53] When the disease was hyped as a formidable enemy, it seemed like an impossible foe for normal people to neutralize. A 1957 Jiangxi report warned that "some, by making snail fever seem excessively dangerous, cause the people to feel afraid of it."[54] As the eradication campaign endlessly lengthened beyond its targeted conclusion, many rural people concluded that the propaganda was right: snail fever was an age-old intractable disease that no government could cure.

In addition to touting new attitudes, campaign propaganda also lauded the Party's new scientific medicine methods and modern doctors while censuring those who sought help from traditional religion. A 1956 comic published in the Qingpu newspaper titled "Don't Look for Gods, Only Look for Doctors" admonished: "After Chen Quanqing's son got sick, instead of taking him to a doctor he borrowed six yuan from the high-level cooperative to go to the temple and have them pray for him. However, his son got worse and when he finally went to the doctor it was too late." After Chen's wife was cured using scientific medicine, "he kept thinking that if he had believed in the doctor perhaps his son would still be alive."[55] These messages denounced the victim for taking a retrograde attitude, unable to grasp what was new in society. Activists cured by the campaign employed the riveting theater of public self-criticism to push others to consider modern medical choices. In Jiangsu's Jiangdu County, Xu Chunhe, an asymptomatic man who had earlier refused treatment, became so sick that he had to give in. Post-treatment he enthusiastically criticized himself in a meeting: "Before, I didn't obey the doctor. The result was that I harmed myself."[56] How these messages were received is unknown, but based on treatment statistics they did not result in people flocking to get treated. In general, villagers and grassroots cadres seemed unwilling to jump on the bandwagon of any campaign or activity simply because it was new. In fact, they demanded the sorts of rationales and scientific proof that the Party was trying to teach them. Ironically, when they were unwilling to take new things on faith, Party leadership blamed locals' resistance on backward thinking.

A second focus to spur participation was based on rationality and efficiency and determined by a cost-benefit analysis. A common campaign slogan codified this as *san suan liang bi,* the three calculations (of bodily health, production levels, and economic situation) and the two comparisons (of the present to the past). Many meetings were dedicated to working out specific calculations of time and money of household-based budgetary analyses to prove that treatment was cost-effective.[57] Unlike scientific knowledge, the logic behind cost-benefit analyses was easily assimilated by rural people. However, the likely reason for this was probably not because of rational enlightenment by the Party, but because villagers were already making these kinds of assessments—weighing the consequences was a survival strategy for people living in precarious circumstances. The novelty lay in adding specific numbers to the decision-making process. Unfortunately for the snail fever campaign, rural people were quite capable of totting up treatment's risks and costs based on daily economic realities, rather than potential future earning power. They concluded that treatment was unaffordable, a situation that remained in effect until 1966 when the government fully subsidized treatment.

The Party focus on rational reasons for treatment reinforced people's belief that treatment did not apply to them. Education advocated treatment so that people could work harder, not so that they could feel better, and definitely not so that they could rid themselves of a pathogen. As a text intended for a grassroots audience explained, "Those who prior to catching this disease could carry 100 jin on their carrying pole, can only carry 70–80 jin when the disease is light, 40–50 when it's a little heavy, 20–30 when it's heavier, and in the end they completely lose their labor power."[58] This made treatment rational for those with impaired working ability, but contrary to propaganda, most early-stage patients were working at full capacity. Neither they nor their leaders could see how the campaign related to them. As one cadre from highly endemic Qingpu put it in 1962, after a decade of education: "The people are all healthy and therefore we don't need health work. You don't talk about health with them and still they can lift very heavy burdens so certainly they don't need you!"[59]

After the start of advanced producers' cooperatives (late 1956), when communities had to pay for the campaign, more educated campaign personnel exploited numbers to prove that community-wide sacrifice was a rational choice. In a 1963 report from Jiangxi's Ji'an Prefecture, personnel told villagers in a high-incidence area that, "based on statistics, absence from work due to snail fever for the year reached 27,538 days. If each person receives 0.8 yuan per day, there was a loss of 22,030.40 yuan. [Of the 1,124 sick people] each person on average paid medical fees of 15.28 yuan. The two losses together were a total of 39,205.12 yuan. This was a huge loss and made people shocked and amazed."[60] Even if spurious, numbers helped put the campaign's costs in perspective. Campaign personnel also wielded statistics to demonstrate that insurmountable problems could be cut into realistic portions of work. A 1956 Qingpu summary report noted: "We figured out that we could make a time estimate, given the amount [of snails] a person can clear in one day's work. It will take five hundred people ten days. Doing this sort of accounting provided great educational benefit to the cadres and people."[61] Once the work was completed, more statistics were trotted out to prove the work had accomplished something. In Qingpu's Chengbei Township, a national test site, personnel created tables that documented the amount of snails, the labor needed to eliminate them, and the work points required to finish the job. Even if such numbers were untrue, making the work seem concrete made it harder for local cadres to demur. It also made snail elimination like any other contract labor job, so that it could be slotted into broader production plans.[62] Regrettably, in the campaign's first decade most grassroots personnel did not have the education to effectively wield statistics. When more personnel could use them, by the mid-1960s, numbers not only helped educators convince communities that participation was a rational choice but also were very important to effective planning.

One downside of statistics was a decrease in work quality. Numerical measures initially focused on who did the most, encouraging people to do a scanty job to win in the statistical sweepstakes. A 1956 Jiangsu report discovered that "people's thinking puts particular stress on the numbers achieved and not on the methods to eliminate the snails or that to actually eliminate them the work must be done repeatedly and meticulously."[63] A decade later, this problem had yet to be solved. A 1965 Qingpu report noted, "Some brigades just look at how much area snail elimination has been done in, rather than whether the snails have actually been eliminated."[64]

Statistical measures of success also encouraged people to choose work they could count. Leaders of kill campaigns encouraged villagers to embark on sanitation by using snails as a proxy, hoping that this would result in cleaning up infectious material. However, since it was difficult to count sanitation activities, it was impossible to gain credit for them. Indeed, a February 1956 report from the Shanghai Health Bureau lamented about the Four Harms kill campaign to eliminate pests: "We must have people do activities like garbage management, rather than just killing the rats. . . . The content of the campaign is mainly counting up numbers so that eliminating the Four Harms hasn't become part of people's consciousness."[65] The extreme focus on numbers to assess achievement contributed both to poor-quality work and to selecting only work that could be counted.

Grassroots innovation and creativity were the final characteristics to break the allegedly rigid patterns of conformity inherent in traditional labor practices. Surprisingly, with the advent of high-level cooperatives, villagers willingly designed new ways of doing things. This impulse seems to predate Communist education efforts and likely arose from the well-honed capacity of poor people to "make do." For many rural people, innovation was probably limited by resource scarcity, time, and risk, rather than by creativity or a closed mind. In more stable cooperatives with pooled resources and risk, the natural inclination to make do probably came into play. Propaganda education, newspaper articles, meetings, and people who gained model worker status based on creativity, among other things, reinforced that innovation was a way to gain recognition, material rewards, and job advancement.[66] As a result, villagers carefully drew attention to their fixes but now called them innovation and scientific experimentation.

Grassroots tinkering steadily increased. Initially, villagers used preexisting items in new ways. In 1956–57, when people in Yujiang could not reach the snails on the sides of irrigation channels, after emptying them of water, they grabbed the snails by standing on stilts, an item intended for plays held during Spring Festival. Around villages, people used chopsticks to snag snails. Realizing that this method missed buried snails, some Yujiang villagers thought of raking snail-laden earth into bamboo baskets, dumping the contents on level ground, and then checking for snails bit by bit. In 1958 in Shanghai, villagers spread calcium carbide, a waste product from factories, and reportedly "killed the snails with great success." After the snail fever prevention station "confirmed these results with its own experiments," this strategy was disseminated widely.[67] Educated Shanghai villagers also created job contracts for snail killing in 1954, and a Hunan team reportedly had twenty revisions to existing campaign procedures by 1959. These contributions, and those described in chapters 5 and 6, suggest that local people not only found ways to make their own work more effective but also involved themselves in broader work-process strategies.[68]

Wan Fengxin from Yujiang County epitomizes this innovative mind-set. Almost sixty when he took over the feces management work in 1956, Wan experimented with adding various mixes of lime and grasses, and he found ways to seal the lid of the night soil vat with mud to speed up the fermentation process so that people would have their fertilizer faster. Wan also contacted cadres to assess their future fertilizer needs, and he tried to organize his system so that his product was ready when needed. His efforts to increase efficiency and productivity are a good instance of villagers' effective use of innovation and experimentation. In recognition of his achievements, the county secretary awarded Wan model worker status, and stories about him were published in the newspaper, encouraging others to follow his example.[69]

Grassroots creativity brought acclaim to the inventors, helped create ownership and pride among village communities, and ensconced grassroots science as the height of modernity and a potential path to social respect and authority. Unfortunately, it had little impact on disease elimination. Reevaluating the overheated assertions of the Great Leap Forward, a 1959 Jiangxi report said, "In the past we were good about developing things that were created by the masses and accorded with real practice, but we were not good about doing experiments on them prior to dissemination."[70] Random kill techniques were sometimes ineffective or devastating for the environment. Semi-educated doctors, quite successful within their area of expertise, often failed when pushed to replace medical knowledge with innovation. Finally, in an effort to increase efficiency, inventions often undermined quality control.

Rural people easily assimilated scientific states of mind such as rational decision making and innovative problem solving, but this did not correlate with enthusiastic campaign participation. In the short term, villagers were perfectly able to do a cost-benefit analysis of campaign injunctions and novel techniques and decide whether they were rational and efficient. Indeed, rational decision making provided a perfect justification for jettisoning portions of the campaign. Nonetheless, emphasis on scientific attributes did teach the significance of the trappings of science, even if not of the science itself. Villagers absorbed the idea that, in addition to ideology, Party propositions were promoted via statistics and tropes of rational efficiency. They learned to couch their choices in numbers, to give them legitimacy, and to explain their fixes in experimental and scientific language to gain recognition. Over time, the attributes of science would became a primary mechanism for signaling both authority and authenticity.

EMBEDDING COMPLIANCE IN
ORGANIZATIONAL STRUCTURES

Implanting motivation in organizational structures, rather than education, proved to be the most effective strategy to achieve compliance and was frequently used in mass mobilization campaigns. Tasks were performed because of social and organizational expectations, pressure, and assignment, rather than understanding or personal choice. Treatment work was promoted effectively using traditional social and familial organization. Snail elimination campaigns relied on structures from the new society. However, such campaigns were unable to attach sanitation and hygiene to any organizational structure, possibly explaining the campaigns' limited success in this critical arena.

Exploiting traditional familial and village relationships and respect for the elderly was an extremely effective way to promote treatment. People resisted treatment, fearing that the doctors were quacks and that painful shots would kill them. Using people's family and peers, having them eagerly recount their own cure post-treatment, not only allayed these fears but also persuaded doubting villagers to "start having confidence ... that the treatment was good" (see figure 8).[71] Such activists were carefully matched with those who were sick, for maximum impact and moral suasion: elders of the same gender were paired, good friends, wives and husbands, elder and younger brothers, fathers and sons. As early as 1951, the Shanghai campaign noted that "the most effective way to get people in for treatment was to get family members to recommend that they do it."[72] Realizing the value of peer activists, some areas jump-started their campaigns by "first mobilizing people who were comparatively easy to talk to and also simple to cure and then using them to convince others."[73] After receiving treatment, worried family members sometimes put loved ones on the treatment list without asking them.[74]

Respected elders were also used to push people into supplying stool samples for disease testing. When Dr. Horn visited a model commune, personnel explained that they used Old Chen to deal with evaders: "Old Chen here ... chases up these Smart-Alecs and gives them a lecture and then they nearly

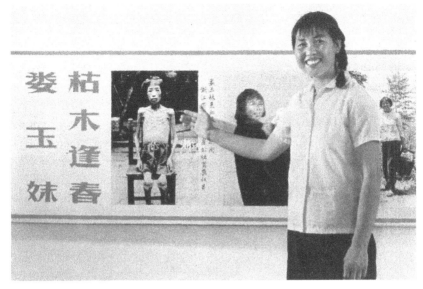

FIGURE 8. Snail fever activist points out her former self, promoting the campaign through personal example. *Qianjunwanma song wenshen* (Guangzhou: Zhongguo chukou sangpin jiaoyihui, 1973), 12.

always send their specimens." "I don't give lectures," said Old Chen. "I'm no good at lecturing. I just tell them what it used to be like here in the old days when practically everybody had a big belly and they soon see the point."[75]

Peers, family members, and elders with life stories similar to their audience were living proof that treatment worked, making them compelling educators. Yujiang's Gongtang Township propaganda sessions sometimes featured Pan Houfa, a man who had snail fever for ten years before being cured. As Pan became incapacitated, his frustrated wife took advantage of the new marriage laws to divorce him and flee with his son and daughter. After receiving treatment, Pan changed from making six to nine work points per day, and he was able to remarry and start a "harmonious household."[76] Women-oriented education efforts featured women talking about borrowing rice and selling off land when their husbands became very sick, a problem solved by treatment. Women also brandished their healthy young sons, a miracle after years of disease-caused infertility.

Successfully treated peers and family members trumpeted the good news, building a sense of excitement, confidence, and victory sorely lacking from other parts of the campaign. When the campaign treated people who appeared to be dying, the impact was even more impressive. After the doctors in Jiangxi's Guangfeng County miraculously treated a patient at death's door, "from then on our authority and trust were raised on high."[77] Reports indicate that peer activists' messages and personal examples were easily understood and very persuasive.

On the prevention side, leaders used the new organizational structures in collectives and mass campaigns to prompt engagement in snail-killing campaigns. People assigned to mass campaign work were offered work points, thereby embedding participation in the work process and removing the choice to refuse. Campaign work was recast as a militaristic exercise, implanting discipline, obedience, patriotism, and value into a seemingly worthless activity. Starting from its earliest medical work among soldiers in guerrilla units in the 1930s, the CCP connected health and physical prowess to military preparedness and racial fitness. The 1952 germ warfare attack that launched the Patriotic Public Health Campaign movement led the CCP to characterize all medical work as the yeomen citizenry attacking the enemy invading germs. Indeed, the very name of the snail fever species in China, *Schistosoma japonicum,* prompted some localities to believe that the disease was brought by Japanese germ warfare during the 1940s.[78]

Snail fever mass mobilization work was framed as a military campaign against "the enemy," who was "staging an armed rebellion."[79] Prevention work involved a "war of annihilation" conducted by "commanders in chief" who planned out their strategy on maps at the "command post."[80] Campaign propaganda was termed "combat slogans." Before a major digging effort, or "bitter battle," "the troops were convened to harangue them before war."[81] This was so that "each person's fighting will make a contribution" and so that they would "persevere in eliminating snail fever with a will like iron and steel."[82] Workers assigned to shoveling were "soldiers" organized into a military structure of battalions, platoons, and brigades and ordered to use strategies stemming more from warfare against fellow humans than those best employed against mollusks. Even consolidation work was framed as part of a long-term crusade. As a Yujiang report put it, "Long time watch; periodic reconnaissance; fight repeatedly; maintain our victory!"[83]

Mass campaigns often went beyond militaristic language and organization to attack a designated "enemy" community member or clique. This provided the campaign with momentum when the scapegoats yielded, and it affirmed in-group bonds among participants and a determination to follow the Party so as to avoid their quarry's fate.[84] Unfortunately, germs and snails did not make for nearly as high drama, so personnel tried another common strategy, turning work into a mock battle between competing brigades.[85] According to a 1957 Jiangxi report, competition "smashes conservative thinking and stops a self-satisfied attitude."[86] Competition was also used to encourage treatment. In Qingpu, recalcitrant villagers "who kept making excuses that they were too busy" were told that "people from other villages are running here to get treatment even though they are busy too."[87] This implied that individuals and villages would seem less capable if they did not get treated and that treatment might be a scarce commodity that should be acquired before it was too late. Not only did the government use mock battles to manipulate people, but people exploited this same strategy to get their efforts noticed. Some Shanghai villagers made small contracts to turn over a set amount of snail-laden land per day, pledging to overcome their laggardly prior efforts, a strategy assuring them of success.[88]

In addition to providing motivation, mock battles were useful because they forced leaders to participate in the campaign to judge who won. Their presence in turn led to "a high level of supervision and monitoring" that greatly increased the efficacy of prevention work.[89] Although a crucial campaign strategy, mock battles had several pitfalls. A 1958 Qingpu report found that strong interunit rivalry "could lead to them [villagers] not working with each other."[90] The bad taste left by feted winners and denigrated losers could lead to constant instability, struggle, and transformation, which Chairman Mao felt was the catalyst for uninterrupted revolution. Additionally, mock battles undercut the already insufficient attention to quality control. Competing groups were unlikely to bury snails deeply enough to actually suffocate them. When high statistical accomplishments gained villagers community-wide recognition, neglect of quality control was validated as a necessary strategy for success.

Unfortunately, the prevention work of sanitation and hygiene was less amenable either to old or new organizational structures. Few family networks were willing to promote alien hygiene regimes. Military framing and mass work under a commander seemed less germane to small surveying or snail-killing groups working in their spare time, and totally inapplicable to solo hygiene habits.[91] Personnel occasionally tried to get villagers to "accuse and denounce" unhygienic neighbors in front of the group. In one case in Qingpu's model test site, people reported an old lady who "was very obstinate and absolutely refused to forgo washing her commode in the river. Eventually she was criticized in a large meeting and had no choice but to change."[92] In Yujiang, this strategy was used to attack people who raised doubts. Report writers felt this "encouraged and mobilized the confidence of the cadres," but the downsides were that it made public dissent dangerous and targeted the unhygienic person villagers could see rather than the dangerous worm they could not.[93]

Compared to other mass campaigns, there were almost no reported instances of public denunciation in the snail fever campaign, mostly because villagers and leaders shared the same unhygienic habits and did not perceive them as problematic. Reports everywhere fulminated about washing commodes in rivers and other sanitation practices for decades. Dr. Komiya, a Japanese snail fever expert, noted that even in 1957 villagers in model areas were still washing commodes in the river and engaging in other unhygienic habits.[94] There was such a strong consensus that old habits were useful and natural and new regimens were incomprehensible and inefficient that even the erosion of privacy in collectives could not compel change. The inability to attach a change in hygienic patterns to a traditional or new organizational structure is one reason why altering such patterns was the least effective part of the campaign.

Nevertheless, permeating the campaign with a patriotic military ethos granted it a vibrancy and validity that it probably lacked on its own merits. Mock battles not only increased output without coercion, or "motivated popular activism," but also led to rewards, praise and a sense of victory becoming the goal rather than the work itself. There was no longer any need to actually understand the logic behind the prevention activities and be motivated by it.[95] When placed in a militaristic light, the snails' constant reappearance was not a failure but an opportunity to demonstrate patriotic affiliation with the New China.

Although impossible without the organization and impetus of militaristic mass mobilization, this structure ultimately constrained what the prevention campaign could accomplish. By their nature, mass campaigns are discontinuous. Both Party members and foreign observers noted that they were "effective as a leadership strategy only temporarily under conditions of great stress." This makes them "totally unsuited to the more bureaucratic politics of a modernizing state" and very bad at tasks requiring continuity.[96] As a Jiangxi report on the October 1959 sixth national snail fever meeting noted, "Some people feel that mass mobilization campaigns can only encompass Sturm und Drang campaigns and not regular work. In fact they separate them and view them as opposite."[97] Many campaigns hit an issue hard, creating tension, relaxed, and then hit hard again. Framing campaigns as mock battles mirrored this structural tendency but made it impossible to justify or even conceive of work as something requiring continuous effort. Yet, health campaigns required uninterrupted work, since the snail population recovered between the large but infrequent snail campaigns. Meanwhile, lackadaisical feces and water management meant that worms were still infesting villagers' water sources. The new body-hygiene disciplines needed to be done at least once and sometimes multiple times per day. Occasionally enacting some of them under the eyes of a leader did not lead to the engrained habits needed to really change the way a person lived. Despite this inherent problem, entrenching snail elimination work in mass mobilization campaign structures was one of the most effective ways to guarantee participation, ensuring that the campaign could function.

CONCLUSION

The Party employed everything from traditional entertainment to microscopes to provide the scientific education that was supposed to motivate participation in health campaigns and to achieve wider societal transformation. However, few scientific ideas were effectively transmitted because of the lack of knowledgeable teachers, incomprehensible language and paradigms, and counterproductive educational strategies. Indeed, campaign reports decades into the snail fever campaign indirectly indicate that many villagers understood neither the concept of pathogen-based disease nor the associated notion of prevention. The inability to transmit the rationale behind prevention helps explain why prevention activities were met with high resistance.

The Party effort to inculcate villagers with scientific attitudes was notably more successful but did not lead to higher participation levels or better campaign practice. Instead, after rationally assessing campaign activities, villagers concluded they were illogical and inefficient and refused to do them. Likewise, while new inventions may have increased participation levels, they rarely benefited the campaign. However, the many scientifically oriented campaigns did convey the authority of science to villagers and taught them to present their work in these terms, possibly leading the Party to an exaggerated view of people's understanding of science and their level of support for the snail fever campaign.

The most effective mobilization strategies had little to do with formal education. Instead, they embedded participation via organizational structures. Exploiting family relationships and village networks worked well for treatment but was not helpful for the campaign's prevention arm. Campaign work assigned by collectives combined with competitive, militaristic mass mobilization structures, ensured participation in unappealing snail elimination campaigns and helped glorify them beyond their apparent value. These methods motivated short-term participation but were unable to promote sustained effort. They also undermined long-term success by encouraging speed over quality. This strategy was least effective at transforming sanitation and hygiene patterns because cooperatives could not promote alternative bathroom habits by assigning them as a job. At the same time, militarized mass campaigns seemed inapplicable to individual hygiene choices, and the intermittent nature of such campaigns made them especially bad at providing the day-by-day enforcement needed to solidify new patterns. Finally, there was a strong consensus that these new hygiene habits were pointless. By the Cultural Revolution, an era exalting the revolutionary masses, hygiene became associated with effete urbanites, making it even easier to ignore. The Chinese countryside would have to wait until children and conscripts learned new habits in school or the army and then had children of their own. Very gradually, this new consensus paired with an updated sanitation and hygienic infrastructure would alter the appearance of villages and the practices of their inhabitants.

By the late 1960s, the snail fever and other campaigns did succeed in introducing the concept of microorganisms to the small number of newly educated village youth. This suggested a new way of looking at a previously invisible world now made visible as much through the lens of the Party as the microscope. However, for most people prevention activities, discussed in the next chapter, remained an incomprehensible imposition by the new government, quietly neglected or undermined for much of the campaign.

CHAPTER FIVE

Preventing the Unpreventable

IT WAS 1956 IN JIANGXI'S Poyang County, and the government had come to provide a village with a new well as part of its many sanitation campaigns to promote hygienic uplift. The snail fever station got to work digging, only to encounter a large problem. "The entire village's women came screaming and beating drums and proceeded to completely fill up the partially drilled well." After that, the women mobbed the Party branch secretary and "gave him a scolding."[1] Villagers were certain that the new wells would doom the community for generations due to destruction of local feng shui. No hole in the ground was worth so much trouble.

The many reports on China's model snail fever campaign by American, Canadian, and European scholars in the late 1960s and 1970s emphasized its popular patriotic engagement and touted its educational and preventative portions as inordinate successes. They described the campaign as a cohesive government endeavor conducted similarly in all places, an example of the new government's ability to make its will manifest at the grassroots level.[2] The reason for these universally positive assessments is clear: archives were unavailable, national campaign propaganda lauding prevention work was the primary source of documentary material, and the sparse scholarly visits were restricted to model communes.

Newly opened archives demonstrate that except for the work of a small group of activists (see chapter 7), popular resistance effectively altered practice on the ground. Despite identical national directives communicated as provincial or municipal mandates, the government was unable to compel localities to perform the campaign in a unitary way, even in model areas. Moreover, although the snail fever and other health campaigns improved sanitation, the former's success at preventing and eliminating the disease was transitory at best. The Chinese conviction that snail fever was mostly eliminated during the Great Leap Forward (1958) and that the campaign succeeded due to low-tech work by the masses, rather than scientific and technical expertise, also prove to be unsupported. Instead, the turning points of the campaign came during and immediately following the Cultural Revolution (1966–71 and 1977–80, respectively) and can be traced to excellent, scientifically based treatment work.

This chapter describes the complex grassroots realities of the campaign's prevention arm during two key periods: 1949–55, when China's Ministry of Public Health conducted early work; and 1956–76, when the campaign was transformed by the participation of Chairman Mao, the collectivization of society, and concurrent revolutionary campaigns. The chapter particularly examines why people resisted and how resistance altered prevention activities in these two periods. The early ministry campaign challenged the prevailing view of people's relationship to nature. It focused on changing community sanitation practices, which entailed cleaning things newly defined as dirt, and on building sanitation infrastructure, which disturbed local feng shui. In the second, more intrusive stage, the campaign focused on altering personal hygiene and bathroom habits and on mass mobilization campaigns to eliminate the snails carrying the disease. The campaign ground to halt from 1959 to the early 1960s, during the famine, and peaked again during the Cultural Revolution, a period notable for its achievements in snail elimination but ultimately not for preventing the disease. The chapter concludes by examining why linking the campaign to production simultaneously supplied motivation and justified the greatest resistance to the campaign.

EARLY PREVENTION WORK: SELLING THE IDEA OF SANITATION

When the Ministry of Public Health began snail fever prevention work, it lacked human and material resources, local buy-in, enforcement capabilities, and even accurate information about disease prevalence. Since MPH did not have the power to goad independent farmers into snail and irrigation work, localized efforts at improving sanitation and drinking water seemed more realistic and corresponded well with concurrent sanitation efforts of Patriotic Public Health Campaigns.[3]

Early sanitation work focused on three activities and tried to institute a fourth. First, campaign personnel tried to stop people from drinking sewage-contaminated local water and encouraged use of newly built wells or other clean water sources instead. Second, campaign workers attempted to stop villagers from washing out their morning commodes in their drinking water. Since fresh night soil was stored in a riverside feces vat that overflowed every time it rained, workers advocated adding covers and moving the vats into newly built shacks away from the river.[4] In places that did not use vats, the campaign encouraged digging a hole that acted as a cesspit to hold all the community's manure. Third, the campaign promoted building and using public toilets, rather than letting people eliminate wherever they wanted. Finally, villagers were encouraged to ferment the night soil for several weeks, creating a chemical reaction that killed snail fever eggs and those of many other diseases.

This seemingly benevolent agenda faced a big challenge: as discussed below, most people did not see a need for sanitation. Feeling that the body's personal products (feces, urine, saliva), garbage, and animal manure were natural and part of the ecosystem, managing them seemed unnecessary and intrusive.[5] Chairman Mao may have shared this view. After his doctor tried to stop him from swimming in Guangzhou's Pearl River because he could see human excrement floating by, Mao replied: "If we tried to follow the standards of you physicians, we wouldn't be able to live. Don't all living things need air and water and soil? . . . Everything has some impurities, some dirt. If you put a fish in distilled water, how long do you think it would live?"[6] If personal products, dirt, and water were fine where they were, then wells, toilets, cleaning, and trash disposal were pointless. As some workers in a big Shanghai hotel restaurant explained, "It's useless to do cleaning because tomorrow new guests will come and mess things up again."[7]

The important corollary is that sanitation activities were considered make-work, a severe indictment in a society that valued productive labor so highly and in a place where people were worked to the bone to make a living. This perspective was backed up by Communist ideology. According to philosophy stemming from Friedrich Engels, "[Labour] is the prime basic condition for all human existence, . . . we have to say that labour created man himself."[8] In China this was taken to mean that any material products formed by labor should be rewarded by community recognition and support in the form of money, goods, or work points. However, sanitation and, more broadly, prevention activities simply stopped something from materializing and did not appear to generate a substantive yield. Therefore, it could be argued that there was no community responsibility to support them. Thus, the highest levels of political thought buttressed the grassroots' inclination to forgo incomprehensible health work if it took away from production.[9]

Because these new hygienic patterns seemed pointless, villagers could not understand why government propaganda education spoke moralistically of creating a higher-level civilization. Some villagers concluded that campaign personnel simply wanted to replicate the customs of their hothouse urban environment in the countryside. As Yujiang villagers remarked after being asked yet again to do a sanitation-oriented prevention activity, "How can people who till the soil be particular about things like city folks?"[10] Though the government followed Western mores and preached that only a clean person was good, villagers felt that one's inner qualities and good works should really matter. Qingpu villagers commented in 1954: "Eating sloppily or wearing dirty clothes won't have a bad result. In fact we can still aim to be a Buddha."[11]

Local government's response to sanitation work varied depending on proximity to big municipalities. In Qingpu, with Shanghai's extensive sanitation system just over the horizon, when it became apparent that occasional Patriotic Public Health Campaign sanitation efforts were insufficient, the county government started a sanitation organization in 1951 with sixty-four units, each in charge of a separate garbage bin.[12] In more typical rural areas like Yujiang, the government neither had a sanitation system nor saw the need for one. No matter where, few individual citizens thought that sanitation equipment was necessary, even when they were offered a loan to pay for it. From 1952 to 1954, Shanghai tried to loan rural families in the suburbs fifty thousand yuan to buy feces vats (equal to about five yuan after the currency was under control). This program did not succeed because families were unwilling to go into debt to buy a shit container. Similarly, Shangrao Prefecture in Jiangxi tried to loan entire villages money for a few vats. However, "it didn't go through because people said they couldn't afford three vats."[13] Sanitation practices seemed so strange that when Qingpu's model Rentun Village decided to stop washing commodes in the river, "other villages didn't believe it and came to see if it was really true."[14] Without acceptance, sanitation efforts were limited to sporadic campaigns and often meant cleaning the village, generally just prior to the arrival of higher-level cadres. Decades into PPHCs, a 1973 Yujiang County report lamented that "many people and cadres think that frequently doing hygiene or sanitary activities is unnecessary and a waste of time."[15] Lack of community consensus that sanitation was important greatly hindered this work even at the height of the campaign.

At the few model test sites where local leadership embraced sanitation work, it was unclear how to encourage these behaviors noncoercively prior to the advent of cooperatives. One strategy was community-wide agreements that shifted enforcement to the community itself. Such pacts often contained long lists of specific injunctions. In Yujiang's Magang Township model test site, villagers made an eight-point agreement that covered all aspects of feces management, bathroom habits, and responsibilities for cleaning the toilets. For example, number 6 stated, "It's prohibited to shit wherever one wants outside."[16] This and other pacts also created rules about appropriately using designated water sources, which led one report to state, no doubt over-optimistically, that the pact "made water management a mass movement."[17] This seems doubtful after examining the pact's sanctions. For example, number 3 stated, "It is forbidden to secretly rearrange the feces vats and to use them before they are brewed," which suggests that rather than eagerly participating in the new hygiene regimens villagers were reshuffling the vats to fool local feces management personnel.[18] Such health pacts worked only when most agreed with their content; they were simply a mechanism to censure the few offenders. Since most people did not understand the purpose behind sanitation and hygiene, there seems to have been little actual implementation even when villagers were prodded into making a pact. Archives do not mention pacts after the early 1950s. Apparently, even model sites had such limited success with this strategy that it was unworthy of further dissemination.

Local personnel also discovered risks in complying with national standards that used methods that had not been tested locally. Yujiang personnel dutifully built the mandated type of wells during a drought and then discovered this was a "northern method that didn't suit our environment and wasted a lot of effort."[19] Jiangxi's Dexing and Yushan Counties also built wells and cesspools and then widely disseminated their strategies to the rest of the province: "But these methods were not too appropriate for other places, resulting in a big loss of money. For example, we built huge cesspools that had very little feces in them. Locals thought they were very inconvenient and also were not used to them, so they ended up not being used. They [campaign leaders] didn't do a detailed analysis of the local situation and just looked at their plans."[20]

The Ministry of Public Health's early personal sanitation work had little lasting impact. Dismay over being forced to clean up a world that was not dirty continued throughout the campaign. The belief that the natural and human worlds were indivisible made it hard to conceive of bodily products as either separable or dangerous. As bad as it was to be asked to adopt incomprehensible new habits, it turned out to be even worse to build a new sanitation infrastructure.

EARLY PREVENTION WORK:
THE CHALLENGES OF FENG SHUI

For the many people who believed in feng shui or environmental geomancy, sanitation infrastructure and prevention work were actively harmful, rather than symbols of a healthier future.[21] Just as *qi,* or vital energy, flows through human beings, it also courses through the landscape. Although many aspects of nature were beyond human control, manipulation of natural *qi* to achieve health, happiness, and prosperity was not. Generally this involved a careful examination of dates, direction, and local environmental features to orient and construct buildings so that they maximized *qi.* Just as well-aligned feng shui could bring benefits, disruptions in local feng shui that cut or impeded the veins of *qi* were thought to underlie many ills experienced by the individual or the community. Since any reconfiguration of the land could have long-term repercussions, rural people were careful about making radical shifts to the environment, particularly breaking new ground. Yet, almost every aspect of the snail fever campaign involved digging: digging wells, toilets, and cesspools; destroying old channels and digging new ones; and even digging up feces vats from the river and reburying them elsewhere.[22]

Hoping that altering the land to suit human needs would give these supposedly fatalistic, apathetic peasants a sense of power, many rural health and agricultural campaigns had a short-term focus of improving production and a long-term focus on taking control of nature. It was hoped that reconfiguring the landscape to meet human needs would allow villagers to realize that they controlled the environment, rather than vice versa, and would spur their transformation into a utopian scientific socialist society. Instead, gauging the many impending digging activities, villagers concluded that the snail fever campaign would probably kill them off. As people in Jiangxi's Poyang County put it, "Digging wells will sever the mountain range, will cause people to be doomed, and will lead to pestilence among the pigs and oxen."[23] People were certain that moving things "could bring a disaster . . . that will influence the next generation."[24]

The intensity of concerns about feng shui varied with geography, economic conditions, and exposure to modern ideas that denigrated feng shui as rank superstition. In the Shanghai region, a flat, relatively economically secure area, people were willing to try some campaign activities despite worry about feng shui. Reconstructing the irrigation system seemed appealing because flooding was the biggest natural threat. The abundance of local water and excellent engineers made this a relatively low-risk activity. In contrast, feng shui was treated very seriously in mountainous, impoverished Jiangxi, where life was tenuous and the landscape had a profound impact on human life. In the vibrant folk religion of 1950s Jiangxi, the energy flows of feng shui were personified as an earth dragon whose veins could be cut by digging and whose eyeballs would be covered if pools were filled. This angry dragon could cause harm in many ways. Realistic fears of drought made reconstructing irrigation a real hazard to sustained agricultural productivity. When the new channels did not conduct water, likely due to incompetent aquatic engineering, people in Jiangxi believed their fears had been confirmed—altering feng shui and impairing flows of *qi* had clear natural consequences.[25]

Villagers and local cadres tried to protect themselves and their communities by maintaining or returning the feng shui to its preexisting state. In addition to refusing to do the campaign work, people seized feces vats at night that had been forcibly dug up from the river and reburied them in their old home. In some areas around Shanghai, people agreed to move vats but demanded a three-year guarantee from the Party that nobody would die.[26] In Yujiang, some places "made a regulation" that the feng shui should "be protected" and that wells and channels should be dug in such a way that "the feng shui won't be cut or harmed."[27]

Prior to coercive advanced producers' cooperatives, methods to achieve digging-based prevention activities were not successful. Some personnel dug wells themselves to shame people into digging. As some villagers put it: "A Shanghai physician dug one well for us. We're embarrassed not to dig a well ourselves." The very next day they dug ten wells.[28] Unfortunately, this was not a strategy that could be sustained. Employing feng shui experts to situate a new well or feces vat was expensive and gave the Party imprimatur to the very "backwardness" it was trying to eliminate. However, the discovery that villagers were more willing to do the work if it was certified by a feng shui expert sometimes led efficacy to triumph over scientific purity. After discovering that persuasion via propaganda education tended to be ineffective, quota-driven personnel were left with little to show for their efforts. In desperation, some personnel hired experts, only to be chastised by higher-level leaders for undermining one of the Party's primary missions.[29]

Local cadres also influenced popular reception to sanitation efforts. Most cadres supported village resistance because they believed in feng shui. Some cadres, seeing the amount of money paid to feng shui experts, appropriated this activity for themselves. A 1952 Qingpu report noted that "each time they [villagers] moved a vat they had to have a feng shui expert check it out." Each siting cost five hundred yuan, so the village paid fifty thousand yuan for its hundred households.[30] In another village, each siting cost one thousand yuan. Some places "established a committee of young village cadres to manage feng shui questions. The young cadres did this in order to corruptly make money off the situation."[31] A few cadres used their leadership to facilitate villagers' acceptance. In 1956, feng shui concerns, reinforced by a leader getting sick, made Yujiang residents reluctant to dig up Dragon Hill: "People were convinced that the disturbed dragon had seized a hold of him." The leader's rejoinder intermingled Western medical ideas (he had earlier received Western medicine for a stomach ailment) and Chinese ones (removing his clothes because he sweated caused his body to fluctuate rapidly from hot to cold, resulting in sickness). Due to his explanation, "people decided that their old [superstitious] thinking was crazy."[32] A leader with stature and personal connection to the problem was effective at transforming local opinion. However, leaders willing to risk carelessly altering feng shui were few and far between in rural places like Jiangxi.

With the onset of high-level cooperatives (late 1956) and communes (1958), villagers had little influence over the work assigned by the hierarchy of leaders. This meant they had difficulty protecting local feng shui, as few could afford to forgo work points because of possible future harm. Later, communes and revolutionary high tides let the CCP experiment with increasingly ambitious environmental reconstruction, completely flying in the face of feng shui. During the Great Leap Forward (1958–61) environmental work meant digging new toilets and wells, reconstructing channels, and filling in swamps to expand cropland. By the Cultural Revolution (1966–76) the goal was "completely altering the environment" by filling every hole, leveling every hill, straightening every channel, and killing a growing number of pests until the countryside resembled (at least in one's imagination) a blank sanitized sheet of paper on which to build the new society.[33] As one Cultural Revolution jingle summarized, "All the fields have become square, the channels an interlocking network, east and west all look the same, north and south have one appearance, the hills are all smoothed out, and the water can both irrigate and drain away."[34] The snail fever campaign helped endorse this extreme topographical makeover by claiming that flat land facilitated finding residual snails and that fast-flowing, straightened channels were a less hospitable environment for them.[35]

Villagers' conception of their relationship with nature formed a major barrier to campaign work. Since humans and nature were inseparable, the notion of moving one part of nature, such as manure, to another part of nature seemed like the ultimate make-work. Moreover, since humans were integrated with their world, their best bet for an auspicious life was aligning with natural energies, not recklessly disrupting them. The belief that changes advocated by the snail fever campaign were more likely to bring death and destruction than future health made resisting sanitary schemes an ethical choice. Real work on sanitation and hygiene awaited the embedded coercive powers of the cooperative system.

CHAIRMAN MAO TAKES COMMAND: MANAGING MANURE AND ATTENDING THE TOILET PROPERLY, 1956–1958

The snail fever prevention station makes everything their own business; they even want to manage people's defecation and urination!

Yujiang villagers, circa 1956

Beginning in 1956, control of the snail fever campaign by Chairman Mao, coupled with transition to advanced cooperatives, ushered in a many decade change in the power dynamics around managing manure and toilet habits.[36] The shared budget of cooperatives simultaneously made sanitation infrastructure more affordable while ensuring that participation was less negotiable. Advanced producers' cooperatives not only built large numbers of wells, public toilets, and septic tanks but also designated feces management personnel. However, the basic stance of the villagers that sewage cleanup was make-work, that bathroom habits were outside the government's purview, and that there was no reason to use a distant water source in preference to one nearby resulted in continuing resistance to the campaign.

Objections to new personal hygiene patterns that reached campaign reports centered around inefficiency and wasted time, an acceptable way to couch dissent. Indeed, drawing water from the well or cleaning commodes at the feces management site did take longer and was more work (see figure 14 in chapter 7). As women from Shanghai put it, "Running back and forth in order to empty out the commodes is a waste of time."[37] It was less convenient to use the public toilet than one's own or a convenient bush—and impossible for men working in the fields. This line of argument carefully mirrored the campaign's own propaganda that promoted participation based on time and labor power. For example, the argument for hiring full-time commode dumpers went as follows: "In this way women's household work burden will be decreased and their energy for production will be concentrated."[38] Similarly, bottom-level reports are filled with villagers' arguments that campaign activities impinged on the time and energy needed for production.

Cultural choices compounded unhappiness about new sanitation infrastructure. According to the blueprints, public toilets were separated by gender and often reflected differences in how men and women were valued. Although men were away in the fields, the male side of the latrine was often larger, including both urinals and more toilet stalls, and sometimes had a winding entrance or privacy screen. These differences reflected social standing, rather than community need, as it was women who helped children and elderly use the toilet. Having the vast majority of the community struggle to use a very few stalls increased irritation, inefficiency, and smell.[39]

Campaign personnel in wealthier areas developed a strikingly effective strategy to work around villagers' views on sanitation. Whenever possible, they assigned hygiene work to someone else, rather than forcing change. Commode washing as a separate job predated the campaign, either as full-time work or in Qingpu, as a sideline.[40] Catching on to this strategy's potential, campaign workers rapidly brought commode workers under government control. Likewise, it was easier to give someone else the job of cleaning public toilets. By 1956, at least in Shanghai and Qingpu, feces management was divided into two types of full-time jobs: washing out morning commodes; and managing/cleaning vats and public toilets, which were often interconnected units.[41] Using small, specialized teams to survey and kill snails was based on similar logic.

Solving feces management by making it a dedicated job had severe limitations, most notably that most communities were unwilling or unable to pay people for jobs that previously took little time and no money. Some communities paid intermittently for commode dumpers at production peaks, to expedite women's coming to the fields, but few consistently compensated those managing toilets or other feces repositories. Communal cesspools exemplified this problem. Cesspools were widely disseminated after 1956, particularly in poorer areas. They were cheap, easy to build, and able to handle a large area's waste disposal needs, but they were especially problematic for snail fever control. Villagers refused to lug excrement long distances merely to dump it in an assigned trench. Moreover, when villagers removed night soil to fertilize the fields, they usually scooped off the top part of the cesspit's manure pile, the only portion they could reach. Consequently, the "clean," well-brewed bottom manure remained in situ, while the top portion, filled with parasitic eggs, was redistributed to the entire region. A further problem was that when accepted, cesspools often acquired other uses, for example, as a reservoir collecting the water from washing out personal commodes. However, the chemical reaction necessary to kill the eggs does not work when night soil is diluted. A full-time feces manager might have mitigated such problems, but few saw the utility of paying someone to preside over a shit hole.[42]

Finally, night soil was the farmers' gold, the main fertilizer that had kept paddy fields producing for centuries. When the time came to apply fertilizer, villagers were unwilling to let a little matter like sufficient brewing time stand in their way. In some areas, people believed that fresher manure was better at helping the plants grow.[43] Throughout China, even model sites dismissed the idea of brewing night soil long enough to kill off parasites' eggs. Most ignored this directive entirely. Others sealed up vats filled with water when monitoring teams came by, assuming that they would not unseal them to check if something was brewing inside. Even when there were feces management personnel, commune members eluded them with tactics like night raids on the feces depot to clear out the fresh stock.[44] In the rare instances when night soil was brewed long enough to kill eggs, the system was often completely overloaded because so much night soil accumulated during the necessary storage period (two weeks during the summer and four during the winter).[45]

For those places that could afford it, off-loading sanitation tasks enabled communes to reach short-term hygiene goals. A 1957 Women's Federation report from Shanghai remarked contentedly, "This work teaches the masses not to wash their commodes in the river and changes a custom many thousands of years old."[46] However, once work reverted to individual women, as it did in Shanghai and Qingpu during the dire conditions postfamine in the early 1960s, people resumed washing commodes in the river.[47] At base, the strategy of making hygiene chores an assigned, compensated job did not alter underlying behavior; it only left top leadership with a false impression of change.

Given this deep-seated resistance, it is important to assess the extent to which sanitation campaigns actually changed hygiene and sanitation. Change was easiest when new patterns evolved from old ones. Because bathroom habits were highly correlated with geography, location became an important predictor of outcome. In places with high water tables, like Shanghai and Qingpu, villagers used commodes and thus were familiar with toilets that moved around. Because toilets were implements rather than locales, there was less resistance to "field toilets" or to manure processing systems composed of big vats, which were simple extensions of the commode concept. Although expensive, the flexible vat-based system could be located at numerous collection points conveniently near people's homes. Ironically, even though initial disease incidence was worse in flat places with high water tables, the campaign experienced the most success in such places because the new sanitary practices were an easier progression from the old.[48]

In areas with low water tables, people used family pit-based toilets and were unaccustomed to commodes. Since a toilet was a hole in the ground, commodes did not qualify as toilets. Fueled by anger over the forcible demolition of private toilets, there was high resistance to public facilities, and field toilets were rarely built because of unfamiliarity and expense. Moreover, when their pit toilets were destroyed, families' lost the contents, which previously were sold when families needed money. Adding insult to injury, their building materials were used to construct the hated new toilets. Not surprisingly, villagers tended to steal back their bricks, stones, and wood at night, leaving the remaining rubble strewn across the new building site. Almost no successful feces management work took place in poor areas with pit toilets, and people vigorously retained or returned to their old habits even when faced with extensive outside pressure.[49] Interestingly, the pit-based system was actually very good at limiting the spread of snail fever, but the associated lifestyle was at odds with the new sanitation procedures.

Populations such as fisherfolk, who lived on the water, presented the biggest geographical impediment to changed behavior but were a key target because they had high infection rates and dumped infectious wastes into water. However, it was almost impossible to provide sufficient propaganda education, gain the control necessary for change, or create a workable toilet system for a population constantly on the move.

Many places provided boats with commodes or forced fisherfolk to buy one. However, having a jug did not actually mean using it.[50] In boats, only women used a commode, while men eliminated directly over the side. As they put it, "We are not used to shitting in a commode and when we try it nothing comes out."[51] Finally, storing large canisters of feces on board to deposit later on land was exceptionally smelly. Fisherfolk would often display the despised commodes and larger feces vats when on shore but use them as versatile containers to store almost anything but shit while on the water.[52] Providing sanitation boats to pick up night soil directly did not solve the problem. "Even though they see the feces boat in front of them, they still dump the commode in the river!"[53]

The large boat-based community in Shanghai was made into an official administrative unit called the Water District, but with a mere fourteen snail fever campaign personnel to reach out to the eight thousand boat people and more than forty thousand boat workers, this strategy failed.[54] Shanghai left small boats outside government control and turned boats that stayed around the harbor into companies slated for intensive control efforts. They were given commodes and required to link up with special feces reception ships at a set time to hand in their daily deposit.[55]

Qingpu ensured that all boats in its large fishing population had a commode, and key harbors established toilets for boat people. A night soil collection boat was dispatched at crucial moments of "collective production."[56] Fisherfolk were issued a feces receipt that entitled them to monetary reimbursement. Given that 2,641 gallons of shit earned only thirty yuan, it is not clear how much incentive compensation provided. Efforts to reach fisherfolk fluctuated: when the campaign peaked, outreach programs were developed; when the campaign ebbed, these were generally the first prevention activities dropped.[57]

Rural Yujiang also had a large boating population that mainly fished outside the county in Poyang Lake. Despite being a top national model, Yujiang was unable to develop programs for this population. Unfortunately, continuous infection from fisherfolk was one of the factors fueling the epidemic after Yujiang declared that it had eliminated the disease in 1958.[58]

The inability to control the fishing community also affected the land-based campaign. Women who were nagged for polluting water sources by washing commodes in the river had the perfect rejoinder. As one woman from Qingpu put it: "I can stop cleaning the commode in the river, but the boat people are still doing it. Doesn't that count as environmental pollution?"[59]

The other arm of the sanitation campaign was changing the sources for drinking water. The limited information in the archives suggests that this work was less successful than efforts to manage night soil.[60] Particularly in mountainous areas with low water tables, even having communes did not make wells economically or technically feasible. Instead, local campaign personnel invented cost-effective alternatives. In Jiangxi, portions of canals and ponds were assigned to specific tasks. In Yujiang, sometimes one pond would be for drinking water, one for clothes washing, one for washing vegetables, one for washing out commodes, and one for watering animals, all with signs stating a pool's particular purpose.[61] This strategy was economical but not particularly effective. A 1957 report from the Jiangxi five-person leadership small group to the national LSG said: "Water management almost everywhere just formalistically divides places into sections and posts signs while the people are still chaotically using the water everywhere. It's not very useful."[62] Even this nominal water management "system" was quite rare. As of May 1957, only 532 households in the entire province had separate pools for drinking.[63]

Impoverished places like Jiangxi managed to build some sanitation infrastructure but were unable to significantly change the bathroom habits of most of the population. Indeed, as a result of local economic realities and priorities, as well as resistance, poorer areas abandoned water and feces management, two major arms of the national campaign. In nonmodel areas in more affluent Jiangsu Province, this part of the campaign was carried out vigorously only at key revolutionary moments.[64] Water and feces management campaigns continued to be a major target of all rural public health work and were written up extensively as a primary objective in barefoot doctors' manuals after the program started in 1968. However, evidence of extensive intestinal worms and diarrhea in rural areas in the late 1970s suggests that these campaigns had not achieved the overwhelming successes reported by the Party.[65] The government claimed that peasant resistance to the new hygiene regimes showed backwardness and reflected feudalistic thinking. However, the new sanitary patterns took more time, more money, and more work, and some also embedded coercive practices for achieving non-health-related political goals (see chapter 7).

ERADICATING SNAILS: THE PREVENTION ACTIVITY PEOPLE PERFORMED

Mass mobilization snail-suffocation efforts became a symbol of the campaign. Snails were executed as vigorously and flamboyantly as possible. This provided an easy measure of campaign efficacy, as snail numbers could be quantified, and reflected the international standard of prevention at the time.[66] In addition, negligible achievements in altering people's hygiene and sanitation practices made snail killing seem easier. Because of scarce economic and technical resources, including molluscicides, the snail elimination campaign in the 1950s became a preeminent example of grassroots innovation and self-reliance, a core value of the Maoist era. Indeed, instilling resourcefulness in the grassroots was a primary purpose for many rural campaigns.

Eliminating snails was a major undertaking. They infested about 14.5 billion square meters of land and could survive on land, under water, and in oxygen-poor conditions. Snails were least noticeable in the winter and summer, because they burrowed into soil for protection against cold and heat. Unfortunately, since fall and spring were peak agricultural periods, farmers had no time to kill snails when they were visible. Instead, they performed mass campaigns in winter or summer, when many snails were buried.[67] Finally, the rate of snail reproduction is density dependent, increasing after some are killed. Snails replenished in ten months when 80 percent were killed and in twenty months when 95 percent were killed, making it difficult for a single annual campaign to keep pace with the snails.[68]

Ironically, at the same time as Chairman Mao's famous campaign against snail fever, concurrent campaigns enlarging irrigation systems and building dams expanded the snails' habitat and vastly increased disease prevalence. Even worse, linking up smaller pieces of irrigation into an integrated system allowed snails to spread miles away, sometimes reinfesting newly cleared land. Parallel campaigns draining wetlands and shallows to create new farmland diminished the volume of lake beds while damaging natural flood control systems. This resulted in more frequent and worse floods that also redistributed lakes' snails to farmland. In addition, with water now available, farmers changed from a summer wet-rice crop and a winter dry crop to two wet-rice crops annually. Natural die-off of the snails during the dry season was discontinued, allowing the snails to proliferate year-round. Although never acknowledged, the natural difficulties of eliminating the snails combined with their vast increase in habitat made the snail-killing campaign almost impossible from the start.[69]

Presented with the challenge of making the snail campaign a model of self-reliance and innovation, local cadres concocted a wide variety of approaches. Qingpu tried herding flocks of ducks and geese along the riverbank, but the

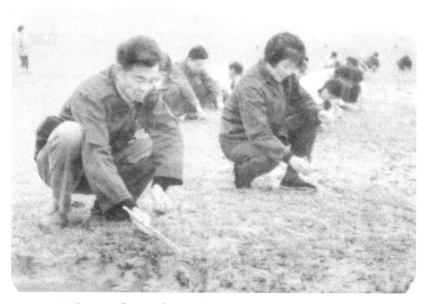

FIGURE 9. Tedious, ineffective efforts to eliminate snails with chopsticks deterred villagers from campaign participation. Unlike in this campaign photo, such monotonous, uncompensated work was generally relegated to women and the elderly. Zhonggong zhongyang nanfang shisan sheng, shi, qu xuefang lingdao xiaozu bangongshi, *Song wenshen: Huace* (Beijing: Zhonggong zhongyang nanfang shisan sheng, shi, qu xuefang lingdao xiaozu bangongshi, 1978), 65.

recalcitrant birds proved uninterested in snacking on snails. Next, people tried snagging snails with chopsticks, with grannies donning their spectacles to meticulously peruse the terrain. A total of 280,000 snails were eliminated in this way.[70] A July 1954 Jiangxi account recorded that, after mobilizing people six times and collecting only 14.8 pounds of snails, "we expended a lot of labor without killing many snails" (see figure 9).[71] Further, as the slippery snails kept popping out from between the chopsticks, the inevitable urge was to grab them by hand. Some previously uninfected people got sick this way.[72] Next, people tried casting hot water on snail-laden land, hoping to boil them into oblivion. However, it was expensive to boil so much water and difficult to transport it. In places with more resources, like Shanghai, the campaign considered purchasing a fleet of steamships whose boilers could be used to conduct scalding maneuvers alongside major riverbanks.[73]

The next tactic was molluscicides. Since chemicals were expensive and often unavailable, some places used industrial waste, which was dumped indiscriminately on fields and in water sources. Luckily, it was used only on a small scale because China's transport system was decrepit and the country's nascent industrial complex produced limited waste.[74] Most impoverished provinces like Jiangxi used lime and teacake, cheap natural snail killers. Unfortunately, even in perfect conditions, tea leaves were only 80 percent effective.[75] When the cost of molluscicides decreased, chemicals were more affordable for richer provinces like Jiangsu. While very effective against snails, factory-produced molluscicides were toxic, unbeknownst to most villagers: the chemicals poisoned aquatic life in a wide swath around their distribution point, negatively influencing the fishing industry and killing animals that came to drink, including villagers' prized oxen and buffalo, and they occasionally killed people. Molluscicides also created kill zones among the grain. Less poisonous molluscicides were developed but were slow acting, allowing snails to move to neighboring pristine fields, enlarging the infected area. Over time, specially trained teams learned to mitigate molluscicides' problems, but not to solve them.[76]

Villages also had to find ways to eliminate snails on vertical surfaces above the water level, where chemicals were less effective. In some areas, people destroyed vegetation along the banks of irrigation and river channels. This strategy backfired not only because it eliminated a key cattle-grazing area but also because people spread the snail-infested grasses on fields as green fertilizer, disseminating the disease. Wealthier areas invented a flamethrowing machine to eliminate snails in reeds and to annihilate those lurking in stone crevices. One campaign leader remembers night work lasting until midnight because the flames were too hot to stand during the day: "The white fire burned everywhere. . . . Sometimes the high temperature even cracked the stones."[77] Although the flamethrowers were impressive, the machines and fuel were very expensive and often unobtainable, and they frequently had mechanical problems nobody knew how to fix. Many teams spent their time making the machines function, rather than eliminating the snails.[78]

The final tactic, suffocation by burial, became the method of choice for eliminating snails throughout rural China. It was cheap, accessible to mass effort, fairly effective, and required only a shovel. Furthermore, because this activity reconstructed the decrepit irrigation system, it seemed a more worthwhile effort to rural communities. Replacing old curvy channels with new straight ones even created precious new farmland.[79] As these large reconstruction projects infringed on private land rights, they were feasible only in the era of higher-level cooperatives. As one article put it, "Peasants always wanted to fill in old ditches and dig new ones for irrigation, but before, new ditches

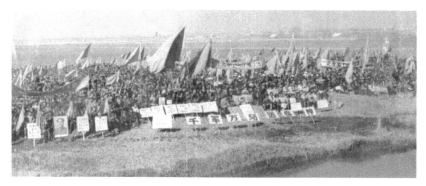

FIGURE 10. Mobilization for a mass snail elimination campaign, Dantu County, Jiangsu Province, 1960s. Photo from the collection of Fan Ka wai.

led to arguments which are avoided with cooperatives."[80] Unfortunately, when avid campaign managers checked work, the twin goals of snail eradication and improved irrigation often diverged, even to the point that snail elimination damaged the irrigation channel (see chapter 3). The result was that "people were angry because they felt they were wasting their energy."[81]

Smothering snails became the campaign's most important icon and was imbued with a wide array of political meanings. It represented patriotic endeavor, dedication to Chairman Mao, and people's willingness to put their bodies on the line to build the new scientific socialist society. The campaign frequently used language that sounded like military theater, such as imagery of the snail as enemy. Participants were supposed to imagine themselves as the newly created yeoman militia cutting swathes through China's age-old foe (figure 10; see also figure 3 in chapter 2). It is probably through these sorts of representations that the snail fever campaign was retroactively transformed into a symbol for all of the Party's benevolent work that helped the masses rid themselves of the ancient evils that had dragged them down.

Yujiang's snail-killing campaign provides a good example of this kind of portrayal. Shu Xiangmao, the vice district head of Magang in Yujiang County, beamed with pleasure as he saw his battle plans unfolding like clockwork. Four thousand people from fifteen townships had been mobilized to the Magang test area. Red flags were fluttering and the village was plastered with red posters and scrubbed to within an inch of its life. In the first battle, fifteen hundred people from seven townships had fought hard but failed to make the standard, the holy grail of success. Now Shu was certain they would conquer the dragon of all irrigation channels, a full six thousand meters long, its watery back glistening, sides peppered with snails, zigzagging through the whole area; with twenty side ditches, it extended its claws until it could deposit infested snails into the smallest nook and cranny.[82]

According to Shu, the key to this impossible task was the methodical planning that only the Communist Party could provide. After getting his orders on January 20, 1956, Shu had only ten days to mount the effort: four to organize and mobilize the surrounding villages, one to position the incoming troops, and five for the four thousand commandos to complete their assault. Shu established a command headquarters and divided his leadership group in two. The Party secretary dealt with logistics, ensuring that the village could feed, house, and appropriately welcome the four thousand incoming soldiers for five days, while his fifteen-person team went back to their villages to promote the cause. Meanwhile, the township head and the prevention cadres worked day and night to map the township, determine the placement of the new ditches, and calculate how many cubic meters of earth needed to be moved. Their project map indicated how to most efficiently distribute the work.[83]

The newly formed battalion marched into the village on January 25 and was welcomed with a huge party on the threshing ground. Everybody chanted slogans, enacted skits, and was, according to Shu, moved to tears remembering the bitterness of the old days. For the next three days and nights, people fought valiantly against their miniature opponent. One group dug new ditches, another moved the dirt, and the last cleaned the snail-infested sidewalls of the old ditches and pounded them down, using the clean earth to suffocate lingering snails. Shu made sure everybody strictly adhered to technical specifications. The county secretary showed up, and all the top leadership ostentatiously got dirty helping the snail crusade. The villagers could not believe it. In just three days, fifty-one big and small ditches, 35,000 meters long, were eliminated; and nine new ditches, 32,000 meters long, were opened up. In only one battle, the whole irrigation system was recreated and all the snails were (supposedly) annihilated.[84]

Well-done snail campaigns not only left behind a big feeling of accomplishment and a sense of revolutionary commitment but also led to impressive decreases in new cases of snail fever. After major burial campaigns in Yujiang County in 1955, infection rates dropped from a high of 49.5 percent to 28.6 percent in Gongtang Township and from 40.9 percent to 8.23 percent in Magang Township.[85] The prevention campaign fared well in the minority of places with access and funds for molluscicides, flamethrowers, and enough educated youth to constitute small groups specializing in snail killing. These groups engaged in snail elimination multiple times per year to keep up with the snail's reproductive rate, and they improved good will by minimizing people's engagement with the campaign. As one 1960 Shanghai report commented jubilantly about pesticides replacing burial techniques, "We only need three people when before we needed 150 people to do the same work!"[86] Similar to delegating hated sanitation work to designated personnel, delegating snail killing to teams allowed villagers to focus on food production, making the campaign more acceptable.[87] In February 1957, with easy assurance in its own affluence, Jiangsu explained that "in big channels it is suitable to use gas fire to kill the snails. . . . This year we have drafted eight boats with gas to eliminate them. Places short of equipment can use chemicals."[88] Wealthy areas were often also able to force nearby urban citizens, students, and the People's Liberation Army to help with their annual symbolic snail suffocation campaign, decreasing rural residents' workload.[89]

However, the vast majority of rural places were stuck with lightning-fast burial campaigns that were highly problematic because they had difficulty maintaining the high standards required for success. Villagers railroaded into the work found that burying snails under at least three inches of earth was onerous, instead scattering just enough soil to make the snails invisible. Because snails like being under about an inch of earth, this sort of "burial" merely resulted in them popping out again. The intense competitive focus on speed and impressive statistics also encouraged people to do a cursory job. As one Qingpu report described in October 1957, "The people don't know how to eliminate snails but do want to earn the most points they can, so they just throw the snails into the river."[90] A 1958 campaign report from Shangrao County, Jiangxi Province, concurred: "Everybody is very impatient. . . . There is a lot of large-scale work but little detailed, high-quality work. You often have fake reports arising. This was a problem, that they want fast results but lack a scientific attitude."[91]

More importantly, the burial strategy was unable keep pace with the reproductive rate of the snails or the increased dissemination resulting from the expanded irrigation system. Wei Wenbo, the scientifically oriented deputy director of the national nine-person LSG, was well aware of these limitations. He warned lower-level campaign leaders and participants that with only a single annual mass campaign, snails would return to their original number in less than a year. Chinese scientists, according to Wei, discovered that snail campaigns were successful only when done seven to eight times per year, with additional routine maintenance. As one big campaign a year was the limit of what popular will and production needs could stand, this was not a message that leaders were willing to hear. Unless people spent all their energy digging, the technical limitations of the only economically viable strategy meant that all their work would inevitably come to naught.[92]

CHANGES WROUGHT BY THE FAMINE AND ITS AFTERMATH

During the great famine (1959–61), the snail fever campaign stopped almost entirely and did not revive during the "recovery period" (1961–65). Loss of personnel, depleted morale, lack of leadership, and changes in agriculture all contributed to the campaign's problems. Prevention personnel either fled campaign work for food production or were transferred by local cadres into production to help the community recuperate. The result was a devastating drop in available personnel. In Jiangsu Province, campaign personnel plummeted from twenty-eight hundred in 1955 to five hundred in 1961, and health departments were usually powerless to recall personnel back to any health work.[93] In relatively wealthy Qingpu, even vaccination work dropped from meeting 100 percent of its goals prefamine to only 40 percent postfamine. In Shanghai, the thirty-nine hundred health workers trained by the Great Leap Forward plunged to only three hundred by 1961. Even the crucially important system for reporting new disease incidence to the government collapsed. Similarly, prefamine Qingpu had at least one group at each commune reporting new snail fever cases, but postfamine, smaller groups were supposed to cover three to four communes.[94] Reigniting prevention work awaited the Cultural Revolution, when the campaign acquired a large number of new personnel.[95]

Popular engagement with the campaign was also exhausted. Since, many villagers and rural cadres had never understood prevention (see chapter 4), participation was motivated by job assignments, societal pressure, patriotism, and faith in the Party. When the famine drained political capital and trust in the Party, few engaged in these apparently senseless activities. A September 1961 report from Qingpu reported: "In the 1950s many people were honestly interested in the campaign. Now almost no one is."[96] Making matters worse, many localities had asserted that snail fever was eliminated during the Great Leap and they held huge celebrations, where people were "blindly happy" because "they thought that after this they'd never have to deal with the problem again." Thus, it seemed unreasonable to be asked to continue divvying up stool samples and performing irritating prevention activities.[97] Faced with a major epidemic of acute snail fever a few years later, leaders could either suppress this fact or lose face by acknowledging that elimination had never occurred.[98] Yujiang, celebrated for its success by Chairman Mao, could not announce that the disease was still going strong. This forced campaign leaders to deal with people who "were convinced the disease was eliminated and won't do work anymore."[99] When pushed, they "became apathetic" and even more antagonistic toward prevention personnel. As Yujiang villagers put it, "The snails have already been eliminated, what are you doing here?"[100] The prevention personnel in turn "felt the work was very difficult and had very bad morale."[101]

Epidemic levels of dangerous acute snail fever, combined with massive snail regeneration after cessation of snail elimination work, confirmed belief that the Party was incapable of eliminating the disease. Summing it up, leaders in 1961 said: "The snails are small, the area is large, and it's hard to find them. We've already been eliminating them for years without a lot of impact. Can we really eradicate them?"[102] After hearing Wei Wenbo's, motivational talk in 1961, a campaign worker commented, "Snail elimination is even harder than dying."[103] By 1963, people in Jiangsu's Kunshan County concluded, "Wait until after we're old; we'll still have to give this work to our children and grandchildren."[104] Interestingly, the global campaign against malaria in Africa and India found similar patterns of resistance to adopting methods for repelling or eliminating mosquitoes. After being promised a quick fix and then seeing long, intrusive campaigns, rural people refused to participate because the methods were expensive and "time-consuming or temporary, or . . . promise[d]—in their minds—marginal efficacy."[105] Like in China, only great leadership could make villagers accept the campaign, and such leadership was rare.[106]

The Shanghai national snail fever campaign headquarters faced its own grave dilemma. After assessing the mass effort of the first campaign peak and resultant epidemic of acute disease, the leadership was unsure how to proceed. Shanghai's official retrospective account of the campaign calls the entire period of intense effort through 1965 "fumbling about to find a way forward [mosuo qianjin]."[107] Faced with little notion of how to proceed, limited political capital, few personnel, a very small health budget, and a stature that was declining in sync with Chairman Mao's other revolutionary ideas, the national government chose to start no new ventures and to diminish its expectations: it made campaign mandates less absolute and reduced standards, suggesting that snail elimination work could be accomplished in "spare time in the morning and evening" rather than by dedicated personnel.[108]

Problems were compounded by agricultural changes. To help recovery postfamine, villagers were allowed small private plots on vacant land, often directly on top of the old irrigation system where snails had just been buried. When people started digging, the snails began popping out again. Monitoring groups were unable to stop people from utilizing snail-laden land, since food trumped snails any day. Private plots also encouraged people to decollectivize manure (see chapter 7). Soon, fresh and egg-laden night soil was once again being dispersed through people's work environment.[109]

CULTURAL REVOLUTION: THE PROBLEMS AND BENEFITS OF REVOLUTIONARY RATIONALES

At the start of the Cultural Revolution, Chairman Mao's attention revitalized the snail fever campaign, using revolutionary zeal to overcome resistance. The simmering tension between scientific and revolutionary decision making that had existed throughout the campaign came to a head during the Cultural Revolution, with revolutionary approaches dominating when political pressure was at its height. Interestingly, the revolutionary excesses of the Cultural Revolution not only impeded the campaign but also helped it to function.

From the very beginning, Shanghai and Qingpu cadres tested and disseminated new practices suggested either by the scientific establishment or the Qingpu test site. Consequently, they were less willing to follow national mandates that seemed contrary to the epidemiology of the disease, resulting in a loose alignment with Party principles—one that was forced closer in revolutionary moments and drifted apart when pressure let up. Indeed, cadres' ability to incorporate scientific practices had a crucial impact on prevention work. A seemingly simple task like dumping earth on snails had variable success depending on expertise. The discovery that snails were concentrated in the first meter of channel banks, rather than the first 1.5 meters, as originally thought, reduced digging work by a third. Upon finding that snails buried themselves when it was hot, Qingpu stopped snail surveying during the summer heat. After campaign workers learned that snails were most mobile at 13–19 degrees Celsius, molluscicides were applied at these temperatures. By tracking snail life cycle and water-flow patterns, Shanghai researchers matched elimination strategies to seasonal configurations and thus increased efficacy. Indeed, Shanghai was able to continue elimination even in the early 1960s, when participation rates were at their nadir, because researchers discovered that almost all infectious snails lived near humans, with the infection rate dropping fourfold at forty meters away from human habitation and becoming negligible at eighty meters. By asking villagers to eliminate snails only within fifty meters of the village, work became manageable, and Shanghai continued the campaign when other places stopped elimination efforts.[110]

Jiangxi, with its high illiteracy rate and limited educated personnel, was more typical in its approach but had the additional legacy of being the site of the famous Jiangxi Soviet (1931–34). Citizens were proud of their revolutionary heritage. As Lü Liang, deputy head of Jiangxi's provincial LSG put it, "We inherited and carried on the excellent tradition of the old revolutionary base, fighting hard under adverse conditions."[111] Mao's populist vision of the masses overcoming everything without highbrow intellectuals telling them what to do was especially appealing in a rural backwater that had limited educational attainments. However, decision making based on revolutionary rationales adversely affected Jiangxi's ability to run a functional campaign. For example, individuals with a landlord background were not allowed to become snail fever treatment or prevention personnel, even though they constituted most of the educated people and Chinese doctors.[112] Consequently, Jiangxi waited more than a decade for the newly built rural school system to produce politically pure educated youth who could carry out the campaign.

Revolutionary consciousness also transformed mass snail burial into a valorous and patriotic activity, making a virtue of necessity while denigrating more targeted approaches. In places like Shanghai, Qingpu, or Jiangsu Province, villagers suffocated snails when funds were insufficient but switched to chemicals when it was economically feasible. As a man from Qingpu said in 1956, "Why don't we just use chemicals, which are easy and cover a lot of area fast?"[113] In contrast, in Jiangxi, the fact that snail elimination via burial was not written down in books and was denigrated by intellectuals and scientists made it even more alluring. Such campaigns appeared glorious because of the ability of human will and labor to overcome the snails. In Jiangxi, burying snails was claimed to be superior to chemicals, a claim never seen in the other study sites or in Jiangsu provincial reports. "In terms of efficacy, burial is best," reported the Jiangxi provincial five-person

LSG in May 1957.[114] Jiangxi citizens' antiscientific bias and glorification of mass digging campaigns led them, according to the biased campaign reports, to take patriotic pride in their work.[115] However, these attitudes also made the Jiangxi campaigns more arduous and less effective than in scientifically oriented places, leaving behind low morale when revolutionary fever subsided.

During the first half of the Cultural Revolution (1966–71), the clash between the scientific and revolutionary approaches became worse, with scientifically leaning areas forced into revolutionary decision making. The association of prevention work with bad categories of people and the heightened attacks on professional science and technical solutions were particularly problematic. Members of the five "black" categories (landlords, rich peasants, antirevolutionaries, bad elements, and right-wingers) were commonly assigned odious work, including feces management. In 1965, just before the Cultural Revolution, a Qingpu report suggested assigning feces management according to popular demand rather than forcing it on people from the five black categories to "make the person more accepted and increase the person's own pride toward the work." The report also suggested giving the person a new title, "sanitation personnel" rather than "commode dumper," so that the person "won't seem so low and will have a respected name."[116] Once the Cultural Revolution began, such proposals were unlikely to be implemented. Likewise, snail elimination work was fobbed off on the bad elements, which according to a Yujiang report, "turns this from honorable work into a punishment for bad people."[117] The increasing association of these jobs with bad elements ensured that normal people would not do them. It also guaranteed that night soil managers would not have the power to halt people pilfering fresh feces, ensuring that snail fever eggs were dumped back on the fields.[118]

An intense ideological battle between Chairman Mao and Liu Shaoqi erupted postfamine, when Mao's more revolutionary mass methods were called into question. These high politics played out in a proxy war in the snail fever campaign, negatively affecting prevention work during the Cultural Revolution. Since this campaign was famous as a positive example of Mao's mass-line policies and community self-reliance, it became problematic to give credence to the sorts of outside experts and technical solutions promoted by Liu Shaoqi.[119] Key high-level leaders—such as Jiangxi's Party secretary, Fang Zhichun, and Wei Wenbo, deputy director of the national nine-person LSG, who advocated a scientific approach—were attacked, associated with Liu

Shaoqi, and called "political gods of plague."[120] Those suggesting methodical snail work were viewed as impeding revolutionary fervor and reinstating hated bureaucracy. Even protective clothing (i.e., cloth wrapped around legs and feet) became a revolutionary issue. When snail fever experts were critiqued and sent down to the countryside to be reeducated, they were forced to relinquish their protective clothing so that they would "fight side by side with poor and lower middle peasants . . . [and] understand [group] devotion above personal concern."[121] Similarly, even though the Qingpu campaign had previously achieved very high elimination rates on one swamp with chemicals, by 1968 the campaign was forced to bury the other four swamps by hand, a process that took over a thousand people two months of grueling labor. Apparently, using chemicals contradicted Mao's tenets of frugality and did not "give full play to the strength of the masses." The Qingpu report carefully does not supply the percentage of snails eliminated by this revolutionary strategy.[122] The result of widespread revolutionary fervor and political pressure was that many new scientific practices, technical improvements, and management strategies were increasingly difficult to implement during the early Cultural Revolution.

On the other hand, revolutionary zeal was extremely helpful in counteracting popular resistance and, oddly enough, in achieving quality control. The revitalized Mao cult made it politically impossible to resist a campaign so closely associated with the chairman, spurring people toward exhaustive effort to eliminate every last snail. Villagers in Anting Commune, Jiading County, near Shanghai, meticulously perused every river in the commune ten times in 1967 alone.[123] This overexaggerated work was carefully totted up and reported so that the commune's revolutionary standards and loyalty would be ostentatiously evident. The superfluous work also helped compensate for the concurrent attack on bureaucratic processes, such as record keeping, and on the prior difficulty of ensuring quality control. Even without records of snail location, endless rechecking enabled people to achieve elimination. While previously it had been good enough to "basically" do the work, during the Cultural Revolution the goal of total elimination buttressed by revolutionary ardor ensured a much more painstaking snail elimination process.

The Cultural Revolution also rejuvenated campaign leadership both by adding large numbers of personnel and by making snail fever mass mobilization campaigns a political necessity for local cadres. Association of all prior failures with the "bourgeois reactionary line, capitalist roaders, and Liu

Shaoqi" made it crucial for even the most cynical leaders to maintain an overtly optimistic attitude and to ostentatiously conduct the campaign as a necessary piece of political theater.[124]

Finally, close to two decades of school building (see chapter 8) resulted in newly educated youth, who as campaign leaders were able to employ scientific tools to plan more effective mass campaigns. The escalating production and corresponding decreased cost of molluscicides made less labor-intensive snail-killing methods available. Trained teams of educated youth did better surveying to find residual snails and were able to use dangerous molluscicides more safely. When revolutionary heat diminished after 1971, many areas took advantage of this fact by carefully framing chemical use as consolidation work. Molluscicides, often used jointly with burial techniques for mop-up, resulted in fewer remnant snails and better morale. Some areas also paid more attention to remnant snails in borderlands by doing joint work between brigades, communes, or even counties.[125] With this symbolic acquiescence to national mandates, many localities deemed their responsibilities to the campaign's prevention arm finished, as neither feces and water management nor hygiene habits were an important part of the Cultural Revolution campaign. Although few regions were successful at long-term snail elimination, they greatly reduced the snail population during the crucial treatment period, significantly decreasing reinfection rates. As will be discussed in the next chapter, this short-term work obliterating every residual snail, mainly from 1966 to 1971, combined with superb work on treatment, was sufficient to create a tipping point in the disease.

THE PROBLEM WITH PRIORITIZING PRODUCTION: THE ULTIMATE LIMIT TO PREVENTION WORK

Linking snail fever elimination to increased productivity was undoubtedly a central reason why this overextended, impoverished government embarked on its snail fever campaign. National leaders felt the campaign would increase production in the long-term, while local leaders worried about short-term losses in productivity, but both judged the campaign in relation to this larger goal. However, subordination to this objective meant that all leaders prioritized production at the expense of disease elimination, jettisoning campaign activities that impeded agricultural work. No rationale, whether scientific or revolutionary, could breach this ultimate barrier.

When maximizing production conflicted with preventing snail fever, production won, even if more people got sick. For example, fresh manure placed in paddy fields was a source of infection. Instead of warning people about the dangers of rice production, the government admonished campaign personnel to "avoid emphasizing that going into the fields to work is a cause of transmission, to make sure peasants don't fear the water."[126] Many decisions not only concealed information that people needed to protect themselves but also directly caused illness. To ensure that land laid waste by the disease was plowed, Jiangxi placed state farms in areas known to be snail fever death traps, resulting in extremely high rates of hospitalization from acute snail fever. Throughout China, communes dispatched members to collect reeds as green fertilizer despite this material's proven ability to cause large amounts of acute snail fever. Even after whole teams were devastated, the very same communes sent them back the next year because nothing could get in the way of improving production.[127]

Likewise, local leaders and villagers refused to perform prevention activities that conflicted with production efforts. Because people thought it would reduce crop yields, night soil was not fermented long enough to kill the parasite's eggs, even though this is the most important aspect of feces management. As a result, infectious material was constantly disseminated into people's work environment. Protective clothing or a salve covering the skin to reduce worms' penetration were sensible, cost-effective tactics for preventing snail fever. However, farmers absolutely refused to wear such irritating, hot garb while working because it hampered the way normal work was done.[128] Fish farming was an important part of food production in rural China. Fish farmers floated snail-infested rice straw on top of the water to provide a more congenial environment. Some campaign propaganda suggested eliminating the straw, but farmers rejected the idea entirely. One of the most effective approaches to combating snail fever was changing from wet fields to dry land, as snails have difficulty surviving without a moist habitat. From the agricultural bureau down to individual villagers, everyone refused to implement this strategy because of unfamiliarity with dry farming, lack of proper seeds, and fear that it would result in less food.[129]

Even slight changes in normal work practice were unacceptable. Food was so essential and in many places so tenuous that it could not be disturbed in any way. In addition, villagers and local leaders were in complete agreement about the importance of food production. There was almost nothing leaders could gain by reducing their community's food supply. Together these groups, along with the agricultural ministry, formed a united front against any aspect of the snail fever campaign that directly affected production, successfully ensuring that key campaign strategies were never carried out.

CONCLUSION

The prevention arm of the snail fever campaign is famous in China and internationally for its purported accomplishments and popular support. This chapter finds that preexisting paradigms about the environment, disease, work, efficient living patterns, and productivity all played a role in how villagers and local cadres interacted with the campaign and were a primary reason why people resisted its mandates.

Prior to the coercive pressure of collectives and the leadership of Chairman Mao, the campaign focused on improving sanitation. As discussed in chapter 4, few villagers understood that pathogens caused disease, making the rationale for many prevention activities unclear. Likewise, since water and feces were natural parts of the environment, most people never grasped why sanitation was necessary. Moreover, concerns about feng shui made many of the core prevention activities seem actively harmful. As faith in feng shui was forced underground, the Party was left with the illusion that its education had been effective and that environmentally oriented campaigns to conquer nature were a good way to empower the people. Yet, despite decades of condemnatory propaganda, beliefs about feng shui remain strong. Following the Sichuan earthquake of 2008, one of the first explanations was that the huge Zipingpu Dam, 5.5 kilometers from the epicenter, must have disturbed regional feng shui, causing the disastrous earthquake.[130] Indeed, feng shui considerations are still an accepted mechanism for critiquing CCP environmental projects.

It becomes clear that acquiescence to and participation in the campaign derived from the level of revolutionary fervor, faith in the Party and Chairman Mao, degree of social coercion, mandatory job assignments, and political capital of leaders, rather than from understanding why prevention activities were necessary or the belief that humans controlled nature. As a result, during the famine and its aftermath (1959–65) and the latter parts of the Cultural Revolution presided over by the Gang of Four (1972–76), mass campaign activities tended to grind to a halt.

Initially, it seemed logical that resistance might center on intrusion into private, bodily business, but in fact it centered on alterations to food production. Even extremely intimate incursions into personal hygiene were perfunctorily performed, and sometimes incorporated. In contrast, since food production was a primary goal of both leaders and villagers, activities with possible negative implications for food production were rarely implemented. The supremacy of production justified upper-level cadres' discarding accurate education and worker safety in the interest of increased production numbers. It equally legitimated communities and local cadres' forming a unified front to entirely resist key portions of the prevention campaign. The forgotten treatment arm, discussed in the next chapter, explores how the campaign succeeded despite great resistance to testing and treatment.

CHAPTER SIX

The Challenges of Treatment

THE SUN WAS SHINING BRIGHTLY when the snail fever surveying team marched into one of Yujiang's backwater townships to collect stool samples, but door after door was shut tight. On that day in May 1953, everybody was in the fields transplanting rice seedlings. Villagers and local leaders did everything they could to avoid these strange outsiders, even though treatment was seemingly one of the most benevolent offerings of the new government. For rural people, it was unclear what person in his or her right mind would wander into a village, procure people's shit, and ask invasive questions. What kind of government got involved in people's bowel movements? People were busy and tired. They gave face-saving excuses of "no time." When pressed, they sent back empty specimen cups or even passed off small children's feces as their own. Equally disturbing, strangers used a weird machine (a microscope) to stare at stool samples. What could they be peering at? Villagers speculated that they were figuring out what people ate. "They aren't coming to check whether people are sick, but to check what our living standards are." Later reports explained that such "obstructionist thinking" did not help to procure stool samples.[1] The opposition of rural people reflects their concern about government intrusiveness into personal bodily matters, a part of the government's wider agenda to gain control over rural bodies to facilitate building a modern scientific socialist society.

This chapter explores how prior understandings of the body now challenged by the state, relationships to the medical profession, gender barriers, and people's experiences on the wards help explain popular resistance to snail fever testing and treatment. It concludes by examining how treatment work during the Cultural Revolution campaign peak ensured the success of the entire campaign despite a fanatical environment and methods similar to those employed during the Great Leap Forward.

TESTING: WHY IT ENGENDERED POPULAR RESISTANCE

Government involvement in collecting stool samples, the primary method for testing for the disease during most of the campaign, was viewed as the most outlandish aspect of treatment work, yet it was the part of the campaign that people encountered first. This section examines the many impediments to testing and how hatred of stool samples affected relationships between campaign personnel and villagers. It explores how technical limitations and popular resistance made it extremely difficult to organize an effective campaign in the 1950s. Finally, it describes the development of a less intrusive and more sensitive skin test. This test, combined with the revolutionary fervor of the Cultural Revolution (1966–71), gradually decreased rural resistance and made the campaign more effective.

From 1949 to 1955, the government had limited coercive power, making it easy for individual households to ignore public health department stool-sample requests or to hide the specimen jar. Older women in particular might send back empty jars repeatedly. Only those who were very ill were willing to be tested. People's distrust and frustration was reinforced because in the face of limited resources, the Ministry of Public Health surveyed and tested repeatedly, without doing broad-scale treatment. When asked for more stool samples, people remarked, "In '51 you came to survey, but didn't give us any treatment. Now you come to survey again, we don't have so much time to waste on this."[2]

In places with few health resources and personnel, prioritizing snail fever came at the expense of treating other diseases that were more important to villagers because they had higher mortality rates. In June 1953, when campaign workers told villagers from Yujiang's Magang Township test site that they were receiving treatment for snail fever so that they would be better at production, villagers remarked: "You've just come to check shit. You don't look at other diseases and don't give any medicine for them. Don't you think sick people [with other diseases] will cause problems or obstruct production?"[3] The global malaria campaign faced a similar reception from rural Africans, where "people cannot understand why malaria should be selected for elimination rather than poverty, hunger, or other diseases or conditions."[4]

In China, providing stool samples seemed especially annoying when people were hungry, often the case in the early 1950s. As an insolvent Yujiang villager put it, "Without any food how can I produce any shit?" When these hungry populations were on the move, as happened often in the early PRC, which lacked the waterworks systems necessary for flood control, collection was even more frustrating. Displaced villagers felt that the new government was more interested in collecting the nonexistent products of their empty stomachs than in filling their stomachs by providing disaster relief, a traditional symbol of benevolent and effective government.[5]

In the second stage of the campaign, 1956–76, the advent of advanced producers' cooperatives and communes and personal control of the campaign by Chairman Mao made resistance more difficult. Stool requests were harder to oppose when land, work points, and benefits were under government control and when top local leaders, rather than public health personnel, conducted the campaign. Some particularly avid places came up with a unique strategy during the Great Leap Forward (1958–59). Chen Hongting, a Chinese medicine doctor, recounted that "if members didn't submit samples, they were not allowed to have dinner in the canteen. The situation improved a great deal."[6] Even then, people eluded national directives because local cadres also had a hard time fathoming why the government wanted stool samples.

The technical limitations of the stool test, revealed over time, enhanced resistance. This easy test, which mainly involves counting eggs under a microscope, was almost universally used. However, even well-trained personnel find less than 50 percent of the cases, and poorly trained technicians find even less. A Jiangxi November 1958 report indicated that a Wuhu District surveying team found 1 percent and 2.3 percent infection rates at two sites, whereas snail fever office personnel sent to verify these results found a 19 percent and 20 percent infection rate. This mistake was broadcast nationwide.[7] Due to personnel shortages and limited funding, such incidents rarely resulted in more training or additional personnel. Thus, after criticism, the same incompetent teams would go out again. The result was that villagers could find themselves tested repeatedly to compensate for inept testing teams and technical limitations of the test.

Some areas decided to increase quality control by establishing mass stool-processing centers. Their testing methods were better, but they lacked accurate record and tracking systems. Often, a person's name was lost in the shuffle, which did not endear the campaign to villagers. For example, in February 1952, a Shanghai report stated that "specific units were in a rush. The results from six thousand people's feces tests were mixed up, wasting people's energy and material resources and certainly slowing down campaign preparations."[8]

Campaign personnel tried to improve efficacy by requiring three different samples. However, securing three samples was even more difficult than acquiring one. Men were away in the fields, children were out playing, and women were busy with work. Each group eliminated wherever they were. Few people were used to shitting into a small jar, and they had no interest in dragging multiple shit samples around with them all day. Even in advanced producers' cooperatives, it was impossible to track down feces. During the day people were out, and at night the whole family used the communal commode in the dark, making it difficult to distinguish specimens. Inevitably, this awful job was palmed off on the lowest-status woman in the family, the daughter-in-law, though her position as a wife of the younger generation also made it morally questionable for her to get fecal samples from elders, particularly her father-in-law. Additionally, women often had to bring specimen jars to the testing center, causing them to lose face in front of their community. In one extreme example, the wife of a cadre refused to do this, was beaten up, and ran away rather than give in. Finally, many women were disturbed by the idea of an unknown male doctor examining something as personal as a woman's excrement.[9]

As the campaign took on revolutionary overtones in the late 1950s, stool testing was supposed to become universal and happen at least yearly, though this does not seem to have occurred in most places. Ideally, those who had received treatment would be tested repeatedly to see if they were cured. Villagers never got used to the process: the more frequently they were asked to provide samples, the lower the participation rate became, the greater the variety of resistance tactics.[10] Since turning in a stool sample was nonnegotiable, people used shit-like substitutes, including stones, mud, and cow and dog manure. Baby stool, the easiest to collect, was sometimes used for the entire family. Because the idea of assembling three separate samples was too annoying to consider, people would generally split one sample in three. Some people, especially women desperate not to be treated, would solicit samples from people who had tested clean and send them in as their own.[11]

Rural Chinese people's unenthusiastic response to stool samples and the new level of government intrusiveness bears a striking resemblance to findings from colonial public health campaigns. Most colonial tropical disease campaigns involved the same invasive questioning, physical exams, and stool samples paired with forcible, often lengthy treatment employing foreign paradigms of health and disease. Colonial subjects' resistance rationales and strategies tended to be identical to the Chinese. During a major cholera epidemic in the Philippines in 1915, when E. L. Munson, a U.S. Army medical corps major, tested people using stool samples, Filipinos experienced the testing as an "invasion of the accepted rights of the home and of the individual" that was "repulsive to modesty."[12] A British Egyptian snail fever campaign in the 1920s and 1930s, discovered that Egyptian villagers, like Chinese peasants, "distributed stools from one member of a household into the collecting cans of the rest; they put buffalo stools into cans; they returned cans empty; they put camel urine and even ditch water into cans."[13] Whether Communist or colonial, invasive state involvement was experienced as an unacceptable intrusion into previously private bodily issues.

Opposition by colonial subjects seems to have been an individual reaction, but in China local cadres often set an example counter to their own regime, empowering community-wide resistance. When asked to help with collection by using his home as an intermediate feces depot, a leader from Qujiang Township in Jiangxi's Yongxin County said, "Due to mass thinking I was unable to get through." However, an investigation established that when villagers tried to leave samples at his home, he violently cursed the villagers and screamed: "What are you doing bringing in such dirty things? What kind of bloody disease are you checking out! Is my home not a latrine pit again?" After that, all of the village's stool samples were "lost" down the cesspool. With great restraint, prevention personnel reported, "This indicates that certain village cadres have a very hazy understanding of snail fever prevention work." Certainly from the perspective of mobilizing the community to provide stool samples, there could not be a more counterproductive example.[14]

Disgust at feces testing was transferred to the testing personnel themselves. Whereas people in Shanghai, Qingpu, and Jiangsu felt that stool testing was distasteful, those in Jiangxi disparaged the doctors themselves, calling them shit doctors (*shi yisheng* or *fenbian yisheng*). Indeed, this problem was sufficiently severe to be reported to the national nine-person leadership small group by Jiangxi's campaign leaders. Speculatively, this extreme reaction may reflect the fact that in rural areas, the most fetid part of the procedure occurred in the villages themselves, rather than in the centralized sites for processing samples used by wealthier cities and provinces. It was also inconceivable to some villagers that people would do such a degrading job. Upon hearing the purpose of a visit from a female doctor, a lady in Yujiang said: "Why is someone young and beautiful like you doing a job like this? Other people will call you a shit doctor!" Even after years of excellent treatment work, in 1965 in Yujiang County some people greeted treatment personnel with, "The shit doctors have come again," while local youths clamped shut their noses and shouted, "You stink like hell!"[15] This popular reaction neither helped treatment team morale nor encouraged a close community relationship.

Rural areas were unable to perform accurate testing in the 1950s due to technical limitations and popular resistance. Unfortunately, testing was a prerequisite for effective campaign planning and resource acquisition. Indeed, many diseased people escaped detection decades into the campaign. Popular discomfort and hostility toward treatment personnel made it difficult for them to function effectively and contributed to their downward spiral of apathy and inertia. These negative interactions made it difficult for the government to convince people that this campaign was for their benefit or that it represented the Party's benevolent care for the people. Instead, some people initially dreamed up conspiracy theories.[16] Later, people either ignored the stool-testing aspect of the campaign or became partially habituated to it as one more irksome, incomprehensible, or even nauseating burden foisted upon them by the Party.

Many of these issues could have been alleviated if the campaign had been able to use the skin test widely. Skin tests were less intrusive, easier to perform, and more sensitive, discovering a higher percentage of cases than stool tests. However, initially the skin test could be used only in urban areas like Shanghai, where the antigen used in the test was produced. This antigen lasted only seven days even at 4 degrees Celsius, precluding its use in rural areas that lacked electricity, refrigeration, or decent transportation to the city.[17] The snail fever campaign in Shanghai, the medical and technical center of the campaign, presaged how effective testing could transform campaign work, a change that in most rural areas would only come to fruition during the Cultural Revolution (1966–71).

Shanghai's early access to skin tests, improved stool tests, and relatively abundant resources and personnel allowed it to do broad-scale testing of whole populations, rather than sample surveying, and to use multiple testing methods on the same individual to cross-check results. This strategy had a remarkable impact on Shanghai's disease detection and campaign planning.

The city's original plan stated that the campaign would treat 30,000–35,000 sick people by the end of 1956. Even though this goal was accomplished, reports still announced that only 45 percent of the sick people had been treated. By using the more sensitive skin test in the 1956 campaign, the city discovered it had 68,000 rather than 35,000 people with the disease. Without accurate tests to precisely grasp the scope of the problem, it was impossible to do realistic planning.[18]

Fortuitously, a new skin antigen was developed in 1964, just before the start of the Cultural Revolution. This antigen lasted more than half a year at low temperatures, enabling the skin test to be used in rural areas. The skin test was gradually disseminated to the countryside and was employed along with the stool test. At the same time, more than a decade's work expanding the rural education system led to the simultaneous appearance of a large cadre of rural educated youth who could act as technicians, organizers, and mobilizers. Revolutionary fervor, combined with the appearance of a less intrusive and more sensitive skin test, gradually decreased rural resistance while making the campaign more effective. Thus, during the Cultural Revolution, rural areas partially replicated Shanghai's early success while mitigating, but never truly solving, rural resistance to disease testing.[19]

TREATMENT: CONTENDING PARADIGMS AND PRACTITIONERS

Even if you execute me, I won't receive shots.

Qingpu villager, 1952

We don't want the government to care about anything. We just want them to not care about having us get treated!

Villagers in Jiangxi's infectious Poyang Lake region, 1957

Treatment was the aspect of the snail fever campaign that seemed most obviously beneficial.[20] Yet many villagers resisted it even under strong duress. Newspapers and reports in the archives claimed that villagers were superstitious and backward, clinging to Chinese medicine rather than welcoming the enlightened scientific methods brought by the Chinese state.[21] However, a careful reading of local campaign reports indicates that in addition to economic impediments, prior perceptions of health and disease and earlier experiences with medical practitioners strongly influenced reception of this campaign. Many rural people refused to participate in the early treatment campaign because it was indistinguishable from a government-run medical scam.

In the 1950s, villagers across China shared a similar practical vision of health. A man was healthy if he could work hard for an extended period of time; a woman was healthy if she could work hard and have multiple healthy children. Since state of health was based on the ability to accomplish daily activities, a low fever, weakness, diarrhea, coughing, or other minor symptoms of chronic snail fever were simply an annoyance, but not a sign of sickness. On the other hand, a big belly, occurring in a small fraction of late-stage patients, indicated illness. According to popular understanding, most villagers had neither snail fever nor any other disease. As one asymptomatic patient from Jiangsu put it, "I can eat, I can work at a job, what disease do you want to treat?"[22] Not surprisingly, this made expensive, coercive treatment a hard sell.

When rural people felt ill, their explanations were unhappy gods, ghosts, demons, and ancestors; disrupted feng shui; bad behavior in a prior incarnation; and bodily imbalance due to excess cold, heat, or wind. Since disease causality was unclear, people tried many cures simultaneously: diet modification, propitiating local spirits, temple trips, the local herbalist, visits by Buddhist/Daoist healing clerics, consuming "cure-alls" like the ash from temple incense, and finally, bringing in a Chinese doctor. The methods chosen depended on economic resources, access, and shared knowledge, but since most illnesses came from the gods or spirits, it made sense to start with the temple.[23]

Traditional treatment for snail fever likewise used a large variety of techniques. According to a likely biased report from Yujiang intent on showcasing peasant superstitions, in Yangjiache Village snail fever symptoms were thought to result from a disgruntled ghost or bad fate. Women spent hours praying and lighting incense, did good deeds to shore up karma, changed ill people's names to alter their fate, and made medicine from incense ash mixed with water. When nothing worked, villagers turned to experts to re-equilibrate regional feng shui. Even an expensive sorcerer, beating his gongs until they broke, was ineffective. One disgusted villager even "threw the village's Buddha into the manure pit."[24] The inability to contend with snail fever by normal means caused a small revolution in Yujiang's popular religion during the Republican era (1911–49). Many Yujiang residents believed that snail fever was caused by a stone lion cliff that bled into the water after people carved him up while building a new irrigation channel during the Ming dynasty, Jiajing reign period (1522–66). While villagers may not have understood the disease's life cycle, they correctly identified water as the dangerous point of contact and irrigation channels as a precipitating cause for a noticeable increase in disease intensity. After local residents determined that the Buddhist temple was useless at curing the disease, attendance dropped and villagers created new ceremonies and frequented other temples dedicated to the sharpening stone that harmed the lion cliff or to the rusty water that resulted. They concocted an expensive ceremony sacrificing pigs and chickens that was conducted by Daoist monks and directed at the dragon king in charge of rainwater.[25]

Prior to the PRC, traditional Chinese medicine doctors provided some of the least utilized and most expensive treatment. Professor Mobo Gao, a native of Jiangxi's Gao Village, explained, "Effective or not, Gao villagers usually do not go to the doctor anyway."[26] Dr. Joshua Horn, who worked in rural China, concurred: "Before Liberation, most of China's peasants had virtually no access to modern medicine and very scant access to traditional medicine. . . . Traditional doctors . . . were closely linked with the landlords and officials. . . . Their scarcity value in the villages enabled them to charge fees which were beyond the reach of the mass of poor peasants."[27] The result was that few skilled practitioners, most of whom had a literati background, practiced among villagers who could neither pay them nor afford their expensive herbs.[28] At the same time, doctors who were stuck receiving villagers' mediocre reimbursement tended to be among the least knowledgeable and competent. According to bottom-level reports and oral histories, villagers generally viewed doctors as useless shysters who exploited and deceived prospective patients, a perspective confirmed by derogatory representations of country doctors in Chinese literature. Many accounts discuss extended family networks paying doctors who may have hastened the patient's death.[29] As a popular saying about locals' perceptions of doctors put it, "If you don't treat your eyes, you won't become blind; if you don't treat your feet, you won't limp; if you don't treat an illness, you won't die."[30] In places like Jiangxi, this general experience is corroborated by Chinese doctors' lack of of expertise. A 1955 report indicated that of 16,731 Chinese medicine practitioners, 12 percent were highly skilled, 45 percent had a very low skill level, and 3 percent were quacks. Thus, close to 50 percent of the available practitioners lacked a competent skill level in Chinese medicine.[31] Unfortunately, in the 1950s in Jiangxi and many other rural areas, experience with rural providers led people to believe that medical care by a doctor was likely more injurious than no care at all.

When the snail fever campaign started in the mid-1950s, it was generally felt that medical teams were pulling a scam, both because late-stage patients were initially excluded from treatment and because wards were empty while urban doctors were supported at local expense. Until 1957, the Party focused on early-stage patients and excluded complicated late-stage patients because of inexperienced medical personnel and limited clinical facilities. Early-stage patients were easier and took less time, allowing doctors to fulfill patient quotas. Most importantly, such patients were less prone to serious complications or death. Realizing that high patient mortality rates would not be a helpful marketing tool, a 1952 Shanghai report admonished, "Safety is the first principle." It advised not giving treatment to late-stage patients, "to forestall accidents that would influence the progress of the treatment work." When patients did die, treatment teams often tried to cover up it up.[32] When a fifteen-year-old Qingpu boy died in 1951, the medical team tried unsuccessfully to conceal him in the hospital and finally gave the family 200 jin (220.5 lb) of rice, announcing, "It is because your family is in straitened conditions that we are helping you and not because of the death of your son."[33] This treatment focus made no sense from rural people's perspective. Seemingly, doctors were only willing to treat healthy early-stage patients and refused to treat desperately ill late-stage patients (see figure 11). Villagers from Yujiang's Magang Township commented in disgust: "Those of us who are sick, you say aren't; those who aren't sick, you say are. Those who have a big stomach you can't cure and say we should stay at home to slowly recuperate. Won't this mean you have nothing to do in your own hospital?" According to a 1953 Qingpu report, disappointed late-stage patients, after being rejected, also "spread their unhappiness" throughout the area, contributing to a hostile campaign environment. From the villagers' standpoint, refusal to treat those who really needed it, while charging exorbitant fees for those who were healthy, not only proved that doctors were incompetent, but also fit perfectly with the people's expectations of a medical swindle.[34]

The empty wards, resulting both from leaders' refusal to take responsibility for the campaign and mobilize prospective patients and from economic impediments to treatment, further reinforced the idea of a scam. In Jiangxi's Boyang and De'an Counties, each physician treated an average of 1.6 and 0.6 people per month, respectively, suggesting a campaign that would never end.[35] Lacking patients, but forbidden to return to their own institutions,

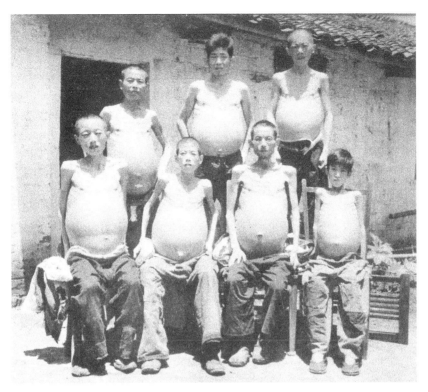

FIGURE 11. Late-stage snail fever. Zhonggong zhongyang nanfang shisan sheng, shi, qu xuefang lingdao xiaozu bangongshi, *Song wenshen: Huace* (Beijing: Zhonggong zhongyang nanfang shisan sheng, shi, qu xuefang lingdao xiaozu bangongshi, 1978), 45.

doctors sometimes lolled around on the wards sleeping, eating, gambling, playing chess and ball games, and they went out to watch local opera performances. A 1956 Jiangxi report noted that after requesting seven times to be allowed to return to the city, doctors began "doing passive work slowdowns"; the report compared them to "Buddhist monks," whose main activity was chanting all day.[36]

Villagers logically concluded that these slothful outsiders had come to steal from them. People from Jiangxi's Wannian County complained: "You, the so-called doctors, really want to eat food you didn't earn. You simply want us to provide for you."[37] Villagers from Qingpu agreed: "Cadres from the snail fever treatment and prevention station are useless and worn out. We wonder if the government has no use for their grain tax and the excess is going to feed these people. Before, cadres just came for food and then left. Now they come for food and then conk out on a bed sleeping, making people even more angry."[38] Villagers, particularly in Jiangxi, had a solution to this problem. Since the treatment personnel were basically ineffectual, why not get rid of them entirely and disseminate their salaries to villagers? Or, if all the treatment personnel were transferred to the village to do production activities, then "we'd be doing better," said the villagers.[39] Campaign leaders repeatedly encouraged doctors and prevention personnel to get involved in production, flood control, and household tasks like feeding the pigs or caring for the children. Since it was not obvious that the doctors served a useful medical purpose, it was only by doing regular work that campaign personnel could "help villagers understand that the campaign is helpful to them."[40]

Government propaganda framed resistance to treatment as a sign of backwardness, but my work suggests two logical reasons why villagers declined treatment. First, a fundamentally different evaluation of what constituted health and disease made the expensive treatment seem unnecessary. Second, past experience indicated that medical practitioners were often con men. The targeting of apparently healthy people for treatment and the lounging urban doctors reinforced this assessment.

DANGEROUS MEDICINE AND DESTITUTE WARDS: THE TREATMENT EXPERIENCE

Once villagers decided or were forced to get treatment in the late 1950s, they did not seem to differentiate between Western and Chinese medicine, despite propaganda reports that decried their superstitious resistance.[41] Western cures simply joined the existing complex medical and spiritual marketplace. People judged their treatment based on its effectiveness and affordability, rather than whether it was foreign, modern, or scientific. However, these new practitioners were problematic: they did not practice medicine according to existing norms; their medicine was dangerous and of questionable efficacy; and the rural wards where they practiced were harrowing. These realities acted as a further barrier to treatment.

Rural people may never have interacted with a skilled Chinese doctor, but they knew the proper procedures for a good checkup. Besides acupuncture, performed with very thin needles, a doctor checked a patient's pulse and mixed and brewed a complex herb mixture specifically designed for each patient that was efficacious in proportion to its bitterness. The new doctors barely checked the pulse and did not brew bitter drinks or perform acupuncture. Instead of these well-respected procedures, they used a strange metallic necklace to prod chests, gave identical medicines through huge hollow needles, wanted stool samples, and most disturbingly asked people to undress and undergo close physical scrutiny, something no stranger should be doing. In Shanghai, doctors also drew blood, which some felt might cause serious bodily harm because blood is a form of *qi,* or essential energy.[42]

These new practitioners also looked wrong. Chinese doctors looked like traditional literati in long robes, and their age was an important determinant of skill level. Urban hospital doctors wore modern Western clothing or worse yet, attempting to look scientific, some wore white, a color symbolizing death. They were also very young, making them incompetent by definition (see figure 13 in chapter 7).[43] Thus, villagers distrusted Western doctors because their appearance and forms and practice of medicine were at odds with people's expectations, rather than because the doctors used Western medicine and assessed disease based on a different theoretical system.

In 1958, during the Great Leap Forward, and after, Chairman Mao insisted that Chinese medicine doctors play a more prominent role, not only as part of mixed teams with Western doctors, but also solo. Although some elders liked their doctors to be "scions of special families," in which "medicine was an art fathers passed to sons," for most people the main appeal of Chinese medicine was not its familiarity but rather that it was cheaper and sometimes allowed people to stay at home. Disincentives were treatment length, often even longer than Western treatment, and fewer subsidies, which resulted in Chinese medicine wards being in terrible condition, with patients at all stages of snail fever packed tightly together. By 1958, villagers in infectious areas with high-quality Western treatment, such as the Shanghai region, had concluded that shots worked, although they were obnoxious and painful. In only a few years, the multitude of vaccination and other health campaigns had normalized physical exams and needles as the correct disease treatment. When these people were finally offered Chinese medicine, some were uninterested because they thought it would be ineffective and a waste of money.[44]

It soon became apparent that Western treatment was painful and dangerous, and the same was true of experimental Chinese medicine. Antimony (tartar emetic), the primary snail fever treatment through 1980, is extremely toxic, comparable to arsenic. In fact, early treatment efforts experimented with arsenic and strychnine. According to a 1958 article in the *Chinese Medical Journal,* which likely described the best care, a normal twenty-day course of antimony had a 4 percent mortality rate.[45] The competence of the person injecting antimony was critical. Misinjection into subcutaneous tissue rather than the vein was intensely painful and could cause tissue necrosis; dosage was also critical, and conditions like anemia were a contraindication for treatment. Most rural practitioners in the early 1950s were either newly trained or minimally retrained Chinese medicine doctors, inexperienced at giving shots, assessing dosage, and treating other complicating conditions.[46] Even though most patients were asymptomatic when treated, about 57 percent had severe negative reactions. Indeed, patients were carefully watched for convulsions, as emergency measures were necessary to prevent death. Negative reactions escalated as the drug progressively built up in people's bodies during the twenty days they were forced to stay on the wards. To make matters worse, early drug production had exceptionally uneven quality control. Shanghai doctors sent to Qingpu in 1950 were encouraged to write down each ampoule's batch number so that "when emergencies happen, it will be easier to investigate."[47]

Restricted access to most drugs compounded problems. Forced by Chairman Mao, pharmaceutical companies produced antimony for rural clinics, but most other drugs, including those mitigating the effects of antimony, were unavailable or quickly used up and never replaced. As one 1956 report from Jiangsu's seven-person LSG put it: "Many clinics are very short of medicine because they don't have money to buy it. This results in doctors treating based on what medicines they have, rather than on what diseases they are presented with!" With increasing focus on maximizing grain production, land and time for producing sidelines like medical herbs also diminished. Thus, even inexpensive, locally grown, palliative herbs used in Chinese medicine became harder to find.[48]

Not surprisingly, many felt worse after treatment than before, saying, "Prior to treatment I didn't have a disease; now I should spend money to get sick?" Given the choice, many stopped treatment midcourse when drug reactions peaked and the patients' economic situation became untenable. Moreover, treatment required people to lie flat on their backs for a month without moving, inconceivable for those who associated well-being with constant work. Some Yujiang residents remarked that "even a good person" after a month of not working, "they are going to get sick!"[49]

While many deaths were due to antimony shots, others were caused by Chinese medicine. Chinese medicine does not have a cure for snail fever. Throughout the campaign, Chinese herbs were successfully used to bolster the bodies of fragile late-stage patients so they could tolerate antimony without dying. Doctors also employed acupuncture to drain people's engorged abdomens and acupuncture anesthesia to remove their spleens. In some cases very ill patients did not survive these procedures. In Chairman Mao's special campaign, political imperatives made it necessary to use China's own medical heritage to cure snail fever, rather than using Western medicine, but this ideal was never achieved. Throughout the campaign, patients were nevertheless used as unknowing test subjects to experiment with dangerous Chinese herbs, a process that increased mortality rates.[50]

The more deaths or extreme negative symptoms, the more difficult it was to convince people that treatment was a good idea. A February 1952 report from Shanghai noted, "It was necessary to try to lessen negative reactions: if they [patients] had light reactions they became frightened and fled the wards; if they had heavy reactions they could die; if that happened it impeded the whole treatment process."[51] Yujiang provides a good example of this dynamic. After 1958, when the disease was supposedly eliminated, local practitioners took over treatment from outside medical experts. One result was that from 1961 to 1965, the patient dropout rate skyrocketed from 5.7 percent under outside experts to 11.5 percent under resident doctors. Although the situation postfamine likely led some to withdraw due to economic reasons, the advent of assistance for indigent patients through the commune system made it improbable that the increased rate was entirely due to poverty. More likely is that local professionals' poor management of the medicine's scary side effects caused many people to flee treatment.[52] As reports of deaths on rural wards started to circulate, some villagers refused treatment because "they were afraid of dying due to treatment and afraid that if they got treated they wouldn't recover to their prior state of health." Even late-stage patients, the only previously enthusiastic group, rejected treatment after hearing the news, because "they think they'll soon be closed up in a coffin and that treatment will make them die directly, while without treatment they might live a few more years after all."[53]

Patients surviving the twenty-day treatment soon found that the cure rate was around 60 percent, necessitating multiple treatment courses to correct unsuccessful treatment and to cure reinfections. Cure rates dropped further as doctors started utilizing "revolutionary" short-course regimens during the Great Leap Forward, which had an efficacy rate below 40 percent. Thus, Qingpu and Jiangxi's De'an County respectively averaged 2.55 and 2.76 treatments per person to achieve a cure.[54] Although the short course was not very effective, it did lead to vast numbers of people being rapidly treated. However, low efficacy also encouraged people to refuse treatment, especially when they had to pay for it multiple times.

In light of a recalcitrant population distrustful of both treatment and doctors, forced treatment increased. Levels of coercion tended to be highest at the beginning of the campaign because the treatment process was unknown, less experienced doctors provided worse care, treatment took close to a month, limited economic support was available, and doctors, intent on meeting quotas, scheduled treatment at inopportune times, such as peak agriculture periods. Tactics ranged from multiple visits by people's immediate leader, by doctors, or even by higher-level cadres, to badger people into treatment; to the purposeful gathering together of an individual's family and neighbors to act as a pressure group; to assigning people without their agreement to report to the ward, like any other work responsibility; and to employing economic pressure "to forcefully command them" by withholding work points until people went for treatment.[55] Once trapped on the ward, people tried "sneakily to go back home. When we [campaign personnel] found out, we would take them right back." The anger from virtual imprisonment on the wards was directed at the easiest target—the outside medical provider. Additionally, "Because patients didn't volunteer to come get treated and felt pressured into it, their family wasn't willing to pay either treatment or board fees."[56] This unanticipated consequence of forced treatment contributed to the campaign's economic woes.

Fewer coercive strategies were necessary during the Great Leap. Villagers were swept up in the revolution, and more received loans from their commune and could depend on fellow workers to cover necessary field labor. By this point, they knew what to expect from treatment and more willingly participated in convenient short-course regimens, men during the winter and women during the summer. However, willingness to be treated did not make the ward experience any more pleasant.

Ward accommodations were very bad. Jiangxi campaign personnel discovered that treating patients in rural village wards rather than distant snail fever stations maximized treatment numbers and was most cost-effective. Although some local cadres' houses were used to treat patients, many felt that if someone died, lingering "bad energy" would pervade their homes. Treatment teams that lacked building skills, construction material, and sufficient money had to establish wards or operating rooms from preexisting temples or ramshackle, abandoned buildings. Most wards were crowded, inhospitable places, and patients had to supply their own beds and bedding, something many poor patients did not have.[57] Treatment mostly occurred during the winter slack season, when rain poured through the roof, seemingly targeting the immobile patients shivering on their sickbeds. Unless ward spaces were fixed and bedding procured, patients tended to flee for home, looking for greener (and warmer) pastures.[58]

Food was also a big problem. When wards were close to home, families brought food. Otherwise, no one had this responsibility. Before the advent of advanced producers' cooperatives and communes, many local grain departments were unwilling to sell food to "outside" people, and when a grain ration was provided, it was rarely sufficient. With communes came a new problem: lack of internal regulations to provide food allocation for workers not earning work points or being treated within the commune but outside the production unit. Dr. Mao Zhixiao recounted that after waiting ten hours in the Guangming Commune director's office to ask for food for his patients, he was told, "We don't even have cash for oil lamps." Dr. Mao explained: "I broke my lips through talking. . . . I told him: 'Let me make clear to you they are my patients—but they are your relatives.' Finally, I convinced him and received the cash for grain." Without persistent doctors, patients were forced to leave treatment to hunt down food.[59]

Infection control was also poor. Needles were reused, few things were washed, and almost nothing was sterilized. At one point, Qingpu personnel used food pots for sanitizing treatment equipment, resulting in high fevers and massive vomiting attacks among patients. By 1958, Qingpu mandated the washing of needles every three days and syringes once a day in hot water. As Qingpu provided some of the best nonurban treatment, one wonders if any infection-control procedures were in place in more typical rural counties. Infections acquired in the hospital were common. Additional illnesses, such as malaria, ravaged the unprotected patients trapped on their rice-straw mattresses, and influenza passed rapidly from patient to patient in the close confines of the ward.[60]

In addition to untenable conditions, villagers had no experience with assuming a compliant, inert persona and lying in bed for a month. Patients were unused to following medical advice, particularly if they believed themselves healthy.[61] In contrast, doctors, especially those from a hospital setting, expected their advice to be respected. When doctors assumed a condescending urban attitude, it became a point of pride to resist them. Wards were often a total madhouse. Patients sang, drank, danced, played mahjong, gambled, and fought. When particularly bored, they took off on collective missions such as tea and liquor drinking, food procurement, or participation in neighborhood entertainment. Women with dependents added very young children and nursing infants to the mix. Since the injections were very dangerous and people who moved sometimes lost consciousness or went into convulsions, doctors were desperate to try to teach people the new role of patient.[62]

Doctors and nurses generally lacked the stature or authority to enforce order, except in the rare case that a nurse came from the community being treated. One strategy used in Shanghai was "telling patients that other patients were well disciplined. This created a competitive feeling to be the best patient, which influenced them to listen to their doctors."[63] One of the most effective and widely used strategies was having patients elect a ward representative, generally an older, respected male patient, whose job was to ensure order on the ward and to funnel requests and complaints from his compatriots. Some wards also had patients and doctors sign a pact that outlined the ward's regulations and established shared expectations.[64]

Campaign personnel and local cadres soon realized that the captive, bored group of patients provided the perfect opportunity to engage in extensive propaganda education. This included singing, storytelling, study groups, some teaching of literacy skills, and reading aloud from newspapers, with a particular focus on patriotic heroes who sacrificed themselves for their country like the frustrated patients were supposed to do. Wards that had an hour-by-hour schedule of medical and educational activities, including meal times and rest periods, had more luck at maintaining order. While these measures helped, the ward remained an uproarious environment. There is little indication that villagers learned this new role of patient. Instead, the switch toward three-day treatment and eventually oral treatment received at home meant that people could avoid the ward almost entirely, a change they welcomed with great pleasure.[65]

AGE AND GENDER: THE ULTIMATE OBSTACLES TO TREATMENT

Elders and women faced particular barriers to treatment. For elderly people, there was the sense that fate had kicked in and there was no sense wasting family resources on a dying proposition. As one older Yujiang man put it:

"People all pass away by the side of the pit. Worrying about whether they have a disease or not—you still want to check, check, check, what are you checking for? If I'm going to die, I'd just prefer to die!" However, since life expectancy was only thirty-five years at the beginning of the PRC, people often thought of themselves as elderly when medical personnel did not. [66] Additionally, some elders had late-stage disease, which the campaign was unable to treat. Even sophisticated areas, like Qingpu, excluded people over fifty-five from mass testing.[67] Such cases waited until the Cultural Revolution for help.

For women, a complex set of bodily issues, family dynamics, and gender roles kept them from treatment. Pregnant and nursing women could not receive treatment because antimony could harm the developing child. Additionally, both malnourishment and anemia were warning signs for a dangerous drug reaction. As in many places, access to food in China was directly correlated to social status. Because of their low status, women as a group were more malnourished and anemic than men. When women exhibited these preconditions too severely, doctors would not accept them as patients, particularly in the early campaign.[68] Further, caretaking duties such as cleaning, cooking, tending animals and vegetable gardens, caring for children, and attending the elderly required constant availability at home and made treatment unthinkable. One summary of Yujiang's campaign explained, "If the woman goes to the hospital to get cured, she fears her husband will have no food, her son won't be cared for, and the housework will be abandoned."[69]

Initially, caring for gardens and large animals impeded men's treatment too.[70] However, with high-level cooperatives and then communes, men were part of a team, with tasks delegated to specific team members, turning agricultural production into a quasi assembly line. Such a system made it easier to organize and control a planned economy where labor was the major input. When a laborer was unavailable, another could be slotted into his job. Thus, with careful organization an individual could be freed up to get treatment without greatly disturbing the work process.[71] However, this streamlining did not extend to home-based caretaking duties. Except for the mother-in-law, there was no one to pick up the slack. And in most families, the daughter-in-law's lowly status was affirmed by performing the dirtiest, most tedious, or physically challenging duties: emptying the chamber pot, hauling huge pots of water, cleaning heavy clothing, or cooking in the heat over the stove. Having elders take on these burdens had a symbolic weight beyond the physical challenges they represented.[72]

A mother-in-law's interest in providing help was often directly correlated to whether her daughter-in-law was worthy—did she work industriously at home duties, bear many sons, and later participate energetically in commune production activities in the fields? Women sick with snail fever were unlikely to meet these standards. Husbands sick with the disease might be infertile; sick sons sometimes spent their lives looking like ten-year-olds. Both problems were blamed on the daughter-in-law. Few mother-in-laws were interested in sacrificing their time, energy, and status for such a useless addition to the family. In-laws were also less interested in paying for a daughter-in-law's treatment. Whereas a son was their social security system, a woman who would not work around the house or bear children bestowed a bad fate on their new household that would curtail the family line. Nobody wanted to waste family resources on somebody like that.[73]

Apart from family dynamics, women themselves did not want treatment. Many women felt that their most important role was to take care of their family's needs. How could they abandon them to an uncertain fate during such a long treatment process? It seemed impossible to encumber family members and neighbors with such an enormous burden.[74] Women also found testing embarrassing. Very few treatment teams had female doctors. Chaste women did not answer personal questions about their body or state of health asked by a strange man. Physical exams that involved taking off one's clothing were particularly unacceptable. In the Shanghai region, in an effort to be "scientific," photographing people's nude bodies sometimes joined these other indignities.[75] Determining that treatment was not only impossible but likely immoral, women invented many avoidance strategies, ranging from tinkering with stool samples, to absenting oneself from testing, to nursing indefinitely. Up until about 1957, those who refused to show up for treatment were usually able to avoid it.[76]

Because treatment groups rarely broke out data by gender, it is difficult to determine whether women were systematically underrepresented, but anecdotal evidence suggests this to be the case. In Qingpu, approximately equal numbers of women and men had the disease, but aggregated reports for thirteen Chinese medical groups in 1956, with careful data on age and sex, indicate that of 505 patients treated, 63 percent were men and 37 percent were women. Additionally, of the 335 patients treated by six Western treatment groups in Qingpu from 1956 to 1957, 75 percent were men and 25 percent were women. Such numbers clearly reflect a sex-based differential rather than disease prevalence. While data are sparse, there is some indication that older women were particularly undertreated, as gender disparity was worse in the age group above forty to forty-five. Old women were either not considered for treatment or were particularly effective at refusing it.[77]

Sex bias abruptly reversed in Qingpu starting in 1957, as a result of membership in high-level cooperatives and communes and pressure during the Great Leap Forward. By 1958, treatment ratios of women to men were 50:50 or even higher. The focus on women likely reflected both ideological and practical concerns. Since the bar had been set at complete disease elimination, it became a point of revolutionary pride to achieve this goal, as well as being a concrete signpost of the new scientific socialist society. In addition, as men were pulled into labor-intensive activities, such as backyard furnaces and infrastructure construction projects, women were required to do some of the heaviest labor for production. This made it essential that they were parasite-free so that they could exert full labor power.[78]

To accomplish this goal, the CCP purposefully interfered in family dynamics and child rearing. Realizing that caretaking was women's greatest hurdle, some local cadres and a large numbers of leaders from Fulian (the Woman's Federation) got involved. Wealthier collectives started a nursery near the treatment ward, and Fulian held propaganda education meetings pushing women to wean babies earlier. This strategy, according to local reports, not only facilitated snail fever treatment but also meant that breastfeeding would not deplete the mother's vigor or prevent a full day's labor in the fields. Most importantly, members of Fulian barged into people's houses, announced that women would get treated, and then negotiated who would take over which duties. The intrusion of Fulian made the decision to help dependent on the Party, rather than on affection or familial power. After watching neighbors targeted by political campaigns, most people decided it was unwise to ignore Party demands after a home visit. Despite the infringement, this was the only way women could be extricated from family responsibilities to receive treatment.[79] Though this had huge benefits for women's access to treatment, the underlying purpose, for women as for men, was to maximize their strength for production, rather than to improve their well-being.

Forced treatment called into question the definition of the fundamental categories of "health" and "disease." People's assessment of disease causality was marginalized when they were forced to get treatment despite believing themselves healthy. This new biomedical paradigm suggested that people's knowledge about disease and their appraisal of their own body's well-being were no longer accurate or were even evidence of their backwardness. This effort to judge what represented a healthy or sick body joined a multitude of other Party efforts to take charge of rural people's bodies.[80] Gaining authority over this previously private realm had two large benefits: greater predictability and control over labor, the main input in central planning; and better ability to frame the Party's intrusive new campaigns as an example of benevolent government. While these larger implications were not clear to most rural people, over and over again bottom-level reports described villagers as pleading that they were not ill, only to have that discounted by the next wave of campaign work.

RESURGENCE OF DISEASE DURING THE FAMINE

The first campaign peak during the Great Leap Forward (1958–59) was closely followed by the famine (1959–61) and recovery period (1961–65). Treatment stopped during the famine and recovery period, except for in a few model areas, and infectious disease of all types increased.[81] China experienced a revival of snail fever, particularly of acute disease, in previously unseen epidemic proportions. This was due to the fairly successful Great Leap treatment effort, which created an infectiously naïve population in an environment that was still highly infectious due to mediocre prevention work and the massive increase in the irrigation system. As a result, in 1960–62 Jiangxi Province alone had 8,363 cases of acute disease, 216 of whom immediately died. Even Yujiang County, the place Chairman Mao had just lauded as the first to completely eliminate snail fever, had a large number of new cases in the early 1960s.[82] Even more disheartening, near the end of 1959 infectious diseases of all kinds were rapidly spreading, a trend that continued during the next couple of years. This was partially due to the famine, since starving people have little resistance to disease. However, it was also because it was easier to collect accurate statistics after people were organized into communes, causing disease statistics to seemingly rise across the nation. Many rural leaders took this to mean that their efforts at improving rural health and sanitation were useless or even counterproductive.[83]

The pause in the campaign and the large drop in revolutionary enthusiasm during the famine gave villagers and local cadres time to assess the efficacy of treatment. It became clear that many people seemed temporarily better and then relapsed, and this rate of recurrence was even higher after the ineffective short-course treatments used during the Great Leap. When those who were not cured were combined with those who were reinfected from the highly infectious environment, people began to doubt that treatment was really possible. As they put it, "Year after year it's tested, year after year it's treated; you can test it endlessly and never finish treating." One report noted that some who personally experienced this phenomenon "think that they have to get treated every year and that it [the disease] will never be treated well. Thus they lose confidence in the work."[84] By the early 1960s, many people had a great sense of futility and were ready to discard the campaign, like so many other peculiar mass schemes enacted during the Great Leap.

TREATMENT SUCCESS: THE CULTURAL REVOLUTION

The Cultural Revolution (1966–76) was one of the most irrational and antiscientific eras in Chinese history. Reports of snail fever campaign activities proudly showcased the sort of craziness that makes it hard to take this period seriously. Despite this, the first half of the Cultural Revolution (1966–71) was the turning point of the campaign. As I recount below, success of the treatment arm resulted from the fact that treatment became almost universal, resistance decreased because of revolutionary zeal, and newly educated rural youth, in combination with the long-term presence of professional physicians sent to the countryside, enabled the campaign to succeed against all odds.

The start of the Cultural Revolution revitalized the campaign but also brought excesses in terms of both drug choices and treatment methods. Dissatisfied with antimony and desiring a drug that was created in China by Chinese, in 1965 many places around Shanghai began experimenting on people with a new oral drug called "snail fever prevention 846." Although somewhat effective, it had long-lasting impacts on the nervous system, brain, and especially memory. From the campaign's perspective, the most horrifying aspect of this drug was that it could leave a lasting negative impact on people's ability to work. Because of this latter symptom, the drug was discontinued in 1967.[85]

Compounding the problems of uncontrolled human drug experiments, a revolutionary perspective extolled the ability of peasants to perform all treatment, including curing late-stage patients. For example, in 1969 campaign personnel in Jiangxi's Boyang County (a nonmodel rural backwater) tried to do a splenectomy (spleen removal). Boyang personnel prepared an operating theater by recycling an old birthing table as an operating table. They also borrowed scalpels and anesthesia, but they could not find a surgeon. Mr. Xiong, a thirty-eight-year-old villager, was convinced that the spirit of Chairman Mao could solve their problems, and he decided to learn how to operate himself and to study acupuncture to compensate for the shortage of anesthetics. Mr. Xiong followed the doctors who were posted to Boyang for a short-term treatment campaign back to the provincial medical school, studied medicine for one month, and then assisted the experienced Dr. Zhu in spleen removal. After only six days, Mr. Xiong determined that he was competent and returned to Boyang as the area's chief surgeon, with Dr. Zhu (thankfully) acting as his assistant.[86]

After hearing accounts like this, few would give much credence to treatment during the Cultural Revolution. Yet, this revolutionary zeal for tracking and treating every patient, whether human or animal, the enthusiastic incorporation of inexperienced personnel, the large number of sent-down professional doctors, and some technical advances were all major determinants of treatment success during this period.

The Cultural Revolution was the first real attempt to treat water buffalo and oxen, a new government priority, signaled by holding a national conference in Shanghai on the issue in 1966. Treating cattle is now recognized as crucial for eliminating snail fever because they are the disease's most important reservoir host and produce one hundred times more manure than humans, causing a high percentage of environmental contamination.[87] However, most areas initially did not understand that treating cattle was important; they lacked sufficient resources for the human population, let alone animals. There were also large technical impediments: stool samples of individual water buffalo were hard to collect, tests for cattle missed a third of the cases, and treatment under the best conditions killed 1.4 percent and only cured 31.5 percent of the cases. A report from Shanghai, one of the few places that began cattle treatment during the Great Leap, said, "Most of what people gained from this training [during the Great Leap] was how to do testing, not actually how to cure the cattle."[88] However, by the Cultural Revolution, new testing methods discovered a third more cases, and a new medicine, Dipterex, was found to be less toxic to animals but still fairly effective. At the same time, as wealthier areas such as Shanghai mechanized, they switched from oxen to buffalo, which were three times less likely than oxen to get infected. In Shanghai, oxen made up a little over half of the cattle (563 in 1,000) in 1960 and less than 1 percent (8 in 1,000) by 1985. Dramatically decreasing the animal reservoir for snail fever caused human cases to decline precipitously. Based on data from 1978, throughout China the campaign treated 78.5 percent of the more than 440,000 sick cattle. While these data are likely exaggerated, they demonstrate that cattle treatment was a key component of the Cultural Revolution snail fever campaign.[89]

Treatment for humans also changed dramatically. Most importantly, treatment became free in 1966 at the start of the Cultural Revolution, enabling everyone to access care.[90] Previously, seeking treatment had been hampered both by individual economic constraints and by assigning limited treatment slots based on ideology or economics, as discussed below. From the perspective of disease control, it did not matter what people were labeled or what their potential labor power was. Without universal treatment, the disease would never be eliminated.

Shanghai, Qingpu, and Jiangsu Province fluctuated between an economic and a disease-based calculus for who should be treated. When treatment slots were extremely limited, the campaign suggested that "young people and those with the most energy for production" should be treated first to maximize the campaign's economic benefits. Starting in September 1957, Qingpu announced that while "we should treat everyone, we should first treat those with symptoms," a scientifically based decision that would maximize disease control. Qingpu established a special treatment group focused entirely on treating the challenging cases of late-stage patients. Experienced Shanghai doctors posted longer term in Qingpu due to the 1957 Anti-Rightist Campaign and the Great Leap Forward undoubtedly helped make these new campaign targets possible.[91] Since professional scientists and physicians were almost always excluded from supervisory positions during revolutionary moments, these campaign priorities likely reflected the newly developed understanding of disease control by educated youth and cadres, as well as their ability to quietly defy the government's drive toward ideological decision making. In the early 1960s, postfamine, Jiangsu struggled to maintain treatment parity so that both expensive late-stage patients and those with good labor power received treatment despite straitened conditions. Except at revolutionary heights, such as the Cultural Revolution, mention of class-based treatment biases does not appear in the Qingpu, Jiangsu, or Shanghai archives.[92] These locales' ability to put science first and treat all infected people is one reason their snail fever campaigns were so successful.

In contrast, places like Jiangxi employed an ideological lens to determine treatment priorities, focusing on workers, peasants, and soldiers' health, and eventually class background. More than a decade into the campaign, Jiangxi still maintained this problematic framework. After the famine, the provincial government told counties that they must first treat those with labor power, a decision based on economics, and then those who were poor or middle peasants. Individuals with landlord or rich peasant backgrounds were not mentioned as targets, which mainly precluded them from getting treatment.[93] When the Party announced that treatment was free during the Cultural Revolution, the whole ideological framework shifted; provision of universal care became the new way to showcase leftist credentials. As a result, places like Jiangxi could continue being ideologically correct while conducting a campaign that suddenly aligned with effective disease control.

From the perspective of potential patients, Chairman Mao's decision to make treatment free and communes' increased effort to supplement work points so that people would not lose much salary removed the biggest obstacles to receiving treatment.[94] The growing use of short-term and oral treatment that could be taken at home without the use of painful shots also decreased costs and resulted in fewer side effects. Home-based treatment greatly facilitated women's access and made the entire process much less challenging to the family and work unit. Once the state covered treatment costs, people's appreciation of the better medical care provided by outside doctors also greatly increased, despite doctors' holding rightist and counterrevolutionary labels.[95]

A second change during the Cultural Revolution was that resistance to treatment by both residents and local cadres for ideological and economic reasons dissipated due to the Mao cult. It no longer mattered whether the campaign was logical or even whether it worked; it was now a matter of faith, or if faith was lacking, a mechanism for a public demonstration of devotion. As more people were successfully treated, untreated peers began to see treatment as normal and necessary. At the same time, attacks on community members, particularly those who had previously held power, and the high level of social instability made overt resistance, especially by lower-level leaders, increasingly difficult.[96]

Technical improvements, such as oral treatment, made treatment both more palatable and easier to administer. There were no injections and fewer dangerous side effects. In addition, short-course treatments were kept at a fairly effective three-day regimen, rather than the ineffective four-hour treatment of the Great Leap Forward. Better testing methods and more universal testing made possible by the commune setting identified a greater proportion of infected people. At least in the Shanghai region, universal testing in 1973 included issuing cards to each person, certifying they had been treated. This made it easier for campaign personnel to track their efforts and much harder for individuals to slip through the cracks.[97]

Finally, the situation for rural medical providers was transformed. Although professional science was devastated, dispatching physicians from both the Western and elite Chinese medical traditions to rural areas facilitated the dispersal of medical expertise. The scale of this transfer was spectacular. Starting in the mid-1960s, almost all graduates of Western and traditional Chinese medicine schools were automatically posted to country hospitals in rural areas. Due to Chairman Mao's June 26, 1965, attack on the Ministry of Public Health in his "Directive on Public Health," in that year alone the urban medical establishment sent 150,000 medical personnel to the countryside; they trained more than 200,000 rural health workers in addition to conducting regular treatment work. By 1972, this number had reportedly grown to 330,000 urban medical workers placed permanently in the countryside and another 400,000 doctors and nurses who visited as part of roving medical teams, a two-year post. The elite of the medical profession led the way, including the president and vice president of the Chinese Academy of Medical Science; the director of the Peking Union Medical College, the country's top medical school; and the director of the prestigious Shanghai College of Traditional Medicine.[98] Following this example, some provinces, such as Anhui, emptied out their entire medical staff from provincial, prefectural, and county medical units and hospitals and moved them to the countryside. By 1972, so many of Shanghai's snail fever prevention personnel and members of the Shanghai Institute of Parasitic Diseases had been sent out that those left in the city reported "having trouble carrying out our own work."[99] The military medical establishment also dispatched more than 14,000 medical teams—over 100,000 medical workers—to rural areas.[100] As top urban medical colleges and research institutions dispatched increasing numbers of mobile teams or transferred personnel long-term to specific rural provinces and counties, permanent medical linkages were formed. These leading institutions then became responsible for improving medical resources and acting as referral sites for their "sister" counties' medical institutions.[101]

Despite many physicians' rightist label, most were still able to practice medicine in the countryside. For example, in 1968 Yujiang received 135 "intellectuals" with medical skills. Provincial leaders' main comment was that "those sent down to the countryside don't include any good people; good people are not sent down."[102] Initially, leaders in Yujiang, a revolutionary stronghold, took this to heart and assigned the transferred medical workers to agricultural production, where they could learn from the peasants. However, within only a year, local leaders felt this "attitude was not right" and shifted the medical personnel to production brigade clinics instead. Since this maneuver successfully passed under the political radar, by 1970 cadres decided that the "conditions there [in the grassroots brigade clinics] were bad and they couldn't really use all their skills," so the medical workers were sent up to commune-level hospitals.[103] Competent medical personnel were such a rarity in rural places that it was difficult letting them go to waste merely to fulfill political dictates.

Importantly, during the Cultural Revolution, medical professionals were posted to the countryside long-term, enabling an ongoing relationship between rural providers and doctors. Two decades of work had vastly expanded the rural school system, creating a large group of educated youth. In addition, starting in 1968, many urban youth were sent to the countryside. The start of the barefoot doctors program in 1968 took advantage of this talent and steered many rural youth and a minority of sent-down urban youth directly into medical work, eventually creating more than a million practitioners.[104] Up to a third of rural youth inducted into this program had prior training as an indigenous herbalist from an older relative, which served as a hidden knowledge subsidy to the barefoot doctor program.[105]

The presence of professional physicians in Shanghai, Jiangsu, and Jiangxi was crucial to enhancing the utility of barefoot doctors and to the campaign's ability to engage in broad-scale treatment, particularly of late-stage patients. The arrival of large numbers of experienced medical personnel made it possible to set up training courses, something that had been challenging due to a dearth of competent instructors. However, many barefoot doctors received barely enough training to function.

The long-term presence of experienced doctors, combined with the many urban personnel in mobile health teams in the countryside, meant that many barefoot doctors had an on-site or occasional mentor and medical supervision, allowing them to serve the equivalent of a medical apprenticeship while starting their practice (see figure 12). Dr. Chung, an expert sent-down urban professional, noted that after running a training course for barefoot doctors, the "teachers were assigned to visit newly-trained students at regular intervals, helping them to solve their problems and to consolidate their medical and surgical knowledge learned in class."[106] Although Mao Zhixiao, a newly

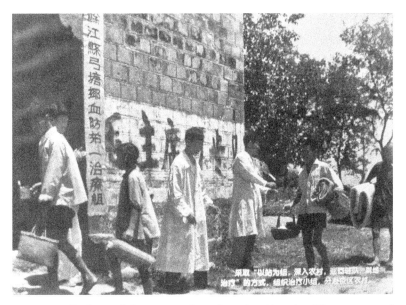

FIGURE 12. Professional doctors sent down from the cities who did treatment and oversaw preceptorships for barefoot doctors made it possible to do mass treatment during the Cultural Revolution. Photo from the collection of Miriam Gross. Picture taken in the Yujiang County Songwenshen Memorial Museum.

trained doctor in Jiangxi's Guangfeng County, had strong revolutionary sensibilities, he waited for the arrival of his assistant director, the experienced doctor Song Jinhui, before embarking on disease prevalence surveys. After examining the late-stage patient whose miraculous recovery would eventually make people receptive to the campaign, Dr. Mao could only find Dr. Han Songling, another professional, to "beg him to specially treat the patient." Even in Qingpu County, experienced and well-trained local doctors waited for expert urban counterparts. One 1966 report commented, "Basically when those people [from Shanghai] come, then late-stage patients are treated, and when they are not there, then few patients are treated or none at all."[107] When a U.S. medical delegation came to China in 1978, they noted that teams of Beijing physicians dispatched to rural areas "provide care and upgrade the skills of the physicians in the country and commune hospitals and of the barefoot doctors in the brigade health stations."[108] Without this sort of guidance, the campaign would have never been able to follow through on revolutionary imperatives to treat every patient no matter how severe the illness. Further research is needed to determine if professional doctors sent to rural areas served a similar role in other provinces besides Jiangxi and Jiangsu.

The barrier to large-scale universal treatment had always been the minute quantity and low quality of rural medical personnel. By combining the many hands of barefoot doctors and the medical expertise of experienced doctors, the government finally overcame this problem, which explains why there was such an efflorescence of health campaigns during the Cultural Revolution. As a result, many places experienced a turning point in the incidence of snail fever. The more cattle and people that were treated, the less infectious material was present in the environment. The ardent attempts to treat every last patient, even those who were unwilling or in the disease's late stages, ensured that the areas immediately surrounding human habitation were clean. Once this was the case, snails could not be infected and the tiny creatures became innocuous. With treatment as the major focus, in combination with short-term snail killing while infectious material was still present, the campaign was able to avoid the intractable problems of altering personal habits or eliminating every snail and still achieve success, finally bringing the disease under control.[109]

Treatment numbers from the Cultural Revolution document the extraordinary success of this part of the campaign. Few trustworthy statistics are available from the Cultural Revolution, a problem made worse because records were burned and, from 1972 to 1978, the Shanghai Institute of Parasitic Diseases was closed, which was the institution responsible for maintaining the campaign's statistics.[110] As a result, I have chosen to judge treatment accomplishments based on statistics collected in 1981, after more stringent scientific norms had been established by Deng Xiaoping. The campaign headquarters in Shanghai reports that the much more effective medicine praziquantel saw wide-scale use beginning in 1980, but it is unlikely that this medicine made significant inroads into rural areas by 1981. Thus the following data reflect Maoist-era work (1949–76) and continuing efforts from 1977 to 1980, all work that would have been impossible without the paradigm of urban and barefoot doctors working together to treat rural patients using antimony. China had 10.6 million cases in 1949 and an accumulated total of 11,335,798 cases over the course of the campaign, of which 3.17 million were treated by the end of the Great Leap Forward in 1959, though revolutionary short courses make it likely that some treatment did not actually cure snail fever. By 1981, China only had 704,982 people infected with the disease. Because very little campaign work happened from 1959 to 1966, most treatment occurred during the early Cultural Revolution (1966–71) and immediately after (1977–80) (see table 4).[111]

TABLE 4 Treatment accomplishments of the snail fever campaign

	Total sick people, c. 1949*	Late-stage, c. 1949	Total sick, 1981 (% of 1949)	Late-stage, 1981 (% of 1949)	% of total population infected, c. 1949	% of total population infected, 1981	Snail-covered land, c. 1949 (m²)	Snail-covered land, 1981 (m²) (% of 1949)
Shanghai[†]	759,287	20,541	6,952 (0.92%)	31 (0.15%)	13.55%	0.28%	166,477,511	67,020 (0.04%)
Qingpu Area	157,232	6,014	1,403 (0.89%)	1 (0.02%)	45.9%	0.02%	74,297,296	110 (0.0001%)
Jiangsu Province	2,465,341	89,947	38,220 (1.6%)	11,504 (12.8%)	21.72%	0.33%	1,393,350,232	5,444,864 (0.39%)
Jiangxi Province	537,337	27,493	52,268 (9.7%)	4,640 (16.9%)	No data	No data	2,367,956,434	495,602,197 (20.9%)
Yujiang County	6,220	335	0	0	26.14%	0	974,630	0
China	11,335,798	357,038	704,982 (6.2%)	48,972 (13.7%)	Not provided	Not provided	14,212,810,372	2,888,494,718 (20.3%)

SOURCE: Qian Xinzhong, *Zhonghua renmin gongheguo xuexichongbing dtuji*, *shangce*, 22.5, 24.5, 28.5, 38.5; *zhongce*, 170.5.

* Numbers reflect accumulated totals of patients, some of whom were found in the 1950s and 1960s.

† Shanghai numbers include Qingpu and nine other counties that were incorporated into Shanghai in 1958.

While all areas had notable success in treatment, those with higher human and economic resources did best. Thus Shanghai and the national campaign test site, Qingpu, originally a county in Jiangsu Province that came under Shanghai control in 1958, reduced ill patients to less than 1 percent of their former number. Late-stage patients requiring the most sophisticated medical expertise were the real test of campaign treatment success. Shanghai and Qingpu both had significantly less than 1 percent left by 1981. Infection rates in the whole population, which are the best determinant of true disease control, similarly were considerably below 1 percent by 1981. Not surprisingly, these resource-rich areas that could afford molluscicides, flamethrowers, and eventually tractors also had atypical success at eliminating the snails. Jiangsu, a relatively wealthy coastal province, showed almost the same achievements with early and midstage patients and cured 87 percent of its late-stage patients. Perhaps the most impressive accomplishments were in Jiangxi Province. Despite its being rural and impoverished, with very few medical personnel, the combination of urban and barefoot doctors still managed to treat 90 percent of all patients and 83 percent of the late-stage patients. Yujiang, the Jiangxi county that made this campaign so famous, achieved total disease elimination by 1981. As expected, about 20 percent of both Jiangxi's and of China's areas where the parasite was endemic remain covered with snails today. Places such as Jiangxi's Poyang Lake, which serve as vast reservoirs for the snails, suggest that the disease will never be completely eliminated. However, as long as high rates of treatment occur among humans and cattle, little infectious material will be available to fuel the disease cycle.

CONCLUSION

From 1949 to the late 1970s, the snail fever campaign embarked on a heroic undertaking to cure millions of people and to test even more. Stymied by poor testing methods, intolerable treatment regimens, limited equipment and medicines, and inexperienced personnel, it was a significant challenge to make the campaign function. Although retrospectively this campaign is described as a patriotic undertaking in which treatment should have been the most personally beneficial part, in fact there was a great deal of resistance by both cadres and villagers. Government reports suggest that this opposition was due to superstitious thinking and attachment to traditional Chinese medicine. However, this study finds that most rural people did not have a problem with Western medicine. Instead, they were dubious about some of the strange new methods associated with Western medical practice and completely distrustful of medical practitioners in general. Once it became clear that the new medicine worked, and once economic and access problems were solved and safety issues mitigated, villagers pragmatically partook of Western treatment while continuing alternative treatment modalities.

Many rural people's complex engagement with the campaign reflected their response to the broader trend of increased government intrusiveness as China transitioned from an empire to a socialist nation-state. The tug and pull between people and Party over who had authority over rural people's bodies was a constant dynamic throughout the 1950s and revealed the state's attempt to institute and normalize its version of biopower.[112] In this campaign, rural people were particularly upset that the government would involve itself in something as private as stool, a distaste that affected their relations with both the campaign and its personnel. Although villagers became partially inured to stool samples, when revolutionary and communal pressures let up, many chose to ignore further demands. Villagers were also disturbed that the Party intruded in family power dynamics. However, this interference was the main factor facilitating married women's ability to get treated. Finally, new ideas about pathogens not only challenged people's understandings about health and disease but also suggested that the Party hoped to assess people's bodily health, rather than leaving such a determination to people's own experiential reality. Party success would not only facilitate government control but also help turn the population into a defined labor input whose daily labor power could be calculated and maximized. In essence, the campaign filled one of the last gaps in managing the labor force so that it was more likely to fulfill production goals.

Even though the campaign is remembered as eliminating the disease in 1958, in reality snail fever, particularly acute cases, arose in epidemic proportions in many places only a few years later. In addition, despite international recognition of China's excellent homegrown prevention methods, the prevention portion of the campaign was never a great success. Instead, treatment, which rarely received much attention, flourished in the campaign's second peak, during the early Cultural Revolution (1966–71), and immediately after (1977–80), eventually leading to control but not elimination of the disease. This impressive accomplishment resulted from greatly improved technical methods and medical personnel's revolutionary eagerness to treat every last patient. This success was greatly aided by the popular obligation to follow Chairman Mao as well as by more palatable medical regimens and diminished economic obstacles, all of which decreased villagers' resistance. Finally, experienced urban professional doctors posted long-term in the countryside mentored the new flock of barefoot doctors, which was crucially important for increasing the latter's efficacy and decreasing their malpractice rates. Together, these factors greatly diminished the amount of infectious material surrounding villages, triggering the tipping point that led to the campaign's ultimate success.

PART IV

Government Benevolence?

THE NONHEALTH BENEFITS OF
HEALTH CAMPAIGNS

CHAPTER SEVEN

Doing the Unthinkable

SCIENTIFICALLY LEGITIMATING PARTY
INTRUSION IN THE 1950S

> Once the mental blockade caused by superstitious beliefs is shattered, the CCP can give a command, cadres figure it out, and the people will be able do it. The [Party] just needs to hold up a ladder and [the people] will dare to go up to heaven.
>
> *Yujiang campaign propaganda, 1958*

IN THE EARLY 1950S, the new Chinese government faced a big challenge: how could it retain rural support while transforming society at the expense of rural people?[1] Initially, the CCP gained respect by evicting foreign aggressors, stabilizing the country, and conducting land reform. However, the government's excess grain procurement transferred the meager rural surplus to support urban industrialization, while returning less than 10 percent of the state's investment to the countryside. This caused some of the rapidly growing population to go hungry and others to sell off their new land due to debt. The government hoped that collective farms would solve these problems by fostering economies of scale, the imposition of modern agriculture, and the ability to conduct a planned economy down to the grassroots.[2] Many farmers who had just gained private land were dismayed at this reversal. The Party's conundrum was how to conduct disadvantageous policies while positioning them as both positive and necessary. This chapter considers whether legitimating change in rural areas through scientific health campaigns, nominally in accord with natural laws, contributed to the Party's ability to carry out its agenda.

Data from the snail fever campaign suggest that many hygiene, sanitation, and parasitic disease campaigns did not have notable success during the 1950s and lost the Party political capital. Why, then, did the Party keep doing more of these campaigns, revitalizing them with even greater intensity during the early Cultural Revolution (1966–71)? Health campaigns facilitated Party control in four ways. First, they joined concurrent political campaigns in redefining the meaning of both superstition and science so that some aspects of professional science and traditional culture were termed superstition. Second, they provided the Party with specific mechanisms to attack traditional culture and the resistance to the new scientific socialist society that seemed a part of that culture. Third, they were one of the most effective ways of developing true grassroots activists who would faithfully promote alien Party campaigns and act as catalysts for rural change. Finally, sanitation campaigns encouraged participation in higher-level cooperatives without the use of force. This chapter suggests that in the 1950s, the nonhealth benefits from the early health campaigns helped ensure their longevity. The next chapter examines nonhealth benefits in the mid-1960s and 1970s.

CONTROLLING THE SCIENCE/SUPERSTITION DYAD: SUPPLANTING PROFESSIONAL SCIENCE AND POPULAR CULTURE

The CCP had an extraordinary agenda for an untried regime. It wanted to construct a country based on new beliefs, behaviors, identities, power relations, and even topographies. To accomplish this makeover, the Party needed to be the arbiter of truth, at least in public discourse, if not in people's minds. In the 1950s, the Party faced two entrenched sources of authority: traditional culture and science. New frameworks of leadership and control almost invariably reverted quickly to traditional relationship networks. Likewise, positioning Party goals as the guiding vision for the new society collided with people's aspirations for a utopia that resembled a more wealthy and equitable traditional society. Science was equally problematic. In the 1950s, the era of *Sputnik,* many Chinese urbanites joined the international community in identifying science as the correct mechanism for modernizing society and achieving strength internationally.

To replace these alternative authorities with its own, the Party embarked on a time-honored Chinese strategy: resurrecting the idea of a superstition/science dyad and then dominating the meaning of these words in public discourse. Starting in the late Qing dynasty (1880–1911), escalating during the New Culture Movement (c. 1915–30s), and reinforced by ideas from Friedrich Engels, superstition and science had been framed as mutually incompatible.

During the New Culture Movement, science was elevated from simply providing technology to being one of the two elements (the other being democracy) necessary to transform the nation, bringing it into the modern era. Much of this change was due to John Dewey (1859–1952), a renowned American psychologist and philosopher who spent two years in China (1919–21) teaching his philosophies of empirical knowledge, science, democracy, and educational reform. Dewey advocated that China replace the "authority of tradition" with the "authority of science."[3] The idea that science and superstition represent opposite domains in constant competition came from this and other New Culture Movement discourse.

These ideas were reinforced by Marxist teachings from Friedrich Engels (1820–95) that represented both science and human societies as materialist processes governed by natural laws understandable by human beings.[4] Those who understood these laws and controlled their material bases should be able to manipulate human social organization to progress in a desired direction. To perceive the true materialist underpinnings of nature and society, traditional cultures and religions believing in ancestors, spirits, and gods must be sloughed off. Like the New Culture Movement, this philosophy made an attack on superstition necessary. The CCP annexed this existing dyad and then redefined the meaning and relationship of "science" and "superstition" so that it could call its own plans and methods scientific, while casting aspects of both science and traditional culture as superstition.

This created a conundrum: How could the Party assert control over science when professional scientists and medical personnel seemingly had a more valid claim to this realm, and their knowledge was essential for grassroots scientifically oriented campaigns to function? How could the very professionals designated as rightists, trying to destroy the new society, be necessary for health campaigns that were a guarantor of the new society? Redefining superstition helped the Party address this problem. Doctors were accused of superstition because their resistance to Party guidance and leadership by the masses demonstrated they were stuck in the past. As early as 1954, Chairman Mao critiqued Western doctors for their inability to accept Chinese medicine practitioners: They "ignore the traditional Chinese doctors' rich experience and obvious clinical effectiveness; . . . [saying] Chinese medicine is 'backward' and 'unscientific' and [they] negate it wholesale. Such an attitude of not recognizing facts and not emphasizing practical experience is an attitude of extremely 'unscientific' arbitrariness." It was a short step from "unscientific" and irrational to superstitious.[5]

In the 1957 Hundred Flowers Campaign, scientists requested professional autonomy, which would place scientific truth above Party authority. Chairman Mao promptly attacked them in the 1957 Anti-Rightist Campaign. During the Great Leap Forward (1958–61) and the Cultural Revolution (1966–76), condemning doctors and scientists as superstitious became common. Usually, they were termed superstitious for adhering to professional standards, such as opposing the dangerous revolutionary medical regimens that might lead to medical malpractice lawsuits. Resistance was used as proof that doctors were unfit for the new society. They held onto "traditional" medical modalities and refused to "emancipate their minds" and embrace the Party revolutionary medical models, such as providing a four-week treatment in only four hours.[6] Attachment to "foreign methods" rather than "indigenous methods" was also viewed as superstitious, as was insisting on working in hospitals with sterile environments, medicines, and equipment, rather than in rough rural wards.[7] The "foreign" standards inevitably involved more time, resources, and money, placing doctors in direct opposition to Chairman Mao's Great Leap motto: "more, faster, better, and more economical results." A 1958 Jiangsu report accused, "It is because the superstitious experts don't believe in the masses that they promote fewer, slower, poorer, and costlier methods."[8]

Terming scientists and doctors superstitious opened a space for the Party to transfer scientific authority to newly trained, revolutionary rural campaign personnel, while allowing the CCP to covertly get guidance from disgraced, sent-down professionals. Likewise, villagers asking for the skills of experts were superstitious for not trusting that the masses' revolutionary science and spirit could overcome anything.[9] Calling scientists superstitious neither miraculously made doctors proponents of revolutionary medicine nor changed the focus of professional scientific institutes. However, it did make it difficult for professionals to put forth a credible competing vision for science in the public domain. Thus, during revolutionary eras the Party dominated how science was practiced outside the laboratory, and it used anything labeled scientific to bolster its power and legitimate its policies as rational choices based on trustworthy data and natural laws.[10]

Trying to unseat traditional culture as the arbiter of cultural norms, relationships, and aspirations was an even thornier problem. On April 24, 1956, in his important speech "On the Ten Great Relationships," Chairman Mao proclaimed that the Chinese masses were "poor and blank." According to Mao, poor people desire revolution because they have nothing to lose, and "blank" people are like "a blank sheet of paper [which] is good for writing on."[11] However, health campaign workers made the predictable discovery that people were poor but not "blank," harboring a complex series of behaviors, beliefs, and relationships that often did not align with Party directives, leading them to inconveniently question many aspects of mandated campaigns. The Party tried to make the people blank so that they would be more amenable to becoming the new Socialist Man. As Maurice Meisner explains, "Mao Zedong, by declaring the Chinese people 'blank,' was driven by a utopian impulse to escape history and by an iconoclastic desire to wipe the historical-cultural slate clean. . . . A new culture, Mao seemed to believe, could be created ex nihilo on a fresh canvas, on a 'clean sheet of paper' unmarred by historical blemishes."[12]

The Party's assault on popular culture gained legitimacy by casting it as holding back the new scientific socialist society. Likewise, labeling general dissatisfaction or resistance to the Party's goals as superstition made it easy to deride alternative perspectives as ignorance. Resistance was framed as superstitious thinking waiting for Party enlightenment, whether it derived from concerns about feng shui, fears that campaigns were unrealistic, or economic and logistical barriers.

Since superstition and science were cast as mutually incompatible, lingering superstition could actually block the assimilation of scientific thought. Thus, a 1956 report on a key snail fever meeting in Jiangxi's Shangrao Prefecture said: "There's a strong relationship between fighting disease and fighting superstitious thinking. Superstition is science's opposite. Some people say that snail fever stems from doing evil in one's previous incarnation and that elephantiasis comes from stepping on coffin boards. If we don't eliminate superstitious thinking, then science cannot gain ground."[13] Losing superstition was credited with enabling people to learn previously inaccessible skills. A 1956 account from Fengxian, a suburban county near Shanghai, commented that the ability of people with limited education to become lab techs was "due to them getting rid of their superstitions." In this vision, science and superstition were in a battle for the minds and hearts of the people.[14] After assimilating science, people were supposed to align themselves with the Party and support its scientific socialist construction goals. Thus, a March 1956 Shanghai report attributed the superior ability of troops versus local villagers to do snail elimination to the troops' technical expertise.[15] Interestingly, their technical expertise consisted of being willing to follow orders to dig faster and deeper. From this perspective, villagers performed worse due to lack of technical skill, rather than because they were being refractory and purposely engaged in work slow-downs. They would, no doubt, become enthusiastic once their technical skills improved.

Although almost all rural campaigns and projects had an antisuperstition component, health campaigns were thought to be particularly effective. Being sick was likened to being in a state of superstition (similar to being in a state of sin). Thus, Qingpu's campaign personnel suggested that Rentun Village had such high rates of snail fever partly due to the prior reactionary government and partly due to "local people lacking scientific knowledge and having very widespread and deep superstitions and customs."[16] This implied that the diseased state of the village was caused by villagers' lack of scientific enlightenment rather than by pathogens.

Health campaigns were also valuable because sick people were thought to have an apathetic, backward state of mind, best healed jointly by medicine and exposure to the campaign's scientific orientation. China was not alone in eliding ill health, superstitious backwardness, and loss of productivity. When explaining the need for a hookworm campaign for the *jibaro* (Puerto Rican peasants) prior to their employment in American coffee and sugar plantations, Bailey Ashford and Pedro Gutiérrez Igaravidez remarked, "There is a hypochondriacal, melancholy, hopeless expression, which in severe cases deepens to apparent dense stupidity, with indifference to surroundings and lack of all ambition."[17] Apparently, curing this disease would be the antidote to a range of personality characteristics assigned to the *jibaro* by the new colonial power. Similarly, CCP reports stated that "snail fever was bad for socialist construction because it causes an extremely pessimistic attitude and leads to people only looking at today, not thinking about tomorrow, just trying to get a bit of food and a little something."[18] These reports also noted that sick people thought that their disease was a barrier to joining collectives and that it was a reason for withdrawing from them. Yujiang's Party secretary, Li Junjiu, concurred, explaining that "after working for a period in the affected area, I felt deeply that snail fever was a great barrier to agricultural development and the collective system."[19] Other Party leaders connected the disease to limited energy for production, unwillingness to pay the state grain tax, and disinterest in joining the army. A 1959 report from Jiangxi summed up these themes: "Previously people just prayed to gods and waited to die. . . . Now [post-treatment] all the past passive elements have been changed to active ones. So one can say that the face of the people's spirit has had a huge change."[20] According to this logic, contact with health campaigns would scientifically heal both people's bodies and their spirits. This scientific uplift would then solve the problem of citizen resistance to Party goals in everything from the grain tax to collectivization to national defense.

Many modern states have grasped the utility of dressing up politically driven public policy in a scientific guise. "As the authoritative knowledge in modernity," writes Susan Greenhalgh, "science serves to legitimize both the exercise of power through policy and the authority of the policy makers . . .; when science speaks in the name of nature, it depoliticizes beliefs and practices that are often eminently political, removing them from the arena of contestation."[21] The CCP followed this well-honed strategy but pushed it a step further by taking control of the meanings embedded in the science/superstition dyad. This allowed the Party to dislodge scientific authority over what was termed science in public discourse and to define traditional culture and aspects of professional science as superstition. Once these preexisting authoritative paradigms were relegated to the superstitious past, the Party-led campaigns automatically represented rational scientific thought. Within this syllogism, there was no valid disagreement with the Party's agenda.

BEYOND RHETORIC: EXPLOITING HEALTH CAMPAIGNS TO HELP ERADICATE TRADITIONAL CULTURE

Health campaigns and other antisuperstition campaigns moved beyond rhetoric, directly attacking traditional culture, especially temples, gravesites, and community festivals. Temples were in direct competition with the Party agenda that people use their minds to comprehend the truth of Marxism and their bodies to build the new society. At temples people squandered scarce resources on superstitious ceremonies; supported indolent priests; propitiated deities, ghosts, and ancestors who competed with Party authority; and reaffirmed bonds to ancestors and family rather than to class.[22] Health campaigns had a particularly effective strategy to supplant temples—repurposing them as treatment wards.[23] This choice was symbolically important because the terrain of the temple, the ultimate superstitious space inhabited by ghosts, was now overwritten by a scientific campaign. Since ghosts were previously thought to cause some diseases, placing a treatment ward among them was also a way to counter prior disease etiologies. Once the temple became a ward, people could no longer worship there. Moreover, both the physical residue of hundreds of very sick people with poor care and the spiritual residue left by deaths on the ward made it much more unlikely that the space would be reestablished as a temple once the ward was closed. Thus, repurposing as a treatment ward was an effective short- and long-term strategy for temple removal.

Many public health campaigns went even further. Lack of building materials was a primary impediment to constructing the needed sanitation infrastructure. Many ancestral and other temples were torn down so that their bricks, stones, and beams could become the primary building blocks of "scientific" toilets. Superstition was literally torn apart and reborn as part of people's glorious scientific future. The fact that temples were being sacrificed for the greater health and well-being of the people made it more difficult to protest their destruction.[24]

During both revolutionary peaks, particularly the Cultural Revolution, the snail fever campaign helped justify eliminating sacred burial land. While it was difficult to persuade people to disturb their ancestors for marginal crop land on a hillside, it was harder to argue with the hidden evil of snails lurking in uncut grasses around grave mounds. Jiangxi's De'an County, Hedong Village, had six hillocks with graves inconveniently cluttering communal fields. In the latter part of the Cultural Revolution, the local Party proposed "driving away the ancient tombs to eliminate the snails." After extensive propaganda education challenging villagers to consider whether they wanted to "leave the old tombs or leave living people," the community decided to "go to war expelling 367 tombs." In the process of destroying putative snail reservoirs, they, coincidentally, increased the land under plow by another sixty mu and erased this "superstitious" eyesore from the community's vision.[25] Since most areas protected by religious or cultural beliefs had freely growing greenery, the snail fever campaign could easily be used to justify eliminating them, simultaneously furthering Party production and modernization goals.

Community-wide celebrations were important mechanisms for creating and maintaining a vibrant popular culture and lineage relations. Health campaigns were used to subvert their original purpose. Many holidays—including Spring Festival, Tomb-Sweeping Day *(qingmingjie),* the Dragon Boat Festival *(duanwujie),* and the sixth day of the sixth lunar month *(liuyueliu)*—included ritual sweeping or washing with water, which purified people or places, showed respect for the dead by attending to their tombs, and swept out ghosts or bad luck from one's residence. Campaign personnel sabotaged these preexisting traditions by reframing them as cleaning the house and tidying up the village. Over time, most original celebrations were washed away by village cleanup days, expanded to incorporate feces management and kill campaigns against various insect, snail, and animal pests. Cleanup days also allowed the Party to attack household taboos and enforce bathing, something nonhealth, antisuperstition campaigns had little luck accomplishing.[26] The result was that reformulating traditional holidays as cleanup days cut down on popular resistance to sanitation (see chapter 5) while using a time for cleaning that would have been lost to field work anyway. Like Christian recharacterization of pagan holidays, Party repurposing of popular holidays realigned their content with Communist goals. The Party was able to assail prior traditions on the very day that should have reaffirmed them and transformed superstitious activities into science by reconceiving their purpose, all with minimal disruption to prior routines and lifestyle choices.

Given the powerful resurgence of popular religious culture during the Reform era (1976–present), it seems likely that antisuperstition campaigns mainly succeeded in driving traditional culture underground. However, among the many campaigns assaulting popular religion, health campaigns were a particularly powerful tool because their benevolent rationale for change made opposition more difficult.

CREATING GRASSROOTS ACTIVISTS

Finding genuine grassroots activists was a big challenge for the Party. According to Gordon Bennett, most mass mobilization campaigns were carried out by activists *(jiji fenzi),* energetic individuals with more enthusiasm than their compatriots, and backbone elements *(gugan fenzi),* mainly members of the Party or the Communist Youth League co-opted or mandated to do the work. Whereas being named an activist was a real honor and was "officially regarded as a 'spiritual reward' *[jingshen jiangli],*" this was not the case for reviled health campaigns.[27] Joshua Horn, a sympathetic English physician, observing the snail fever campaign at a model site during the Cultural Revolution, recounts that a snail elimination work group leader described the work as "trying," noting, "The children, too, used to annoy us. At first they didn't understand what we were doing and they used to walk along the bank laughing at us and asking us why we didn't do proper work like the other grown-ups instead of playing about in boats all day. I sometimes felt like asking to be transferred to ordinary agricultural work."[28] Many villagers' feelings about the new sanitation regimes led them to make withering remarks and treat campaign personnel like pariahs. For example, in Yujiang, a passerby insulted an elderly lady working on toilets, saying, "She must be a landlord's wife." Only by having the most sullied class status imaginable could she be stuck with this sort of work.[29] During peak revolutionary moments, campaign work was a punishment for bad elements, requiring true dedication to continue. Nonetheless, health campaigns produced some of the Party's most dedicated grassroots activists, making it interesting to consider who became activists, and why.

Initially, youth and women were targeted by campaign propaganda and Fulian, the national Women's Federation. Youth were admonished to take a leading role because they represented the new society. Women were selected because they symbolized the most backward elements of the exploitative old society, making their participation in a modern campaign a great victory certain to empower them. Ironically, campaign organizers also thought that women, with their less powerful status and supposedly more pliable nature, would be easier to coerce. Finally, these activities were envisioned as a new version of cleaning and caretaking, tasks associated with women.[30]

Despite campaign leaders' efforts, few young and middle-aged men contributed to ongoing prevention activities, mainly participating in short mass mobilization campaigns.[31] Men felt that production was their primary role and did not want to dissipate energy in prevention work. Moreover, sanitation-oriented prevention activities were cleaning, which was a woman's job. Because such campaign activities provided limited reimbursement, like other women's work, men were less willing to contribute to them. In contrast, snail killing while rebuilding irrigation channels often received some compensation and was mainly done by men.[32]

Most genuinely voluntary grassroots activists in the snail fever campaign came from three groups: young women, elders who had watched their families die from the disease, and late-stage patients cured by the campaign. Women's participation is particularly impressive because their campaign work was not only unpaid; it was often dirty, tedious, conducted in their spare time, and devalued by being termed "helping out." Generally, the snail elimination strategy given to women, children, and elders employed chopsticks and was thought of as cleaning up the village. When men did not do a thorough job burying the snails, women and youth were often sent to do uncompensated cleanup work involving heavy digging. Collection of the "wild" feces scattered around the village was another minimally or unpaid job slated for women. Women's patience and perseverance were expected and evaluated as normative behavior.[33] Interestingly, according to archival records, on the rare occasions when men took on women's work, they were viewed as special leaders. When an elderly Yujiang man took over feces management work, he was portrayed as heroic for sacrificing himself for the greater good. Indeed, a surprising number of the few men who did this work gained model worker status.[34] Given this milieu, it is impressive that women were still interested in these activities. Many women agreed that the campaign activities were in their natural work and spatial domain and that therefore they should control their implementation rather than outside men. In addition, some young women, who were disempowered members of the community, used public health campaigns, where there was little competition from young men, to gain status outside the preexisting hierarchies. Active engagement in CCP social construction work could be a route to more or better opportunities both inside the village and beyond it.[35]

Elders were the second group of activists. Their role was supposed to be "speaking bitterness" storytelling, comparing the bad old society to the wonderful new one. However, in prevalent disease areas where children and grandchildren often predeceased them and their lineages died out due to disease-caused infertility, elders were often highly motivated to throw their authority behind the campaign and to actively contribute to prevention activities nobody else wanted to do. As the dynamics of local resistance and avoidance unfolded, campaign personnel seem to have willingly incorporated elders despite the lack of higher-level directives mandating their inclusion.[36]

A final group of activists were late-stage patients cured by the campaign or people whose late-stage parents or children were saved.[37] Patients recognized that skilled city doctors would never have come to the countryside without the CCP, a further reason to be thankful to the Party. In contrast, since patients in the early stages of the disease perceived themselves as healthy and forced into treatment, they were often critical of the campaign. Because this campaign treated far more early or asymptomatic people than late-stage patients, the number of activists it produced in the latter category was a small but nevertheless very effective minority.

Individuals who knew their lives or families had just been saved in a health campaign were tied to the Party by loyalty and indebtedness. This bond was fostered by the Party's insistence on physicians becoming "people's doctors" whose main purpose was personalized caretaking. In China, caretaking was a defining principle of family bonds and a primary way of showing affection.

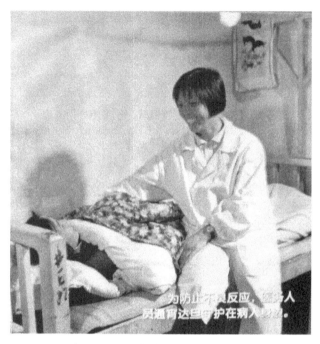

FIGURE 13. The Party's medical representative looking after the people like family by helping them with intimate caretaking needs. Photo from the collection of Miriam Gross. Picture taken in the Yujiang County Songwenshen Memorial Museum.

Previously, nursing had been assumed by family members. When medical personnel took on the responsibility of cleaning the ward, boiling drinking water, washing patients' feet and bodies, helping them go to the bathroom, finding them needed food, giving them the quilt off their own beds, and taking care of their children or animals when they were not well, it made a very strong impression. Campaign accounts repeatedly refer to this not as infection control, good medical care, or even appropriate nursing, but rather as "treating the patients like family" or "as close to the patients as family members" (see figure 13). In the admittedly propagandistic bottom-level reports, it is the caretaking undertaken by the Party's medical representatives that garners some of the strongest response.[38] As one Shanghai villager put it: "Prior to treatment we were very afraid because physicians from Shanghai definitely have a bad disposition. But now we've found they care for us even better than relatives. This sort of doctor only comes because they've received training from Chairman Mao."[39]

This awareness downgraded the doctors as solo actors and turned them into chess pieces whose caring acts redounded to the Party and Chairman Mao. In one Qingpu family, after seven different family members had been treated for snail fever by 1956, the mother said: "If we didn't have the CCP, our family wouldn't exist. Now I completely welcome them as if they were family."[40] As one sixty-year-old woman put it after the campaign treated her family members, "If Chairman Mao is taking care of our bodies' health in this way, then we should exert ourselves too."[41] While health campaigns did not create a population of loyalists among participants in prevention activities or among the majority who thought themselves healthy, they did generate a group of very dedicated activists among the "saved" who were predisposed to promote the Party's nonhealth objectives to the wider community.

Peer activists were a vital repository of good will and an important catalyst for socialist construction efforts. Villages where disease was prevalent and that were a major campaign focus sometimes had higher enlistment rates in all Party activities. Cured people were more willing to join early cooperatives, pay taxes, and sell their grain at artificially low prices on the newly nationalized market. While data are anecdotal, the more that treatment was subsidized, the more willingly people supported the Party in nonhealth domains.[42] Qingpu's famous Rentun Village as of 1951 had only 341 residents, but according to a 1965 report, at least one person enlisted in the army every year. In contrast, a village of comparable size with less disease that had neither energetically engaged in health work, nor received treatment from the government, "didn't have even one person enlist."[43] In 1953, after the government provided free treatment to people in Longhua District, on the periphery of Shanghai, the distrustful relationship between the people and the Party was transformed. Villagers' compliance in paying grain taxes rose from 20 to 80 percent, and the whole area fulfilled its tax responsibilities. Even more surprisingly, villagers changed their position regarding the nationalized grain market. As they put it: "When the government shows loving concern for us peasants' health and treats our diseases, we all support the government state purchasing and marketing monopoly policies. We guarantee we will not sell the grain to private smugglers."[44]

While unlikely to be true across the board, villagers benefitting from the snail fever campaign felt in debt to the Party and were therefore more open to potentially detrimental activities. By 1955, the nationalized grain market was an accepted fact, but it was variably used. Yet, after the campaign came to Jiangsu's Jiangdu County, people "actively sold off surplus grain . . . to greatly thank the Party and government."⁴⁵ The campaign also encouraged people to believe in the government enough to try early forms of cooperatives. In Shanghai's snail-infested Longhua District, post-treatment villagers sent a letter to the newspaper, *Xinwen ribao,* thanking the Party, Chairman Mao, and health personnel. In it they publicly pledged to "resolutely increase mutual aid teams and cooperatives . . . to support the construction of national industry . . . [and] to repay the Party and Chairman Mao's loving kindness."⁴⁶

Even a single activist could make a huge difference to the CCP's community reception. By 1954, Qingpu resident Ma Jincai had gone to twelve private doctors in Shanghai and Kunshan, exhausting all his cash and even forcing him to sell a precious cow. With government-sponsored treatment, he spent only a small amount of money and his snail fever was cured. He was so moved that he said: "Whatever the government tells me to do, I'll do. We must definitely listen to what Chairman Mao says." Ma enthusiastically educated his community and encouraged them to get treated. He went on to sell two thousand jin of grain to the government on the nationalized grain market and mobilized all his neighbors to sell theirs too. He threw himself into the early cooperative movement, joined the people's militia, and became a people's militia model. Here was a case where the Party succeeded in creating a personal bond of loyalty and obligation. This one individual acted as leaven, causing his whole neighborhood to view the Party differently and to give it the benefit of the doubt.⁴⁷

During this era, a multitude of health campaigns reached out to different populations in need. Rural people were aware that without the Party they would never have had access to treatment and subsidies or the skilled care that actually cured disease. To fulfill their personal debt and loyalty owed the Party, a newly conceived powerful family member, they supported socialist construction activities. Their activism was also motivated by the honest belief that the Party could accomplish miracles. Their conviction and dynamic support often continued despite injurious rural policies, undoubtedly helping the Party accomplish its rural reconstruction goals.

CAJOLING PEOPLE INTO ADVANCED PRODUCERS' COOPERATIVES

One of the Party's hardest challenges was coaxing people to join advanced producers' cooperatives (late 1956) without losing significant rural support.

After finally gaining private land, farmers were extremely unhappy with permanently transferring it to the cooperative.[48] Propaganda, community pressure, and coercive strategies urging participation were incorporated into many campaigns, but health campaigns were an important, but understudied, component of Party strategy.[49] Health campaigns employed both the obvious tactic of linking health care with joining cooperatives and the more covert strategy of holding people hostage through their manure.

Chairman Mao promoted APCs by identifying them as one of the only ways to solve rural ills, especially disease. In his December 27, 1955, "Second Preface to *Upsurge of Socialism in China's Countryside*" he wrote that as a result of the cooperatives, "many of the most serious diseases that are harmful to people, such as schistosomiasis and so forth, for which people in the past have thought there were no treatments, can now be treated. In short, the masses can already see their great future."[50] High-level collectives and the health campaigns were often portrayed as inextricably linked. As a representative from Anhui summarized at a national meeting, "Treating snail fever is also guaranteeing the work of launching the cooperatives."[51] While this is likely an overstatement, the health care opportunities suddenly possible with group resources were a concrete manifestation of the radiant future offered by the CCP.

Importantly, APC-associated medical treatment could also be employed as a coercive measure to force people to join. In Jiangdu County, Jiangsu Province, the government suggested "first treating cadres, youth, and peasants who are organized in order to benefit production and the cooperative movement."[52] Since there were far more people waiting to be treated than treatment slots available, the subtext was that without supporting the Party by joining cooperatives, health benefits would not be forthcoming. A similar strategy was tried with fishermen. Party propaganda pointed out that fishing put families at high risk for waterborne diseases, a problem that could be solved by joining land-based collectives. If the fishermen were unwilling, then their families should be settled safely at a collective, where they could help the Party bring their family members under control. When treatment was made free in 1966, the Party used the campaign to persuade fishermen to join fishing cooperatives, something they had till then avoided. The Party made the supposedly universal free treatment conditional on guarantees from fisherfolks' communes. Independence, the Party seemed to be saying, had real costs.[53]

Many of the Party sanitation campaigns were especially helpful at pushing people in to APCs because they legitimated CCP takeover of night soil, the

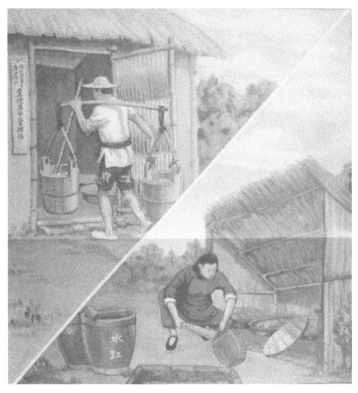

FIGURE 14. Poster promoting the new night soil management system that brought fertilizer under Party control and made solo farming increasingly difficult. Zhejiang kexue jishu puji xiehui and Zhejiang weisheng shiyanyuan, *Xiaomie xuexichongbing guatu* (Beijing: Renmin weisheng chubanshe, 1956), poster no. 8.

main rural fertilizer.[54] Such campaigns included Patriotic Public Health Campaigns and campaigns against parasitic and waterborne diseases. The Party promoted feces co-ops as a way to encourage cooperative farming, but most people were uninterested and resisted. To counter resistance, the government announced that night soil co-ops were the only way to clean up villages and eliminate the parasitic and waterborne diseases that had been preying upon the people (see figure 14). Once the government gained control over night soil, it became exceedingly difficult for farmers to remain independent. By collectivizing night soil in the name of improving health, the government also ensured that all available fertilizer ended up in communal fields. As the Yujiang government explained when trying to eliminate private toilets that served as households' fertilizer reservoirs: "Independent households still maintain their own feces cellars. This form isn't suitable for collectivization."[55]

The Party began the hotly contested battle to capture night soil as early as 1952. In suburban areas around Shanghai, manure vendors made money by paying villagers low fees for night soil, turning it into better fertilizer, and selling it for profit. This job was so lucrative that the 1952 Five-Anti Campaign against capitalists and the bourgeoisie labeled marketing manure a "feudalistic exploitive practice," and venders were called *fentou* (shit heads). After the vendors "received education" during the campaign, "they admitted their guilt." Since they were guilty, local Party leaders felt free "to take their means of production by force."[56] By the end of the campaign, manure vendors were almost entirely cut out of the rural economic system.

The Party also justified a February 1956 takeover of the profitable Shanghai night soil market by claiming that only the CCP sanitation personnel's replacing the existing system would ensure that clean, egg-free feces would be distributed to the greater Shanghai area. Previously, the market was controlled by secret societies and a network of household feces collectors and distribution boats. The new personnel were supposed to simultaneously assume collection duties and stop peasants from collecting, while urban residents were instructed not to sell to peasants anymore.[57] Forcibly ousted from their long-term jobs, former feces collectors engaged in a small-scale street war over shit. As the market became tight, desperate collectors began brawling in the streets, "jeopardizing the social order." Some showed their anger by "using both hands to chaotically smear sludge all over the walls" and some "intentionally" left covers off drains, a hazard that soon collected a quota of falling children and bicycles. When former collectors encountered their replacements, the situation exploded, including hospitalizations after the old collectors beat up the new ones with their shoulder poles. Clashes filled the municipal reports, and in one place such conflicts "even became a routine occurrence."[58] From the government perspective, social unrest was troubling, but the political implications were worse. The old collectors, primarily peasants, demonstrated to the public that it was acceptable to beat up representatives of the Party. They also made it obvious that peasants, workers, and cadres who should have been aligned harmoniously in one leading class in fact had many conflicts of interest. Despite this transitional period's many problems, in the name of snail fever, this crucial marketplace was brought under Party control.[59]

Meanwhile, when various sanitation-oriented public health campaigns started in the countryside, there was a vacuum waiting to be filled by the

Party-appointed feces management co-ops. Enterprising individuals started fertilizer ventures in the guise of cooperatives, which were actually money-making scams. As these co-ops controlled more and more fertilizer, they became similar to an unregulated monopoly. Many up-and-coming grass-roots cadres were quick to take advantage of this situation. The government tried to control prices "to take strict precautions against embezzlement," but it lacked enforcement mechanisms. As late as 1957, this problem had yet to be solved.[60]

Grassroots reports from all areas reflect anxiety about state control over fertilizer. One account explained: "Feces management has a lot of worry associated with it. People are afraid they will be taken advantage of and won't have enough fertilizer . . . and then their own land won't grow well."[61] Many tried desperately to safeguard their fertilizer stock in feces vats or household pit toilets. Cadres often had to "force people" to destroy their toilets, which "made people even more upset."[62] Once toilets were demolished, some villagers tried to hold on to their excrement by secreting it in plain sight. This resulted in new regulations, for example, that people "cannot store human feces in private pig pens."[63] Soon, pens were moved out of the courtyard and collectivized, making it increasingly difficult to resist the new order. In Qingpu, where the vat-based system was easier to take over than private toilets, villagers still tried to elude the new cooperative system by "secretly moving their small feces vats into the house." It was better to have night soil pervade one's living space than to lose the possibility of independent fields. Some places slowed this process by refusing to surrender land for a feces depository. Few people wanted large amounts of other villagers' smelly night soil near their residence. However, with the start of advanced producers' cooperatives, the Party was able to apportion communal land for projects that were not supported by group members.[64]

Farmers who tried to remain sole proprietors were pressured to participate in a feces management program and then found they were discriminated against. Once they put excrement in, there was no record system to ensure that they got the same amount out and every reason for the co-op to preferentially give most of the fertilizer to its own group members. As independent farmers in Jiangxi's Shangrao prefecture discovered in 1953: "There are some people who would like to grow some vegetables. Now that all the night soil has been given to the co-op, trying to use it is extremely inconvenient."[65] Villagers sometimes even had to "steal out the manure from the collective site to do their own farming."[66] Shanghai's retrospective account of the snail fever campaign noted that once the campaign forced every three households to use a single shared vat to manage their night soil, "it solved the problem of people calculating the costs of entering the cooperatives versus doing what they pleased with the manure."[67] Places that could afford commode dumpers closed one of the last loopholes that had helped people resist collectivization. Because commode dumpers' salaries depended on all night soil reaching the communal pot, these workers assiduously showed up every day at villagers' doors to collect the family commode. After this, it became almost impossible to hide away large quantities of fertilizer.[68] As the momentum to create more and more cooperatives swept society, inability to access fertilizer became a very effective motivation for the last holdouts to join up.

Even those in low-level cooperatives—where farmers shared tools, animal, and labor but retained private ownership of land—eyed fertilizer apportionment carefully. Many felt that a household with more adults supplied more feces than one composed mainly of children and should be given a larger quotient of manure in return. Since it was impossible in a mainly illiterate society to track inflows of night soil by individual or by family, some areas developed guidelines for how much excrement a person of a certain age could be expected to produce per month. This allowed for an automatic calculation of what each family was due. Once high-level cooperatives started, private plots were eliminated and careful reckoning of night soil stopped.[69]

The intimate connection between night soil and individual plots becomes evident after the famine (1959–61), when villagers were again allowed private plots. They immediately refused to add their night soil to the communal pot, instead hoarding and distributing it to best benefit their own land. In Jiangxi, pig pens kept protectively inside the house and household pit toilets reappeared, maximizing the ability to keep control of fertilizer. A 1961–62 Yujiang survey postfamine discovered that only 20 percent of the people were still using the public toilet; 50 percent of the public toilets still existed, but people had reverted to their own toilets; and 30 percent of the people had used the chaos of the famine to destroy the public toilet and return to using their household toilet. Although a major push to reconstitute public toilets occurred in the early Cultural Revolution, a similar situation reoccurred by 1973, when external chaos allowed villagers free reign.[70] Even the Qingpu test site, an area with an exceedingly high snail fever infection rate that had received some of the most effective propaganda and had managed to retain a modicum of feces management, apparently dismantled its system during the famine and refused to revive it during the recovery period. A 1961 village survey of 152 households, conducted after people received private plots, found that 150 of them asked that management of night soil be returned to the individual household. It was better to get sick from snail fever than lose control of night soil again. As one report noted, after people received private plots, they were "unwilling to hand [feces] in and [instead] keep it at home." In many places, villagers even refused to allow anybody else to wash out commodes, for fear that they would lose access to fertilizer. It was crucial that every bit of a family's excrement go directly to their own fields.[71]

In summary, the Party used collectivization of both fertilizer and health care to encourage people to join co-ops. While the collectivization of fertilizer was not enough to achieve this aim, it did make it challenging for villagers to refuse. The minute that private plots were reinstituted and Party influence waned, villagers dismantled collectivized feces systems and reasserted control over this crucial resource, demonstrating that they perceived feces co-ops as a significant barrier to solo farming. It is less clear whether access to health care was effective at pushing people into co-ops, particularly because in the 1950s most treatment was still paid for privately, making it unaffordable. However, as motivated activists newly saved by one health campaign or another started backing cooperatives, the assurance of treatment and elimination of age-old diseases was likely one of the co-op system's few obvious advantages. Promises of good health offered consolation for the loss of precious private land and likely encouraged people to resist such a seemingly benevolent system in quieter ways.

CONCLUSION

In the early to mid-1950s, the Party had to carefully position its rural reconstruction efforts to minimize loss of rural support. The scientific rationales embedded in health campaigns were an important mechanism for facilitating and justifying early Party consolidation. By making its goals that were otherwise detrimental to rural people seem scientifically valid and essential for well-being, the Party encouraged villagers to adopt a wait and see attitude. Such a stance was extremely helpful to the Party, because it could then avoid using force while continuing to consolidate power.[72]

By dominating the definitions of superstition and science, assigning science to itself and superstition to traditional culture, the Party made its attack on folk religion an essential requirement for building a modern society, rather than an egregious assault on the people. The result was that obliterating temples, burial mounds, and religious holidays—which supposedly kept villagers trapped in the past—and re-creating them as wards, public toilets, and cleaning days, thus guaranteeing a healthy future, demonstrated the Party's enlightened scientific guidance. Having assumed the mantle of science for itself and proving itself worthy by carrying out health, science, and modern agriculture campaigns, the Party used this same authority over definitions to denigrate professional scientists, thereby removing them as a contender for scientific authority, at least in the public sphere. Each protest by scientists about revolutionary variants of science, technology, and medicine just demonstrated that scientists were relics whose time had passed. The upshot was that this successful assumption of the mantle of science, a claim greatly facilitated by health campaigns, helped legitimate the Party, sidelining all possible competition for authority and power, whether from scientists, gods, ghosts, clerics, traditional leaders, or lineage heads.

The multitude of health campaigns that saved ill people turned the Party into a figurative family member and created personalized bonds of indebtedness with the state. Individuals who were activated in this way served as catalysts for socialist construction goals in every arena; they often loyally supported the Party and encouraged giving it the benefit of the doubt even when new policies or campaigns were clearly detrimental to rural people.

Finally, health campaigns in general and sanitation campaigns in particular were an important mechanism for ushering resistant people into advanced producers' cooperative without the use of overt force. Only collectives provided the resources necessary to guarantee health care—and only if people joined would the government be able (and willing) to minister to the people's needs. Perhaps even more important were the persuasions embedded in government monopolization of rural fertilizer stock. Supposedly, only by cleaning night soil of parasites and other diseases could rural people finally slough off the burden of illness that had kept them stuck in the past. Such a compassionate action made it harder to complain that the same maneuver also made it extremely difficult for sole proprietors to remain outside the collective system.

Together the rhetorical and substantive use of science within health campaigns helped vindicate problematic campaigns, generate activists, and substantiate coercive measures that greatly facilitated early power consolidation and positioned the Party as the arbiter of truth. The next chapter examines how dissemination of scientific practices in health campaigns to educated youth facilitated Party control at the grassroots level in the late 1960s and 1970s.

CHAPTER EIGHT

Scientific Consolidation in the Late 1960s and 1970s

IT WAS 1958, the height of the Great Leap Forward. The Party was busy dismembering professional science in the wake of the 1957 Anti-Rightist Campaign, and achieving "greater, faster, better, and more economical results" by replacing a slow-moving, mechanistic bureaucracy with the rocket velocity of mass mobilization campaigns. At that very moment of revolutionary fervor, something very strange was happening on the ground. The Party was using grassroots scientifically oriented campaigns as a training ground to disseminate the tools that underpinned both science and rationalized bureaucracy.

Franz Schurmann classifies bureaucratic organization as either human or technical in his work *Ideology and Organization in Communist China.* Human organization is based on networks of connection between people linked by values, tradition, or ideology. Technical organization (scientific management) or Weberian rationalized bureaucracy focuses on technical concerns to maximize efficiency and selects staff based on their skills, ensuring appropriate behavior via universal laws and norms. Party organizational strategies during revolutionary moments have been placed firmly in the ideological and charismatic camp of "human bureaucracy," suggesting that rationalized technical bureaucracy reappeared only during the Reform era (1976–present), partly due to a reassertion of the value of professional science.[1]

This chronology raises interesting questions. If bureaucracy was dismantled during the Great Leap Forward and Cultural Revolution, and government planning was decentralized to the grassroots, how did the national government ensure that its goals were actually carried out in the vast hinterland? Revolutionary eras coincided with the creation of large communes with thousands of members, whose efforts needed to be coordinated into mass mobilization campaigns, often with a self-consciously scientific bent. How were rural, poorly educated cadres able to create plans and organize these complex endeavors without bureaucracy? Given the denigration of professional scientists, how was a scientific perspective still able to infuse these campaigns?

Chairman Mao pursued few crusades as enthusiastically as that against bureaucracy.[2] However, my archive-based study reveals that while Mao was busy dismantling elite technical institutions, he was at the same time promoting technical skills to rural cadres, believing these skills essential to effective planning and mass mobilization campaigns, successfully making them both "red" and "expert." Skills were taught to educated youth in many scientific campaigns, with the snail fever campaign serving as one example. Because a minimal education was a precondition for assimilating such skills, Shanghai, with its reservoir of educated youth, was able to begin this effort in the 1950s. In contrast, most rural areas reaped the benefits of scientific skills only in the mid-1960s, when more educated youth were available to these communities. Of course, youth educated to the elementary or junior-high-school level still had limits. Professionals remained essential to carrying out complex medical work and training rural youth as barefoot doctors and technicians. Within these parameters, I argue that a scientific and technical tool kit empowered rural cadres to carry out work in domains and on a scale previously inconceivable.

It is a major contention of this study that science and scientific tools also provided a critical mechanism for the Party to make its will manifest at the grassroots level. When rural cadres collected fixed, state-mandated data and then reported them in front of peers and superiors, these cadres' efforts were channeled into enacting Party goals and mandated required campaign processes without force or bureaucratic oversight. I call this process "scientific consolidation." It is important to note that the "scientific" ideologies and practices of the Maoist-era Party were distinct from science in its normative definition, which has as its goal an understanding of unsolved phenomena based on unbiased, reproducible experimentation.[3] Instead, Maoist-era "grassroots science" focused on performing field investigations to resolve pragmatic problems. By dissecting information gathered locally and exhibiting it as statistics, the Party hoped that the analyst could come up with novel, rational, and realistic solutions that would move the society forward. The CCP initially felt that because of these inquiries' specificity of place and time, they did not require detailed baseline data or a control group, or need to be repeatable or even objective; each inquiry simply had to effectively resolve a problem. While some standard scientific practices were unevenly inserted later, grassroots science was more successful at supplying a scientific veneer than at achieving science itself. Grassroots science joined Marxism and Mao Zedong Thought as an ideological legitimation of the Party's effort to construct a scientific socialist society. Thus, grassroots science had as its goals an ideology of progress that would lead to China's global success; an experimental and innovative mind-set that the Party would propagate among the masses; rationalized, scientific planning that gave the Party authority as an agent of societal transformation; and the medical, scientific, and technical knowledge necessary for campaign success. Only this last idea partially overlaps with a normative understanding of science. This chapter explores how educated youth learned science in the form of tools for scientific planning and how these tools influenced early power consolidation efforts by the Party.

The phenomenon of scientific consolidation during the PRC has not been the subject of prior scholarly inquiry. Scholars have dissected mass mobilization campaigns—the major mechanism for large-scale work during revolutionary periods—but have asked neither how grassroots cadres gained the skills to conduct these complex campaigns nor how using these skills supported efforts of the Party for wider control.[4] Some works have discussed the problems of decentralizing planning to the grassroots and the impediments caused by rural leaders' lack of education and statistical knowledge. However, how educated youth acquired technical skills in the 1960s and the effect of this on rural consolidation have not been explored.[5] The seeming impossibility of gaining bureaucratic skills during a period when the bureaucracy was under attack, along with the consistent assumption that a modern technical bureaucracy was not allowed to function until the Reform era (1976–present), may explain the lack of consideration of scientific consolidation prior to my work.

This chapter first discusses the establishment of scientific management as the modus operandi of the CCP. Drawing on archival information about the snail fever campaign, it explores the challenges of teaching new scientific ideas and skills and the introduction of "scientific performances" as an avenue to demonstrate scientific prowess. The chapter then shows how acquisition of technical skills by rural youth made the snail fever campaign possible. The chapter concludes by examining how acquisition of these tools, coupled with public presentations of campaign achievements, simultaneously empowered and constrained new rural leaders, providing a new state control mechanism called scientific consolidation.

INTRODUCTION OF SCIENTIFIC MANAGEMENT BY THE CCP AND ITS IMPLICATIONS FOR EDUCATED YOUTH

Originating in Frederick Winslow Taylor's 1911 book, *The Principles of Scientific Management,* the doctrine of scientific management laid out new theories of modern business organization and managerial technique, aligned with the goals of efficiency and productivity. Scientific management is a specific application of the premise that when nature is broken down and classified, it can be understood and reconfigured for human ends. Taylor applied this notion to mapping the component parts of people's labor. Time and motion studies by Frank and Lillian Gilbreth and others used practical experiments, statistics, measurements, charts, and graphs to rebuild each piece into the most efficient way of doing a portion of work. This technique broke up the work process so that each worker became skilled at performing one small task. It also carefully sequestered those doing the manufacturing from those proficient in management. The result was a strict division of labor characterized by cooperative effort, a disciplined labor force, standardization, efficiency, and limited input from workers into the management process. Taking America by storm and famously utilized by the Ford factory, this process influenced up-and-coming Chinese business and industrial moguls who brought large numbers of scientific management texts to China and began to apply them under the Nationalist government during the 1920s and 1930s.[6]

Meanwhile, the ground was being laid in China for a broader application of the utility of classifying and reconfiguring nature. During the 1920s, John Dewey gave lectures in Beijing encouraging Chinese intellectuals to integrate his view of science with their work as leaders of a modernizing society. According to Jessica Ching-Sze Wang, Dewey advocated "an experimental, scientific method of inquiry in solving social problems . . . [and science as] a method of intelligence for coping with problems and difficulties in ordinary life, rather than as a collection of objective truths." As Dewey explained, experimental knowledge was "not to produce useless or 'ornamental' knowledge." Instead, its purpose was to "make knowledge and practice more practical."[7]

The future Chairman Mao likely learned about Dewey from Professor Hu Shi, Dewey's student who was a leading member of the New Culture Movement and with whom Mao studied while working as an assistant librarian at Beijing University. By July 21, 1919, in his report "The Founding and Progress of the 'Strengthen Learning Society'" in Hunan, Mao emphasized that "adopting John Dewey's Philosophy of Education" was necessary for the "reform of Hunan" and that "there is no telling . . . how great the benefits might be."[8] Mao began his own scientific investigations, which culminated in his May 1930 *Report from Xunwu.* In Xunwu County, Jiangxi Province, Mao personally collected local data, processed the information as statistics and tables, and used it to do planning and as the basis for achieving larger strategic goals. During the same month, Mao wrote his essay "The Importance of Investigation," later called "Oppose Bookism," in which he said: "You can't solve that problem? Well, go and investigate its present situation and its history! . . . All conclusions emerge at the end of an investigation of the circumstances, not before it."[9] In this essay, theoretical or book knowledge was the opposite of true investigation, as it prevented an authentic understanding of actual conditions, real people's needs, and effective strategizing.

It seems possible that Mao's understanding of the nature of practical science was quite influenced by Dewey and these early experiences. Importantly, the grassroots science Mao promoted often involved encouraging rural leaders to gain the skills to do their own investigations so that their plans had a basis in reality. This helps make sense of Mao's confusing assertion during the PRC that he was promoting science at the same time that he was assaulting the professional science establishment. By attacking bookish, theoretical professional science and bureaucracy during revolutionary periods and replacing them with indigenous innovation and grassroots planning based on locally collected data, he was making his vision of science manifest. When the Party took up the mantle of science, it also tended to focus on experimentation as a practical method for solving problems, rather than as the seemingly abstruse efforts of professionals in academies.

The importance of scientific management to successful, speedy development was reinforced when the Soviet Union, China's primary international model, reintroduced the doctrine intertwined with socialism during the 1950s. After encountering scientific management, the Russian revolutionary Vladimir Lenin declared, "We must organize in Russia the study and the teaching of the Taylor system and systematically try it out and adapt it to our purposes." Leon Trotsky found Taylorism equally appealing. According to

Thomas P. Hughes, in addition to the control over both work process and workers inherent in this system, Trotsky particularly admired that it led to the "restoration of discipline" and "leadership by experts." When drawing up their first five-year plan in the 1920s, with the help of American scientific management experts, Soviet leaders directly applied Taylor's and Ford's strategies for productivity on the factory floor to planning for the country as a whole.[10]

Leaders of the CCP imported almost every aspect of the Russian version of scientific management save one: guidance by technocratic elites. Chairman Mao thought it was imprudent to leave this powerful tool in the hands of professional scientists unbound by ideological constraints of the Party. Instead, all scientific management and planning were to be mapped out by the Party itself, justifying its leading role while simultaneously helping it consolidate power. Scientific management was particularly appealing because it promised increased efficiency and productivity both in the factory and on the farm. It provided the scientific tools to do planning with a particular focus on timing (or speed) and statistics (or production quotas). It promised a fair degree of predictability and control of outcomes, implying that the CCP could have power over a small part of the future. Scientific management encouraged discipline, standards, and conformity among workers at the expense of independent action. Because it was framed as scientific and modern, resistance could be construed as backwardness needing correction via propaganda education. Similarly, the statistical proofs, charts, and graphs required by scientific management lent Party goals a rational, scientific veneer. This made Party mandates seem indisputable rather than erratic versions of ideology or personal choice.[11] Finally, the Taylorist paradigm affirmed the rightful place of planners and managers as directors of the entire enterprise. As long as Party members made work plans and organized the movement of society, they were automatically legitimated as the proper leaders in a system based on scientific management.

There was an inherent contradiction in basing CCP programs on scientific management while simultaneously striving to eliminate bureaucracy. The planning process required universal standards buttressed by identical data collection forms, careful copying of model practices, map making, meetings, and standardized reports to attest to statistical accomplishments. These elements were all quite similar to bureaucratic practices—and they accomplished analogous purposes. They encouraged people to do the work while ensuring some degree of unified outcomes. It is difficult to promote scientific management without also bolstering bureaucracy. The Party solved this problem by disseminating the tools of bureaucracy to a wider group at the grassroots level, but this decision created a new set of problems.

Chairman Mao wanted workers and peasants to develop innovative work processes to unleash rapid economic development, nurture local self-reliance, and cultivate a new sort of person suitable for the scientific socialist society. These goals contradicted standardization, a central tenet of scientific management and a planned economy. Identical work practices made work easy to manage and plan for local cadres and facilitated transparency for higher-level cadres trying to oversee work at a distance, especially in an era where few people had sophisticated accounting skills. Standardization also ensured that nonmodel units would precisely replicate the efficient methods of model sites. Random innovation would undercut these efforts and likely lower efficiency. In fact, according to the mantra of scientific management, work became scientific and more likely to lead to rapid economic progress only when unified work models were achieved.[12] Thus, it was unclear whether grassroots innovation was the key to progress or a major factor impeding forward momentum, leading to an ambivalence reflected in many of Mao's writings.[13]

The focus on statistics that characterized almost all CCP work also had inherent contradictions. In his speech "Methods of Work of Party Committees," Mao explained that it was essential to gather numbers and "make a basic quantitative analysis," because without figures people will "make mistakes" and will also "decide problems subjectively and without basis." In "Sixty Points on Working Methods," Mao required leaders to provide people with "both primary and processed source material" at meetings so that people would not just "rubber-stamp" the Party's conclusions. Yet in the same document, Mao suggested that cadres should control data and present only those things that clarified the Party's opinion.[14] It was thus unclear whether quantitative data should provide an objective measure or simply substantiate Party goals.

Despite this ambivalence, Chairman Mao forged ahead, encouraging grassroots leaders to learn scientific tools because they were essential for guiding the new society, saying that if cadres did not master science and technology, "we shall not be able to lead." In the July 1955 "Conversation with Security Guards," Mao suggested they study both cultural matters and general scientific knowledge such as math, physics, and chemistry. As he put it: "If you earnestly raise your literacy level somewhat, you will then be able to master scientific knowledge, do more things for the people, and serve the people better. . . . We need a great many intellectuals who come from the ranks of the workers and peasants."[15]

Mao's devotion to developing rural cadres had the potential to backfire (see chapter 2). Rural cadres were indebted to their local communities and the Party establishment was far away, giving rural cadres great power and limited oversight. Moreover, their lack of the education or the scientific tools necessary to plan increasingly complex and large campaigns, especially in a strange area like health, made it extremely unlikely that they would willingly lead such efforts. Educated youth, the later incarnation of rural cadres, were even riskier. Their education and entitled status in the Communist system made it easy for them to side with their communities against government demands, perform unwanted work in a dilatory manner, and wait until the next campaign wiped out the current one.

During the Great Leap Forward (1958–61), most rural leaders had yet to assimilate scientific tools, a fact that helps explain why mass prevention activities for the snail fever campaign were limited outside of model areas. The nonmodel areas that did carry out mass snail fever eradication efforts may have been helped by the rural *xiafang ganbu,* whereby 300,000 higher-level cadres at the commune level were sent down to basic units, some to be reformed, others to strengthen local leadership. In his study on the Maoist-era organizational system, Harry Harding concludes that sending down these more accomplished administrators was a primary way the Party compensated for the dearth of local cadres' planning skills, a gap that was especially obvious in the face of the increasingly complex campaign work during the Great Leap.[16]

By the mid-1960s, a vast expansion of the rural education system generated many rural educated youth. At the same time, acquiring higher status was increasingly difficult because older leaders, or *lao ganbu,* clung to their positions and competent *xiafang* cadres filled many openings. For youth wanting to better themselves, there was a clear pathway to success. Aside from being born with a good class background and getting a basic education, youth needed to join the Communist Youth League and be an activist in Party campaigns.[17] Demonstrating the skills to organize and lead campaigns was an excellent way to break in to the system. While many rural campaigns employed scientific tools, health campaigns made a concerted effort to teach them, generally by sending youth out as a special team under experienced leadership. During the Cultural Revolution, it is likely that the attacks on old leaders offered educated youth unprecedented opportunities to seize power.[18] Once youth were in power, their more sophisticated ability to wield the tools of scientific management helps explain the efflorescence of large-scale mass mobilization campaigns in many domains.

INTRODUCING SCIENTIFIC TOOLS TO EDUCATED YOUTH

The introduction of scientific tools was a major focus of government efforts to promote scientific endeavor to educated youth. However, the concept of scientific tools was difficult for rural cadres and educated youth to assimilate, not only because of lack of education, but even more importantly because scientific tools implied a new way of conceptualizing the world. As discussed in chapter 5, many rural people believed in *qi,* the vital energy that flows equally through people and the landscape. In this conception, according to Robert Weller, "there is no fundamental distinction between the human and physical worlds, or between culture and nature."[19] If people are inextricably intertwined with their environment, then it is very hard to think of nature as an external "other" that can be separated into constituent parts, counted up, and analyzed and experimented on. Such an approach could lead to results that appear to be outside of the natural order. Therefore, in the PRC teaching scientific tools was as much about learning a new paradigm for people's relationship to nature as it was about a specific skill set. In addition, few places had sufficient experienced personnel to teach and lead thousands of teams of educated youth. There was very limited classroom training and team leaders were at best only slightly more knowledgeable than the youth they directed. The result was a very slow assimilation of new skills and the worldview behind them. In this section, I examine the introduction and evolution of the major tools in this skill set: statistics, forms and records, evaluation, and experiments.

Statistics

Among scientific tools, none was more important than statistics. Harking back to his own studies, Chairman Mao believed numbers could quantify every aspect of the human or natural world. As he put it, "Every quality manifests itself in a certain quantity, and without quantity there can be no quality."[20] Statistics could pin down amorphous phenomena to bring them under human influence and define the limits of any activity. Having gained an understanding through statistical measures, people could make appropriate plans to transform the status quo.

Luckily, this almost magical tool was among the most accessible: villagers could learn to write numbers without embarking on the larger enterprise of full literacy. Quantifying the surrounding world was apparently simple, requiring only totting up numbers. Unfortunately, determining which numbers should be gathered and counted was no easy task. In the snail fever campaign, rural surveying teams that rapidly traversed large territories with bad roads were unable to collect stool samples from millions of people or accurately count billions of snails. The solution was to sample a subgroup, but choosing an unbiased sample was beyond the skill level of most villagers. Initially, teams gathered the data easiest to collect, or simply asked village heads for their observations on the previously unnoticed *Oncomelania* snail fever vector. Flooding increased sampling difficulty, forcing some teams to float around in boats, snagging snails only a few millimeters long to try to gain accurate snail estimates. A 1955 report from Jiangxi's Shangrao Prefecture remarked that "some groups didn't check the snails' distribution, density, or positivity rate. . . . They sometimes check only a couple of villages so that we can only do a very rough estimate of an area."[21] Because of sampling errors, large numbers of snails were still being found years into the campaign. In 1957, Jiangxi's Wannian County reported that that it had six thousand, not two thousand, mu of snail-laden land.[22]

Determining the fraction of snails and people that were infected was also challenging, because of both inexperience and lack of understanding of sample bias. Although the normal snail infection rate is about 1–2 percent, with a maximal rate of 5 percent, inexperienced personnel found an astounding 69.8 percent rate of snail infection in an October 1954 survey of Yujiang's Xifan Township.[23] As a result, the work scope grew to encompass all snails, rather than the small percentage near human habitation likely to be infected. Determining the rates of human infection was equally problematic. Teams usually tested only the few big-bellied people who thought themselves sick, which could lead to an underestimate of disease prevalence. However, if teams extrapolated from this biased sample to the whole population, the incidence of disease could be overestimated, as shown by a 1951 test of 409 Qingpu youth aged eighteen to twenty-eight. It reported a 90.4 percent incidence in an area later proven to have a 40–60 percent infection rate. As a

September 1956 report from Jiangxi explained, "Survey reports are based on estimates that are quite imprecise and cause people to have doubts about the work."[24] Evolution of data requirements compounded sampling problems. Initially, workers simply reported whether a place had snails, often without being taught how to identify them. Later, they had to create detailed maps demarcating different types of terrain and water and annotate the relative amounts of snails in each zone. Eventually, sophisticated test sites had to assess snails per square foot, their relative riverbank distribution, and even the percentage of infected snails.[25]

Once data were successfully collected, teams had to learn what constituted a useful statistic. Knowing there were 100 sick people or 100 snails was pointless without knowing the size of the total population. Were 100 ill out of 1,000, or 10,000? Survey groups predating the 1953 national census could not compare their sample of sick people to the entire population, as the numbers did not yet exist. Moreover, survey teams often did not record the location of sick people, because they did not understand the relevance of this information and because data forms were not in common use. Finally, teams often could not visit all areas in the allotted time, leading them to obfuscate where data were collected so they could assert that their sampling covered all of their assigned areas.[26] Thus, it was difficult to judge either disease severity or location. Even high-level reports at national conferences detailed numbers without commenting on technical difficulties. People may have thought that these skewed statistics were valid simply because they were numbers. Alternatively, the extreme nature of the numbers may have been so useful for garnering support that it was better not to draw attention to their being an artifact of the collection process.[27]

In the late 1950s, some grassroots groups realized the problems caused by the lack of baseline data. Shanghai, Qingpu, and Jiangsu, which had higher education levels and more educated youth, began including baseline census data in 1956–57, contextualizing sick people as a percentage of the total population. Many of their reports added new information, such as sex, age, occupation, and disease stage. This greater sophistication was due to four factors. Mao's sponsorship gave the snail fever campaign greater political stature. Formation of upper-level cooperatives and of the household registration system in 1955–56 made baseline demographic data more accessible.[28] Finally, educated youth in these areas increasingly grasped statistics, as evidenced by their improved ability to exploit them to mobilize villagers in snail campaigns (see chapter 4). In rural Jiangxi, similar changes did not happen until the 1960s, coincident with more educated youth and knowledgeable team leaders being able to teach members how to do the work.

Forms and Records

The generation of large amounts of numerical and mapping data created a set of new problems. Nobody could remember the details of large data sets or last year's numbers, making it impossible to track change over time. A 1952 report from Shanghai noted a second problem: "Often, people's statistics were not prepared well and did not agree with each other. Since there was no set form, people sent in what they thought was important—which was often different from each other. The result was [that] overall statistics could not be done."[29] Forms and record keeping were an obvious solution. However, except for test sites, there is every indication that they were neither used nor even conceived of in the 1950s.[30] Campaign leaders did not identify forms and records as a necessity, as they were almost never mentioned in prefectural, provincial, or national meetings or in broad-scale campaign plans.

Lack of records was problematic for snail elimination and disastrous for treatment work. Without records pinning down snail location, a 1956 report from Shanghai discovered that "previously, scientific technique and the mass movement were not combined enough. . . .When doing snail surveying, areas that had snails were treated as if they didn't have snails, and areas that didn't have snails were treated as if they did."[31] Because each incarnation of the campaign was conducted de novo, it was difficult to assess progress or to see changing trends in location or density.

Far worse was the situation on the wards. Most rural doctors, particularly those who had been itinerants, had previously managed only a few patients at a time. Suddenly they were confronted with fifty or more patients and multiple medical providers. It would have been difficult for one overworked, exhausted individual to remember specific times, doses, and negative drug reactions; it was utterly impossible to pass on this information in a timely manner to other team members. Individual shots of tartar emetic should have changed dependent on a patient's weight, level of anemia, malnutrition, and a wide variety of other diseases discovered in an initial physical exam. However, in the absence of patient records, this information rarely affected the actual course of treatment.[32] A July 1954 Qingpu report noted, "Some people have already finished their treatment but did not receive enough medicine to complete the process; others are in treatment and have already exceeded the dosage for the whole regimen." Without individual records, it was impossible to track the gradual accretion of negative reactions and stop the medicine in a timely way, leading to many unnecessary deaths. Despite this, there was no mention in any 1950s rural ward report that this utter chaos prompted providers to keep individual patient charts.[33]

Lack of records also made it difficult to judge progress toward overall disease elimination. People were tested and treated multiple times over the years, and personnel could neither evaluate relapse rates nor determine total numbers cured because a person treated five times might be counted as five separate people. Yet the idea of records was so strange that though personnel could identify their knowledge gap, they could not figure out the cause. For example, a high-level report from Jiangsu in 1956 said that "it is not clear who has gotten the disease again post-treatment" but decided the reason was that "statistical work has been done badly." In grouped statistical data, information about a single person is inevitably lost; only individual records could have solved this problem.[34]

For most newly educated youth serving as campaign personnel, forms and records were alien objects. They were tedious and some of the data required were inapplicable or impossible to collect, leading workers to conclude that upper-level leaders were simply creating make-work for the peons below. However, some long-term campaign personnel began to realize that forms and records were useful and started to try them. This process was disrupted during revolutionary peaks (1958, 1970–71).[35] Grassroots cadres with no inclination toward forms had the perfect excuse to jettison them when Mao attacked bureaucracy and promoted speed above all else. In some cases, the government forced people to stop keeping records. A September 1958 report from Qingpu noted: "The government decided that keeping case records was wasting a lot of time on red tape that could more effectively be spent treating people. So we first changed from using a six-page case record to a one-page case record and then decide to eliminate them entirely."[36]

The Great Leap in 1958 made it politically impossible for campaign leaders to require using forms, necessitating another mechanism for achieving standardized, fixed targets for high-quality work. The campaign leadership chose to establish guidelines for three levels of accomplishment that set specific benchmarks for percentage of the population disease-free and number of snails per square foot. Standards were disseminated in the newspaper, at meetings, and through propaganda education. Townships or communes that achieved these benchmarks were feted at meetings in front of their peers and sometimes received material rewards. In Qingpu, townships that achieved the highest standard received one agricultural boat or two bicycles, T-shirts for cadres, a banner, and a certificate of merit; townships that reached the third (lowest) level received only the T-shirts, banner, and certificate. The government's use of numerical standards established that seemingly amorphous work could be evaluated and that using statistics was the primary way to assess accomplishments. These standards also indicated that treatment and snail elimination, rather than other prevention activities like water and night soil management, were the most important. While the creation of numerically based standards likely fueled exaggerated campaign numbers, they also made clear that learning how to wield scientific tools was an essential component for success.[37]

In the early 1960s, the changed political climate enabled places to acknowledge the need for forms and a record system. In areas like Qingpu that had run lengthy campaigns, tracking residual snails and recalcitrant or relapsing patients made the need for an accounting system very apparent. A September 1961 report from a non-test-site area recounted that in 1956, personnel had killed snails wherever they ran into them without recording their location: "At that time the snails were plentiful and widely distributed. After the numbers decreased, we started doing sampling. By 1958–59, the snail density decreased dramatically and there were only pockets of them left. We had to change the way we checked for snails." The solution, the report's author suggested, was to start a new card to track snail distribution. Because keeping records was so strange and had been attacked by Chairman Mao as wasting time and as the domain of bourgeois intellectuals, the author spent most of the report explaining why records were necessary: "First, this information can save effort and resources. Second, a comprehensive system means . . . it may not be necessary afterward to do a complete survey each time. . . . Third, . . . the location of the snails will be totally clear so that anyone can go out and eliminate them without needing special skills. Fourth, . . . we can save molluscicide because we will pinpoint the area where it will be used, . . . and we can do long-term investigations. Fifth, by having a comprehensive system, we can provide later scientific analysis with data."[38]

During the early 1960s, many places began not only using forms or developing card systems but also creating a comprehensive data system to retain this information as records. The Cultural Revolution interrupted this systematization process. Forms and records were discouraged and even the national snail fever campaign headquarters was forced to burn most of its records.[39] However, many grassroots campaigns had decided they were essential. Information cards, which skirted the edge of being forms and records, were quietly used during the Cultural Revolution and contributed to the snail fever campaign's greater efficacy.[40]

Evaluation

The collection and retention of data via forms and records also facilitated the systematic evaluation of work. However, the idea of evaluating work was just as strange as forms and records. Work was either done or not. If the effort had been expended, then the work must have been accomplished and there should be nothing left to evaluate. This basic stance was corroborated by campaign propaganda, which assured villagers that a single big effort to eliminate snail fever would be all that was needed. Even test site personnel had trouble recognizing the need for evaluation. A 1956 report at Qingpu's Chengbei test site, among the best in the country, explained that campaign personnel "generally think that eliminating snails once should solve the problem. They don't go to check the efficacy of their work. . . . They're even less likely to recheck changes in the test site's snail situation at a set interval." Test sites that did evaluate whether they had actually decreased snails were lauded for this impressive accomplishment.[41]

During the Cultural Revolution, revolutionary enthusiasm somewhat compensated for lack of evaluation. Leaders of treatment work could circumvent the disinclination to evaluate cure rates by using the vastly expanded group of educated youth to conduct universal annual or semiannual testing, thereby identifying those who had been treated but not cured. The prevention arm faced greater barriers to gauging true snail elimination. Here again, educated youth helped by conducting repeated snail reconnaissance missions in the same territory, an indiscriminate but thorough method that facilitated bumping into residual snails.[42]

Employing scientific tools correctly turned out to involve more than totaling the numbers to make simple statistics. Learning how to change a holistic vision of the world into constituent parts that could be manipulated, sampled, compared, and evaluated involved a paradigm shift that took many years to teach. By participating in scientifically oriented campaigns, teams of educated youth learned how to collect and process data and then use it to generate simple work plans. The next step was to use data to create basic experiments, a manipulation of observed reality that had been inconceivable before.

Early Experiments

Chairman Mao, perhaps reflecting both on Dewey and his own investigative experiences, hoped that normal people would not only use scientific tools but also design simple experiments to solve problems, rather than relying on traditional methods parlayed by elders. At least in the snail fever campaign, rigorous grassroots experimental science proved to be more dream than reality. Test sites tended to be among the few places that tried experiments, but even these were highly variable in their sophistication, reflecting both the education levels of campaign personal and cadres and the availability of educated youth.

To experiment with new ways to perform a task, the work process had to first be described and dissected, and the ability or inability to do so reflected the education level of the group. In highly educated Shanghai, a 1952 village report from a non–test site provided meticulous instructions for switching vats and brewing times based on whether it was summer or winter, so that snail eggs in the feces would be killed off. It also specified necessary equipment for public toilets and detailed how they should be managed. In more poorly educated Yujiang's Magang Township, which served as Jiangxi Province's scientific test site, a June 1953 report documented its entire feces management program as "digging a cesspool."[43] Over time, personnel at the Magang test site became accustomed to the idea that every aspect of what one did had to be measured.

A further evolution came with the realization that even careful collection of raw numbers was of limited utility. A 1955 report from a non–test site in Qingpu explained, "They did testing and collected the data, but didn't actually analyze it in any way so it would be useful!"[44] Early analysis generally compared two analogous strategies to see which worked better. Would-be researchers then tried to calculate the divergence in the results. Numerically based comparison allowed people to assess subtle gradations of difference and gauge the relative success of multiple methods at once. It also prompted people to invent precise research questions and then develop experiments that could answer them. Chengbei Township, Qingpu's main test site, provides an example of this progression. In the early 1950s, Chengbei campaign workers thought that achieving accurate statistics qualified the township as a test site. Next, they realized they had to determine changes in snail density and infection rates, which required delineating previously undifferentiated space. They marked out squares so that scattered snails could be counted, enabling determination of population density. Two or more squares not only led to a more realistic snail count but also was the springboard for experiments.[45] These data allowed personnel to pose questions about how geography affected snail infection rates and the relationship between disease and the human population. For example, how did the degree of water contact affect the seriousness of infection? How did the disease influence pregnancy? Researchers also assessed the crucial question of the disease's impact on people's work capacity and realized they had to compare people of the same age, sex, and constitution.[46]

Chengbei workers started adding control groups in 1956, because they discovered that comparing the effects of different molluscicides and treatment regimens was difficult without baseline data. When testing the efficacy of two chemicals (arsenic calcite and 666), hot water, and burial at eliminating snails, they found that snail numbers dropped by 65.3 percent after arsenic, by 87.6 percent after 666, and by 46.9 percent in the control group. However, some decrease resulted from snails crawling outside the experimental field to escape from the poison. Moreover, the experiment occurred in August, when snails naturally buried themselves to escape the heat, suggesting that "elimination" might have simply resulted from snails being invisible to the snail counter. Campaign personnel concluded that they could not determine the actual cause of the drop in numbers.[47] Chengbei began using human control groups in 1961. Researchers tested the efficacy of a three-day treatment at three test sites, using patients of differing disease intensity versus a control group. Those receiving medicine had a 60–69 percent cure rate compared to a 41–67 percent cure rate in the control group. Researchers concluded that the medicine was not effective.[48]

During the Great Leap Forward, test site work fed into a larger agenda. Many provinces took seriously Chairman Mao's injunction to bring science to the forefront. Campaign leaders in Jiangsu and Jiangxi Provinces mapped out an extensive snail fever research agenda that assigned specific projects and research questions to institutions and responsible individuals. Extra money was available for places willing to participate in research. Jiangxi even encouraged participation by its many snail fever prevention stations, providing funds and indicating that expenses for research and experimental work were now an acceptable budget category at the health bureau. Professional institutions performed much of this work, but test sites like Qingpu and Yujiang played an active role, and county-level snail fever stations staffed by educated youth also contributed.[49] This agenda of grassroots experimentation was revitalized during the Cultural Revolution when the presence of greater campaign resources, educated youth, and professionals sent down to the countryside made it possible again.

SCIENTIFIC PERFORMANCES

Original scientific research was limited to a few elite sites, but "scientific performances," starting in the late 1950s and coming to fruition during the Cultural Revolution, were a different story. Scientific performances dressed up regular campaign work with statistics and a nominally scientific framework, or repeated experiments already done to prove that a campaign mandate had worked in one's own area. Such performances were encouraged and sometimes required as part of Chairman Mao's effort to disseminate science; to "taste the pears," or directly experience phenomena; and to reduce "compulsory instruction" and "rubber stamping."[50] After describing how performances spread and evolved, this section will discuss their value to both government and grassroots cadres.

Scientific performances were promoted through propaganda education, model sites, scientifically oriented model workers, and the media. Newspapers and journals played an important role by ascribing some discoveries made by scientists to the masses and by hyping routine campaign practices as astonishing examples of grassroots scientific innovation.[51] These narratives made science seem easily attainable and fueled the tendency toward scientific performances by according them as much or more recognition as experiments by professional scientists.

Scientific performances were also embedded in government plans. In a September–December 1957 plan for Qingpu County, districts were instructed to "experiment on the efficacy" of various testing, treatment, and snail-killing methods, all of which had already been comprehensively explored in test sites around China, including Qingpu's own.[52] The odd result was that during peak revolutionary moments, instead of following Party dictates, local campaign personnel would first try out the mandated method to "prove" it and only then would follow through with the work.

In yet another strategy, units were forced to produce an annual research paper. In 1955, Shanghai campaign leaders announced that the following year, articles "introducing their [units'] new research accomplishments" would not only be written by scientific research departments; in addition, said the leadership, "every small group under the research committee must also separately write a special article too."[53] Starting in 1956, Shanghai, Jiangxi, and Jiangsu began publishing books that collected the provinces' research articles on snail fever. Although many were written by professional research institutes, quite a few were by the growing network of grassroots test sites, county-level rural snail fever stations, and a few communes. Forced to produce a paper for the annual provincial meeting, many localities dutifully went through this scientific exercise. A striking number of these papers precisely redid experiments that had already been done repeatedly.[54]

Yujiang provides a particularly sophisticated example of a scientific performance using teacake, an effective molluscicide used in Jiangxi since the early 1950s. August 1954 experiments in Yujiang had previously tested teacake amounts, settling on 150 pounds per mu as best, and campaign workers discovered that water level was the key factor behind efficacy. Despite this knowledge, in July 1957 Yujiang's Dengfu state-run farm ran an elaborate experiment testing teacake efficacy by placing varying amounts of snails and either cooked or fresh teacake on twenty-four pieces of land. There was no control group. The conclusion was that teacake was good, that 150 pounds per mu worked well, but that people should adjust the amount depending on their area. In fact, teacake has an efficacy above 90 percent, making it difficult to differentiate the effects of different amounts and of fresh versus cooked teacake. Additionally, snail numbers have little impact on teacake efficacy. Finally, the experiment was not designed to test the most important determinants: temperature and water level. Thus, this "experiment" was crafted so that the test site could successfully confirm old results while adding a scientific legitimation to normal practice.[55]

Scientific performances were incorporated as a necessary part of political showmanship in areas presenting themselves as models. Although burial was established as the main mechanism to eliminate snails in Yujiang in 1954, campaign personnel dutifully reestablished burial efficacy every year. In 1956, Wu Zaocun, the county Party secretary noted that "many places were doing tests to eliminate the snails. I wanted to do this too so I can 'taste the pears.' I went with some medical personnel and tried the smother-snails technique. My conclusion after this test was that smothering works well." Even in 1958, after most of Yujiang's campaign was over, its county committee was still "repeatedly inspecting and investigating. They decided that burying the snails was the main method to be used."[56]

Chairman Mao's insistence that personal experience was the only real way to learn intensified the tendency toward scientific performances during the Cultural Revolution, eventually leading to its codification as a training method. In 1973, the government mandated a new medicine, Dipterex, for treating water buffalo. Instead of starting treatment, Qingpu personnel conducted their own experiments on sixteen cattle and concluded that it worked, and then they held a large-scale training for all personnel to directly participate in the experimental process: "They did an experimental treatment of thirty-two cattle with great success, leading to personnel welcoming the new treatment. After this it was used all over Qingpu."[57]

Places unable to enact scientific performances reframed normal campaign work as innovative and experimental. When workers found snails, they were doing "investigative research." When Shanghai personnel chatted with women to determine why treatment was refused, they were "participating in research." This propensity came to its logical conclusion in grassroots monthly or quarterly campaign reports during the Cultural Revolution, where a "discussion" section, vaguely modeled on a scientific paper, replaced sections titled "popular reactions," "author's opinion," and "existing problems" in earlier reports. Treatment work was stylistically revamped as medical case reports, even though patients were treated using government-mandated procedures. Finally, despite employing standard methods, many grassroots reports were written like technical guides for other campaign teams. However, these routine reports were intended solely for government consumption and were thus an example of an easier type of scientific performance.[58]

Scientific performances were of great value to the government. They were used to demonstrate that China was successfully heading in a modern scientific direction under Party guidance. The government seems to have believed that extensively publicizing grassroots' innovation and "experiments" helped legitimate Party rule both domestically and internationally. Scientific performances also solved the contradiction that Chairman Mao had created in the Chinese version of scientific management. Mao encouraged comprehensive planning by the Party, which succeeded only if work was standardized and followed Party guidelines. Simultaneously, he encouraged innovation at the grassroots level, which inspired people to try new ways of doing things outside of Party control. Scientific performances encouraged villagers to "innovate" by conducting experiments according to standardized methods that achieved identical results and inevitably reaffirmed Party guidance. Additionally, scientific performances depended on a prominent display of meticulous work methods. Because the Party ensured that far-flung cadres followed mandated methods, rather than past slipshod approaches, quality control rather than mass quantity was encouraged and rewarded.

For educated youth, scientific performances, like a high-school science lab, provided an effective mechanism for learning basic scientific techniques and practicing scientific tools that could later be parlayed into general planning work. They were also a good way to decrease resistance to new techniques. During revolutionary eras, framing routine work as scientific while blatantly wielding scientific tools was a way for these youth to make a political statement that demonstrated support for progressive Party goals. It was also an effective strategy for positioning oneself as a model worker (or area), which, if successful, could bring benefits in every domain.[59] Using scientific tools, innovating new work methods, and enacting scientific performances were so important in getting ahead that educated youth sometimes demanded that they become an integral part of routine campaign work. By 1962, educated cadres from Qingpu, when asked to follow normal campaign procedures, were "dissatisfied" because they were "doing simple stuff for a long time." They wanted to "become experts" and "couldn't see it happening that way." They were also "unhappy that nothing had been set up to help them achieve this goal."[60]

Rural scientifically oriented campaigns were a crucial way for the Party to broadly disseminate scientific tools to the next generation of leaders. Employing these tools and executing scientific performances suggested new, efficient approaches to work; partially compensated for the poor quality control of mass campaigns; taught youth how to develop plans in alien domains; and, in some cases, offered new ways to solve problems. Finally, these campaigns and associated tools were successful at convincing many people that science, however defined or executed, was a crucial way to elevate work, a validation that could potentially become a route to personal and national advancement.

THE TRANSFORMATIVE IMPACT OF SCIENTIFIC TOOLS ON GRASSROOTS WORK

Snail fever was rapidly brought under control in most places soon after the Maoist era ended in 1976, a finding substantiated by surveys indicating vastly fewer sick people and cattle and a very low new infection rate.[61] This success suggests that the campaign functioned exceptionally well during the Cultural Revolution (1966–71). Yet many of the practices, particularly in the campaign's prevention arm, that had not worked during the Great Leap (1958–59) were retained during the Cultural Revolution. What *had* changed was the new phenomenon of educated youth wielding scientific tools conjoined with a massive new wave of professional medical personnel sent to the countryside for an extended time. Once a rural area finally had educated youth who were using scientific tools, this campaign, and likely most others, was entirely transformed in terms of engagement level, administration, education, technical, and eventually, medical expertise.

Documenting the specific practices of this new group of leaders during the Cultural Revolution is very challenging because campaign reports during this period were composed almost entirely of numbers interspersed with quotes from Chairman Mao. One way to explore the impact of educated youth on the snail fever campaign is to examine the rare places like Shanghai and Qingpu where educated youth were available in the early 1950s, when campaign reports were considerably more candid. The Shanghai suburbs and Qingpu, like most areas in the 1950s, had limited leadership from local political cadres, insufficient funding, few personnel to overcome the snails in one of the most infected areas in China, and prior to collectivization, negligible ability to coerce the populace. However, this region did have relatively high education levels and a ready supply of teachers and medical workers. As I document below, both areas surmounted resource limitation and local resistance by training large numbers of educated youth to be the major motivational and work arms of the campaign.

Shanghai and Qingpu's first big advantage was having enough high-level health personnel to lead special teams, which could demonstrate new skills in action. This process telescoped the time and deepened the sophistication of educated youth's absorption of this new knowledge. After receiving extensive classroom training, teams of ten educated youth were dispatched with an experienced leader and data manager to hunt down snails. Teams drew up maps and kept account books that assiduously tracked each day's data. Suspicious data led to immediate supplementary training. All the maps and data were reported to leaders and formed the basis for future snail assault plans.[62] By the end of their surveying, educated youth had assimilated a wide variety of mapping, data-gathering, and statistical skills and had seen how such raw data were turned into plans that were the basis for all government work. Similar training was given to youth so that they could act as medical assistants on the wards. Such youth were able to rapidly tackle basic technical work, and they supplied the massive number of trained hands necessary for running an effective scientifically oriented campaign.

As early as September 1951, in preparation for a large-scale snail fever treatment campaign, the Qingpu County committee organized its relatively abundant health workers, teachers, and grassroots health personnel as a propaganda team and gave 410,000 hours of scientific education to the community. By March 1952, the county committee and government had organized more than six thousand grassroots health workers to launch large-scale snail fever treatment work in the spring, under the guidance of a professor from Shanghai's First Medical College. The county also established a county-wide "health council" in 1952, with 549 members, that extended consciousness about public health to the wider population.[63] In the same time frame, Shanghai trained grassroots health workers to do the unskilled labor and baseline mobilization needed to make the snail fever campaign effective. By 1956, Shanghai had enough trained educated youth that it could dispatch twenty thousand of them on snail surveying and elimination missions. Shanghai also mandated that every five to ten households select one grassroots health worker to receive twenty hours of classes. Once trained, these individuals monitored neighbors for appropriate sanitation practices, provided basic training for family units, and selected and trained three to five "activists" to help build the campaign. This suggests that Shanghai's system was able to spread new health ideas beyond designated personnel to the broader village community. Training of locals as grassroots workers continued throughout the Shanghai and Qingpu campaigns.[64]

Both Shanghai and Qingpu developed a pyramidal structure comprised of three levels of campaign and health personnel: a large number of educated youth acting as grassroots workers at the bottom; Chinese medicine doctors and nurses with additional training in the middle; and a small number of doctors trained in Western medicine, from hospitals, at the top. An obvious advantage to this system was that because educated youth handled mobilization and other baseline campaign work, middle-tier medical providers spent most of their time providing clinical care, and top-tier providers could focus on clinical supervision and guidance.[65] However, there was another critical advantage. Bottom-level campaign workers, who were trained at very little expense in simple scientific education and quantification tools, were village inhabitants. Thus, they provided a constant local voice to promote and organize the campaign. Peer education not only was much more effective than instruction by occasional outsiders (see chapter 4) but also seemed less intrusive than the state's forcing people to engage in a strange campaign. Together, these factors contributed significantly to campaign success.

In some areas of Shanghai and Qingpu, educated youth's grasp of scientific tools was strong enough that they were able to insert the snail fever work into annual agricultural production plans. The government hoped that when leaders fit health work into production plans, they would be encouraged to discover the campaign's requirements and some basic methods for doing the work. In addition, through this planning process, the government imagined that large blocks of apparently impossible work would be cut into smaller pieces that seemed more feasible. Planning also pinned accountability for work on particular individuals or departments and often made them responsible for obtaining funding, labor, and materials. As a 1956 Shanghai snail fever work plan advised lower-level units: "Make plans with separate parts where you can hand out pieces to people who will be responsible for working on them until they are done. This has the advantage that it's easy to check on the work and it will mobilize the masses to be more enthusiastic."[66] Once leaders figured out how to assign work to individuals, they were able to enforce compliance by connecting it to work points, the salary unit in collective life. According to a 1956 account from Qingpu's Chengbei Township, a national test site where the campaign was part of production plans, each production brigade was told it could not earn all its work points unless it killed a certain number of snails every day (an amount that varied by region). Each lower-level production team doled out kill counts to individuals who had to exterminate their snail quota if they wanted their salary.[67] Chengbei personnel reported that this was a very successful way to meet campaign goals.

This optimistic strategy of government control for the snail fever campaign failed almost everywhere else during the 1950s. Annual directives produced by the national and provincial campaign headquarters are filled with repeated injunctions to integrate snail fever into local production work plans; and local snail fever reports on work accomplished are filled with plaints and excuses for why snail fever was in fact never included.[68] Lack of compliance partially reflected the conundrum embodied in this strategy. It was impossible for cadres to make plans that would simultaneously teach them plan making. Until local cadres mastered the tools of scientific management, making campaign plans and including them in broader community work plans was unlikely to happen, explaining why it was hard to gain accountability for campaign work during the 1950s.

By the 1960s, Shanghai and Qingpu's many educated youth were able to form special teams with greater technical skills, replacing mass mobilization efforts when locals were disinclined to go snail hunting. As one retrospective account remarked, "The best way to counteract this [resistance leading to poor-quality work] is to give education emphasizing quality and to get a special team to do the work."[69] When the Party's political capital was low after the 1959–61 famine, and the "masses" refused to do the work, places with educated youth could entirely avoid confrontation by delegating all the campaign work to them.

This early trained talent became the building blocks for Shanghai's pioneering role in national public health. In 1965, Shanghai revved up for the next political convulsion, the Cultural Revolution, by rapidly training forty-five hundred paramedics, mainly drawn from the original thirty-nine hundred grassroots health workers educated during the Great Leap Forward. These paramedics became the prototype for barefoot doctors, allowing Shanghai to field barefoot doctors five years earlier than most other areas. These barefoot doctors trained twenty-nine thousand health workers, vastly expanding Shanghai's capacity to do medical work. During the Cultural Revolution, when many professionals were no longer allowed to guide the snail fever campaign, educated youth had assimilated enough of a scientific worldview and had gained sufficient technical and treatment skills to plan and direct the work, albeit with quiet direction from disgraced, sent-down physicians.[70]

By the Cultural Revolution, mass school building had changed the landscape in many more typical rural places. Schooling created a body of educated youth who had mastered the basic tools of scientific management by serving an unofficial apprenticeship in the special teams that were part of scientifically oriented campaigns. Concerted attacks on the old guard during the Cultural Revolution allowed educated youth to take leadership roles, in which they could alter work processes without much opposition from superiors. They learned how to assess the location and sometimes the density of snails and to report their findings as statistics, charts, and graphs. With the help of scientific tools, people like Mao Zhixiao, a newly trained barefoot doctor in rural Jiangxi Province, were able to plan mass campaigns: "We drew up maps of the affected area that included over two hundred ponds and ditches. . . . Every day I marked on the map what was needed, how many people, and how much time. Based on the map, I'd assign the cadres to lead their teams."[71] When Joshua Horn, an English

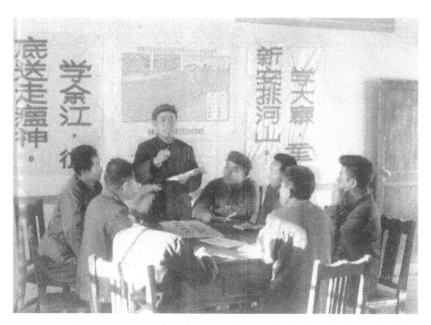

FIGURE 15. Campaign personnel used maps and set standards from books to plan their attack on the snails. Zhonggong zhongyang nanfang shisan sheng, shi, qu xuefang lingdao xiaozu bangongshi, *Song wenshen: Huace* (Beijing: Zhonggong zhongyang nanfang shisan sheng, shi, qu xuefang lingdao xiaozu bangongshi 1978), 59.

doctor, visited a snail fever prevention station in the late 1960s, he noticed that the walls were covered with maps and charts and that personnel made use of both books and ledgers (see figure 15). By the Cultural Revolution, scientific tools had been integrated into the work process and were used to great effect.[72]

This transformation is also validated by the content of bottom-level campaign reports, which were strikingly different during the Cultural Revolution than the Great Leap. The new reports included more "precise" numbers, for example, 52.37 percent instead of 52 percent. The use of some simple forms or cards resulted in data's having an increasingly standardized presentation. Rather than simple bar graphs, charts and graphs of all types proliferated. Finally, the new reports contained an unbelievable quantity of numbers and statistics, to the point where words sometimes disappeared entirely. While some of these changes were due to the dangers of honestly reporting any problems and the need to explicitly portray grassroots work as scientific, and thus revolutionary, they were also due to educated youth's use of scientific tools carried to its logical extreme.

SCIENTIFIC TOOLS INTERTWINED WITH PUBLIC
PRESENTATIONS: A NEW CONSOLIDATION METHOD

Teaching and disseminating scientific tools generated sufficient personnel to perform basic technical and medical work and enabled effective planning and organization of complex campaigns. However, scientific tools alone were not sufficient to spread a campaign to reluctant regions. To create pressure and transparency, the Party introduced "public presentations." Combining public presentations at meetings and model sites with scientific tools was an extremely effective mechanism for government control of the hinterland. Scientific tools delineated every step of the work process, while scientific performances combined with public presentations forced cadres to be transparent about their methods in addition to their accomplishments. Peer pressure, possible loss of face in front of superiors, and concerns about appearing "backward" by failing to meet new statistically based achievements that had become neighborhood norms all added impetus to campaign work. Those who reluctantly complied were rewarded by recognition from superiors and the media, extra resources, and possible career advancement. As a result, many rural cadres decided that even unpopular campaigns were an unfortunate necessity.

At mandatory meetings, local leaders submitted and presented work reports to peers and superiors. This was a powerful method of ensuring both compliance and consistency, especially when campaign requirements and methods were codified as statistics, graphs, and maps. Local cadres were pushed to gather data lest they look incompetent in front of their number-wielding peers. Even though statistics were likely exaggerated, they gave the campaign concrete benchmarks with clearly defined work processes. Realizing the efficacy of meeting reports, the 1955 Shanghai three-year plan increased the required number of reports of work progress for units lower in the political structure, which were reluctant to spend scarce resources on the campaign. Whereas each district "concretely reported progress and problems" at monthly meetings and sent reports twice monthly to the city's seven-person leadership small group, township-level areas were mandated to meet and provide reports every week. Places with high illiteracy in the 1950s, like Yujiang, could not depend on a strategy that required writing, but they did have meetings to encourage leaders to do work and share successful strategies. In 1956, the Yujiang County's five-person LSG was required to hold a meeting once a month and to report at half-monthly intervals to the county committee. Yujiang also held eleven snail fever meetings in 1956 and six in 1957 to solve concrete problems. The county secretary presided at important meetings so that local cadres had to report to their principal superior.[73]

The snail fever campaign was especially effective in using national meetings to promote local compliance. Because of high-level sponsorship, snail fever was one of the only diseases with annual national conferences. The need to report on one's work in front of large groups of peers and high-level superiors goaded people into having numerical accomplishments to report. The message and spirit of such meetings were eventually conveyed to the grassroots via a meeting ripple effect. Attendees at the national meeting held provincial meetings; provincial "bigwigs" then held prefecture-level meetings, and then county and finally township meetings disseminated the spirit down to the grassroots. The ripple of meetings and critique prompted renewed short-term intense campaign activity, producing more reportable data. Even if the snail fever campaign drifted into malaise, it was forcibly brought to the forefront of local agendas at least once a year.[74]

Model test sites were the second core persuasion strategy. This approach, combined acquisition of scientific tools with public presentations, which were made more potent because they demonstrated dedication to the revolutionary cause. According to Gordon Bennett, model test sites, or "key points," were selected for mass mobilization campaigns because they represented desired outcomes and could be used to train personnel in their "advanced" methods. Once trained, visiting personnel and cadres were supposed to return home and establish their own key points or model sites. This was called *yidiandaimian,* or "expanding the point to the plane."[75] Chairman Mao mapped out this strategy in his 1958 paper, "Sixty Points on Working Methods," saying that "leadership . . . [should] organize tours for cadres and the masses to see and learn from advanced experience." By "compare[ing] the advanced with the backward under identical conditions," "the backward" will be encouraged "to catch up with the advanced." The result would be a cycle that endlessly "evolves from disequilibrium, to equilibrium and then to disequilibrium again," wrote Mao. "Each cycle, however, brings us to a higher level of development." By visiting test sites, cadres would "raise the technological level, popularize advanced experience and encourage competition."[76] The snail fever campaign used this approach widely, creating a hierarchical network of tests sites at the provincial, county, district, township, and commune levels. Each new model served as a dissemination point of methods based on scientific tools for lower-level cadres and could also be used to signal new campaign directions. By the end of 1963, Jiangxi had launched 321 test sites.[77]

Test sites ensured grassroots compliance in many ways. Visiting model sites communicated "the rules and requirements and the stages involved" and was an invaluable way to teach cadres how to wield scientific tools to accomplish campaign work. Bottom-level reports noted that "those who did not go [to model test sites] are much worse in night soil management and in snail elimination."[78] On the flip side, test sites motivated participation by reluctant cadres, who lost face and political merit if they remained less technologically savvy than peers who worked under similar conditions. Being labeled backward, apathetic, or even a rightist in a revolutionary era was not a good career move. Some of the most resistant places were purposely selected as bottom-level "models" in their region. For example, when the nominal efforts of Jiangdu County in Jiangsu Province stopped entirely during the famine and had not restarted by March 1963, the county was designated as a special area and a model test site. Since proving model status depended on presenting achievements to peers and superiors on-site, the eyes of the Party and peers were brought directly to the county's fields. Frequent visitors made residual snails and ill people hard to hide. Model status compelled the community and its leadership to accept the campaign as a main responsibility and to dedicate resources accordingly. Forcing places to assume test site status was recognized as such a good way to deal with intractable local leaders that a 1957 report from Jiangsu advised, "Places that haven't done any feces management yet should all create a test site."[79]

Model test sites performed another significant function: the reintroduction of quality control. During the Great Leap Forward and Cultural Revolution, most of the scientific and technical establishments and bureaucratic and management structures that ensured quality control were eliminated. Once watchdog agencies were purged, local leaders had every reason to neglect quality in favor of speed, a tendency bolstered by the competitive element in mass mobilization campaigns. Model test sites, where scientific performances were at their peak, were very good at counteracting this inclination by making adherence to standards and statistical benchmarks the new goal of competition. By dissecting the snail fever work with statistics, combined with scientific tools, it was possible to numerically compare each stage or specific work process and campaign achievement. The more cross-visiting that occurred, the more the model sites helped to regularize work standards and methods regionally. Once higher regional norms with a statistical basis were established, leaders looked incompetent unless they made some effort to do campaign work (see table 5).

TABLE 5 Newspaper report publicizing each Qingpu township's snail fever survey and treatment progress, July 24–26, 1958

	Numbers Tested				Numbers Treated			
	Total population	Stool samples tested, July 24–26	Accumulated number of tested people	% of population	Approximate number of patients	Cured people, July 24–26	Accumulated number of treated people	% of sick population
Whole county	288,723	9,070	186,665	64.65	105,659	8,916	40,646	39.51
Xujing	13,139	309	11,002	83.73	7,995	88	1,382	17.28
Beisong	13,240	801	11,013	83.80	6,712	396	2,070	30.84
Pingdang	10,130	763	9,184	90.66	6,448	748	2,831	43.91
Chonggu	20,574	214	16,899	82.13	10,209		1,669	17.94
Guanyin	20,168		15,606	77.38	11,611	746	3,161	27.17
Baihe	20,374		14,986	73.55	8,687	530	3,925	45.18
Xinqiao	14,330		13,445	93.82	8,210		7,863	95.70
Zhaotun	14,060	2,000	12,637	89.88	7,007	2,666	5,827	83.16
Huancheng	16,857		11,562	69.81	10,585	743	3,125	29.42
Yelong	13,908	2,042	12,767	90.18	8,106	486	1,870	23.06
Shengang	15,664		6,516	41.84	3,202	210	530	16.55
Maodang	10,264				385		19	4.93
Zhengdian	8,962				129		28	21.70
Xiaozheng	9,572				92		2	2.17
Jinze	9,942	545	6,097	61.32	4,174	625	942	22.56
Xicen	8,016	810	6,423	80.12	1,141	422	1,010	87.64
Dasheng	8,547		5,041	58.97	3,508	260	1,045	29.79

Xiangta	9,188	569	9,970	108.51	3,473	455	1,247	35.90
Chengxiang	20,884	897	12,837	61.47	2,266	453	1,752	77.31
Liantang	11,729		3,374	28.76	120		14	11.66
Zhujiajiao	7,175	120	7,306	101.82	1,599	88	334	20.9
Shagang								

SOURCE: Reprinted from "Ge xiang xuexichongbing pujian zhiliao jinbubiao," *Qingpu bao*, no. 205, August 2, 1958, 3, translated by Miriam Gross.

NOTES: Township-level charts comparing testing and treatment accomplishments that were published in newspapers increased transparency and set regional norms during the Great Leap Forward and Cultural Revolution. Data here are verbatim from the Qingpu newspaper. Blank cells indicate no data. When newspapers published mass campaign numbers, townships such as Shagang that did not participate were left blank. This illuminated their lack of participation, making them lose face in front of the whole county.

Increasingly, specific benchmarks garnered from scientific tools allowed units higher in the government hierarchy to ensure compliance from afar even without model sites. In 1958, Jiangsu Province linked up "city with city, prefecture with prefecture, and county with county." Each pair or group was supposed to "sign agreements and launch friendly socialist competitions." Such agreements incorporated new statistically based yardsticks and mutual visiting, making it harder to hide inadequate campaign work. When educated youth were available during the 1960s in Yujiang, production teams had to assess themselves and compare feces management work to others every month, using three evaluative criteria.[80] Once differences between areas were numerically codified, "competitions" were sometimes institutionalized. When Shanghai was unable to motivate the contagious counties around Qingpu to be equally avid, it established a formal county-based group so that errant leaders could frequently visit Qingpu. The group "held meetings at fixed times" and was supposed to do "united work," to "mutually verify" each other's survey results and to "spur each other on" by great achievements. As a result of this tactic, "most of the lagging counties caught up."[81]

CONCLUSION

Most studies of modern Chinese history, sociology, and political science reach a strong consensus that the height of human organization occurred during Mao's revolutionary peaks and that rational technical bureaucracy only reappeared during the Reform era. Instead, this work finds that during revolutionary peaks, at the same time that professional bureaucracies and scientific establishments were attacked, the technical skills of bottom-level cadres were strengthened so that they could effectively organize complex mass mobilization campaigns. This duality reflects Chairman Mao's belief that scientific management was essential for grassroots strategic planning and that it was practical grassroots science that would help China make a great leap toward scientific socialism.

Despite Mao's dreams, rural youth educated at a middle-school level were usually incapable of higher-order science or replacing professional doctors. However, by participating in specialized teams in scientifically oriented campaigns, many educated youth changed their view of nature from something integral to themselves to an externalized object that could be manipulated and experimented on for human benefit. By the Cultural Revolution, educated youth had mastered scientific tools and other technical skills, giving them the ability to develop complex community-wide plans in domains that would otherwise have remained inaccessible. At the same time, scientific performances supplied leaders with a stepping-stone to career advancement and made quality, rather than quantity, the goal of campaign work. This more scientific worldview led educated youth to sustain some scientific processes, ideas, and goals despite revolutionary pressure. Once large groups of educated youth took over education, health monitoring, mobilization, organization, supervision, and bottom-level technical and medical work, the limited pool of sent-down doctors could focus their attention on treatment and training and acting as preceptors for the educated youth who had become barefoot doctors.

The importance of disseminating scientific knowledge and tools went beyond any particular health campaign. This study suggests they were a crucial mechanism for legitimating the CCP's leading role and framing its subjective policy choices as stemming from objective scientific processes. Scientific tools also helped the Party control the new group of rural leaders and make its will manifest at the grassroots level during a time of decentralization. Although such tools gave new leaders unprecedented power to transform society, they also acted to constrain behavior along lines that both matched Party goals and mandated campaign processes. Over the course of campaigns, exactly which statistics had to be collected were codified, which helped delineate the entire planning process. The creation of statistically based universal standards and the public exhibition of numerical accomplishments made it clear that scientific tools had to be used to effectively carry out this campaign. Numerically based standards could be easily evaluated by higher-level cadres and made it challenging to fill reports with equivocal narrative descriptions of accomplishments. The more that local leaders gathered predetermined categories of numerical information, manipulated them to get required standardized results, and publicly presented them in meeting reports or test sites to number-wielding colleagues and superiors, the less space they had to find their own way of doing the campaign, or to not do the campaign at all. The overwhelming leadership of educated youth who had fully assimilated scientific tools and planning processes is one reason the campaign during the Cultural Revolution was such a clear success. Wielding scientific tools publicly not only encouraged uninterested leaders to fulfill campaign goals but also channeled them into the mandated processes laid out by campaign leaders, without the Party having to employ either bureaucratic oversight or overt force.

Today, scientific tools combined with frequent reports of statistical accomplishments are still helping the Party maintain control in a system of fragmented authoritarianism. "The Numbers Game," a recent article in *Science,* explains that numbers may make leaders *(shuzi chuguan),* since that is the major way that people's performance is still judged, but "outright cooking of the books is rare." Because data must be reported monthly or annually, Yong Cai, a demographer at the University of North Carolina, Chapel Hill, explains in the article that "it's very difficult to fake something in a systematic way without being caught."[82] Scientific consolidation via frequent, publicly presented statistics from cadres wielding scientific tools is a Maoist legacy that is still going strong.

Conclusion

FEW HEALTH CAMPAIGNS ARE AS famous in China as Chairman Mao's war against snail fever. This health campaign joined others to cause a profound change in human life over the Maoist era: from 1952 to 1982, the average life expectancy increased from thirty-five to sixty-eight years; infant mortality decreased from 250 to 40 deaths per 1,000 live births; and the overall population increased from 582 million in 1953 to over a billion in 1982. By 1981, close to 95 percent of the people and many of the cattle infected with snail fever had been successfully treated. This and other Patriotic Public Health Campaigns reshaped village sanitation by building more than sixty-five million public latrines and digging innumerable wells. Finally, these campaigns introduced key public health and personal hygiene practices, developed a core group of grassroots health workers, and began a conceptual shift in the way people viewed nature and disease.[1]

These fairly credible statistics, collected before and after the statistical inflationism characteristic of the Maoist era, document impressive accomplishments, mainly in rural areas, where most people lived. So striking were these achievements that the Maoist primary health-care model was disseminated around the world—in the 1978 World Health Organization Declaration on Primary Health Care at Alma-Ata—as a potential solution to health care in poor developing countries. The defining characteristics of the disseminated Maoist model were committed local leadership that effectively utilized rural resources and strengths; mass health education that led to broad popular participation and local innovation; a multitude of grassroots health workers, such as barefoot doctors; and a focus on affordable, low-tech prevention activities rather than expensive treatment. This model was touted as a bottom-up campaign with limited involvement of or need for experts, costly state inputs, or extensive national guidance.

Despite its renown, the snail fever campaign, and more broadly the Maoist primary health-care model, has undergone a creative reconstruction from the very start, such that its true challenges, accomplishments, and methods have been lost to memory.[2] While some of the reasons for success appear to have been unknown, others were purposefully obfuscated to uphold ideological underpinnings. For a campaign that symbolized patriotic participation under wise Party guidance, it was not helpful to document either significant resistance among grassroots cadres and villagers or a notable lack of cadre leadership. Similarly, in a campaign famous for bringing uplift through scientific education, it was problematic to realize that the campaign transmitted few educational messages and that the Party's pedagogical strategies made this problem worse. Finally, for a campaign representing the ultimate example of local innovation and self-reliance, it was not useful to acknowledge that most of the key techniques came from foreigners, that local inventions often undermined the campaign, and that the inability of the impoverished government to fund its own mandates often made campaign work impossible.

Unlike the ideologically correct Maoist medical model that was circulated around the world, archives show that the actual Maoist model was very effective and resilient enough that it not only overcame rural scarcity and resistance, but also compensated for problematic government campaign choices. The model had four components: persuasion and coercion of both the leaders and the participants, extensive government inputs, local knowledge and administration, and mass effort. Below, I first summarize why this model was so effective at overcoming the impediments to rural medical work, and then I discuss how the long-term government commitment to fighting the disease worked together with the model to achieve success.

Despite propagandistic representations of enthusiastic involvement, few local leaders and villagers wanted to participate long-term in this campaign or to learn why prevention activities were necessary. Thus, a combination of ideologically based persuasion and structurally oriented coercion was necessary. Belief in Mao and Maoism, patriotism, and a sense of revolutionary progress all motivated engagement even when interest and understanding of health campaigns were lacking. Instead of directly compelling people, successful campaigns structurally embedded coercion so that people found themselves participating. To co-opt leaders, the campaign relied on leadership small groups, mandatory meetings, reports, and site visits that successfully transferred responsibility, encouraged quality control, and moved campaign work into the unavoidable category of politics. To co-opt participants, the campaign exploited collectives, which assigned campaign work as a regular job, and militaristic campaign structures premised on discipline, obedience, and the sense that the work was part of a greater battle for survival. Other campaigns also used the household responsibility system and neighborhood committees, all of which ensured that surveillance and participation were not a choice.

These health campaigns could not function without extensive government inputs of money, knowledge, and transfer of skills, despite constant references to self-reliance. Therefore, campaigns flourished when treatment was fully subsidized and money was provided for doctors, drugs, equipment, and new medical institutions, and they waned when these necessities were not provided. Thus, when funding was focused on a specific disease, the campaign had a much better chance of success. National funding also signaled to lower-level political leaders that local financing had become a political necessity and that depending solely on health department resources was not wise. The result was a monetary multiplying effect, with lower-level units up and down the hierarchy providing additional resources. Likewise, the transfer of urban doctors and other medical personnel to the countryside provided an extensive knowledge subsidy for rural areas that lacked the expertise necessary for effective treatment. Since treatment, rather than prevention combined with education, tended to be the actual key to success, such high-level medical knowledge was particularly essential. Finally, the key campaign role played by rural people would not have been possible without the medical, technical, and administrative training supplied by medical personnel transferred from the cities.

Local knowledge, administration, and mobilization were essential to these health campaigns. Local herbalists, Chinese medicine doctors, and barefoot doctors were incorporated as an inexpensive medical corps who, once trained in effective treatment strategies, provided nursing and medical support services. This enabled experts to wield their skills to greatest effect while still utilizing the medical knowledge of local medical providers. Educated youth were also harnessed to provide cheap administrative and mobilizing capacity and local knowledge of terrain, people, and resources. This was possible because of the skills these educated youth acquired participating in special groups in scientific campaigns. Local input was crucial to help modify standardized campaigns to local conditions and to supply local labor and resources, because government funding was never enough.

Finally, mass effort, usually trumpeted as critical because it focused on prevention and facilitated rural buy-in and uplift, was helpful, but not for these reasons. Instead, mass effort acted as another coercive strategy, making individual resistance stand out and prompting nominal compliance. Mass work was also massively redundant, partially compensating for the lack of records and quality control in these broad-scale campaigns.

In addition to helping pioneer the Maoist medical model, the snail fever campaign was striking because support by top CCP leaders rarely wavered and their interest was greatest in areas of the highest endemic disease among the hardest to reach populations. Although the first decade or more of many Maoist health campaigns, excluding vaccination work, demonstrated few obvious achievements and frequent loss of scarce resources and human capital, Chairman Mao decided to keep trying. On the face of it, this was a surprisingly unrealistic choice in an era with limited latitude for failure. Yet this tenacity ultimately allowed these campaigns to succeed

What accounts for Mao's persistence? One part of the answer seems to lie in the many nonhealth benefits of health campaigns, which predated improvements in public health. Most benefits seem intimately linked to these campaigns' stature as grassroots or mass science campaigns. Data from this work demonstrate that grassroots science played a core role in three ways: it legitimated the state's authority; it was a mechanism for rural empowerment, albeit not one desired by most rural people; and it was a new way to control the countryside, which I term "scientific consolidation." Together these elements helped the Party reconstruct its vast hinterland and maintain hegemony in a decentralized era. These benefits to the Party ended up unintentionally buttressing failing health campaigns and gradually building the skills rural people needed to make them successful.

Grassroots scientific campaigns had great ideological potential because they helped the Party counter the power of international science and traditional society. By establishing grassroots science as genuine science in public discourse, the Party was able to attack professional scientists while simultaneously claiming that scientific authority underlay its capricious policy choices. Similarly, grassroots science campaigns could attack traditional society by justifying the obliteration of traditional holidays, temples, and burial mounds and by helping move people into advanced producers' cooperatives. When rural people resisted this assault on traditional practices, the CCP claimed that its rationales and methods stemmed from grassroots science and thus natural law.

Grassroots science campaigns were also used to empower people by altering their relationship to the natural world and, even more fundamentally, to their bodies. By pushing people to reconstruct the topography into mass-producing farms, the Party directly countered beliefs about the dangers of disturbing local feng shui (environmental geomancy). Similarly, by ignoring villagers' own assessment of their well-being and forcing treatment, the Party would supposedly empower villagers with the reality of their own healthy bodies. In actuality, by nominally basing land reconstruction decisions on science and disease assessment on microbes, the Party had a scientific rationale to ignore villagers' own understandings, eroding one of rural people's few areas of power. Together, these changes solidified state control, maximizing Party power over labor, production, and humans' relationship to the land, an essential move for a planned economy.

Finally, scientifically oriented campaigns enabled scientific consolidation, a novel mechanism for achieving and maintaining Party control in a decentralized era. Prior research has described the Maoist era as employing a human bureaucracy. This study finds that elements of technical bureaucracy along with grassroots science were disseminated to rural cadres, even as professional bureaucratic and scientific establishments were assaulted. By the mid-1960s, rural educated youth—the next generation of leaders—learned scientific tools, including basic statistics, mapping, modeling, standardization, and simple comparisons of work processes, termed "experiments," due to a decade and a half of school building and serving on special teams for scientific campaigns. These tools, which also underpin scientific planning and bureaucracy, enabled youth to organize mass campaigns, demonstrating their skills and strengthening their bid to obtain future leadership positions. However, the more these new leaders collected statistics delineating pieces of a campaign's work, the more difficult it was to avoid the goals and work process laid out by the Party. As it became mandatory to report work in written and oral forms and to mutually visit campaign sites to observe work in situ, rural cadres were forced into a previously unknown degree of transparency. These new skills, which made red youth expert to a limited degree, help explain how the Party was able to carry out complex mass campaigns in a decentralized era without the use of force. They also clarify how leadership, and organizational and scientific improvements on the ground, increased health campaign efficacy, despite employing treatment and prevention strategies that had failed to work earlier. These attributes explain why the snail fever campaign succeeded and why the Maoist medical model worked in environments of extreme scarcity, limited prior local knowledge, and negligible local commitment.

Next, I place this campaign in historical perspective. First, I compare the snail fever campaign to the contemporaneous global malaria campaign run by the World Health Organization. I find that the idiosyncratic choices in the Maoist campaign also characterized those of the malaria campaign, but that the malaria campaign lacked the components that made the Maoist health model successful. Then, I explore why the famous, politically sensitive snail fever campaign managed to fail during the Reform era (1976–present), coming to the conclusion that failure occurred mainly because the campaign lacked the Maoist medical model. I end by showing that a rejuvenated Maoist medical model led to the success of the 2003 campaign against SARS.

SNAIL FEVER VERSUS MALARIA: A STUDY OF MUTUAL FOLLY

Although the Maoist-era snail fever campaign was ultimately a great success, I have documented in this work that the government's views were so problematic that they almost caused the collapse of the campaign. Interestingly, global campaigns by the World Health Organization (WHO) during the same post–World War II period exhibited some of the same problems as the snail fever campaign, though not to such an extreme extent. Here, I document the eerie similarities between Mao's campaign against snail fever and the WHO's global campaign against malaria, another endemic disease. The malaria campaign was started in 1955 with American funding, revitalized in 1998, and reconstituted a third time in 2007 by the Gates Foundation.[3]

Maoist health campaign goals were based on economic and ideological rather than scientific rationales. Thus the CCP's primary motivations were increased productivity and a socialist consciousness. Similarly, the goal of the international malaria campaign during and after the Cold War was to augment rural productivity in order to fight the spread of Communism and to provide a ready market for American goods.[4] Like the Chinese campaign, this would ideally "change the overall social-psychological attitude [of rural people] to one more conducive to 'progress,'" where progress and capitalism were viewed as interchangeable, just as the Chinese equated progress and Communism.[5] The assumption that eradicating a single disease would provide a magic bullet for economic advancement and cure both an entire range of rural ills and profound social and structural inequities was characteristic of both campaigns. Both the CCP and the Americans used this propaganda to position themselves as liberators and "outside experts" who wielded technological solutions that tended to place rural populations and developing countries "in a position of dependence and in need of guidance and assistance."[6]

Mao's belief in the masses, and his need for plans suitable for large-scale mass effort, led campaign leaders to seize upon the overly simplistic goal of totally eradicating, rather than controlling, an endemic disease on a bizarre seven-year time table. Likewise, the malaria campaign, propelled by the creation of DDT and funding from the United States and the WHO, persuaded itself that it could eliminate the world's mosquito population. When this, like Maoist kill campaigns against various insects, proved impossible, eradication of global malaria became the goal. Worried about increased mosquito resistance to DDT, campaign advisers urgently pointed out that "time is of the essence" and put the campaign on an eight-year schedule, with four to six years years of spraying.[7] The beauty of this idea was that malaria, which has been described by experts as a "thousand different diseases and epidemiological puzzles," could now be eliminated simply by spraying a single substance everywhere.[8]

This one-size-fits-all solution made the effort simple to plan, but almost impossible to implement because, like the snail fever campaign, it ignored impoverished grassroots realities, ill-trained rural personnel, local administrative incapacity, and the complex ecology of both the disease and its vector.[9] It also ignored sociocultural differences—rural people were thought to live in "timeless communities" that were essentially identical. In strategies reminiscent of the snail fever campaign, experts snubbed local knowledge about disease, believing that villagers ignorant of Western disease concepts could not make a contribution. Local scientists were demoted to "native informants" who only provided information about "local fauna and flora" and not control strategies.[10] In the CCP campaign, rural people were placed in the roles of both timeless backward villagers and native informants who could identify local herbs. While the Chinese government gestured at incorporating indigenous know-how, in fact it jettisoned the complexity of local knowledge because it assumed that all rural expertise would be simple common sense. Similarly, grassroots scientific performances nominally adapted campaign practice to local circumstances while in fact legitimating the national campaign headquarters' conducting an identical campaign everywhere.

Finally, attachment to ideology and one-size-fits-all solutions led both Mao and the malaria campaign to sideline experts who disagreed with them. Once "a solution was sought in oversimplification and standardization," the global malaria campaign leaders, like Chairman Mao, began to purposefully ignore the scientific consensus that the campaign was impossible.[11] Malariologists pointed out that extraordinarily rapid development of DDT resistance by mosquitoes, facilitated by mass agricultural spraying as part of the Green Revolution, not only doomed the campaign, but also made it very questionable as a public health intervention. Like snail fever, low-level malaria infection helps prevent acute disease. Experts worried that if treatment removed this protection while ineffective prevention work left behind a highly infectious environment, the campaign could actually trigger worse malaria epidemics. Unfortunately, just like the similar snail fever epidemic created during the Great Leap Forward, these concerns turned out to be prescient—the result of the antimalaria campaign has been unprecedented global epidemics of malaria.[12]

Leaders of the malaria campaign were so certain of their technological solutions that they not only ignored but also attacked experts, resisting experimental work that might have challenged campaign leaders' conclusions. Directors of the global campaign suggested launching the campaign "without awaiting the outcome of further experiments."[13] Later, in this and other campaigns using DDT, promoters suggested that "basic research" was of "no immediate value."[14] When scientists proposed establishing study sites to see if campaign treatment and prevention strategies were affordable and whether they would actually work, they were accused of being "conservative" and "defeatist" and even immoral because they did not want to "save the lives of native children."[15] Similarly, the CCP excluded and denigrated scientists who insisted on legitimate basic research by claiming they did not care about the masses.

The malaria campaign propaganda strategies that resulted from this antiscientific stance were also remarkably similar to those of the CCP. Like the Chinese government, malaria campaign leaders hid scientific disagreements so that local governments would "only find clear statements and nothing whatever which would deter them from taking action."[16] The WHO and the U.S. government replaced stringent science with mass enthusiasm, in turn built by transforming the health campaign into a patriotic military engagement against domestic enemies (i.e., insects) that was a continuation of the international war (i.e., World War II) that had just been won. DDT was called the "atomic bomb of the insect world."[17] Just as the CCP's kill campaigns dressed up bugs, pathogens, and rats in the olive drab of American soldiers, U.S. posters promoting war against various insect vectors pictured the pests with Italian, Japanese, and German heads. Like the CCP, the U.S. and WHO became so caught up in their own rhetoric that they tended to develop insect eradication strategies more suited for battles against humans than bugs. This oratory also reinforced the human "position of dominance" in relation to the natural world.[18]

Once the malaria campaign was painted as a war of eradication, the logical correlate was that when the battle was over, the disease would be gone. The U.S. government and later, global donors divvied up the extensive funding and support necessary for eliminating the disease. When the international community, like lower-level Chinese authorities (but unlike the national Chinese government), realized that the campaign was based on false premises and required unlimited long-term funding, most global funding came to an abrupt stop and enthusiasm for campaign work diminished precipitously.[19] The peaks and valleys of the malaria campaign, like those of the snail fever campaign, undercut disease control and efforts to educate and alter hygiene and sanitation patterns.

A final, regrettable similarity between the campaigns was their refusal to learn from mistakes despite decades of time and multiple campaign peaks. The Maoist campaign kept hammering away using the same unworkable prevention techniques aimed at complete eradication of a vector that was impossible to eliminate. Likewise, the 1998 incarnation of the malaria campaign decided that the simple, standardized solution of treated bed nets would solve the global problem, even as scientists pointed out that many mosquitoes bite in the early evening, anthropologists discovered that some of the alternative ways that local people used the nets undermined their purpose as mosquito protection, journalists reported on the nets' use to catch fish, and rural poverty ensured that most people could not afford nets.[20] The Gates Foundation's 2007 version of the malaria campaign is apparently following the time-honored strategy of "stifling a diversity of views among scientists," while taking a "vested interest . . . [in] seeing the data it helped generate taken to policy."[21] In other words, the current campaign is still caught up in its own ideological correctness at the expense of complex grassroots realities and impartial scientific conclusions. The campaign is still looking for simple, unvarying solutions to complex real-world problems that make funding easy and success scarce.

This point-by-point comparison of the roughly contemporaneous malaria and snail fever campaigns reveals their surprising similarities. It is tempting to blame the skewed policies and goals of the snail fever campaign entirely on overwrought ideology, Maoist excesses, or even Communist governance. Instead, it appears that vertically oriented, top-down health campaigns that disseminate the science and technology of developed countries or urban elites to the hinterland often embody the same fallacies, whether they are conducted by Mao or by the WHO. Where these campaigns differed was in the long-term engagement of Mao's government and in the Maoist medical model. The "global" campaign dropped sub-Saharan Africa, the place with the highest burden of malaria, when things there seemed difficult.[22] Likewise, when resistance to DDT and other problems caused the malaria campaign to fail, global funding diminished until new technological strategies were developed. In contrast, the Chinese government persevered despite more than a decade of comparative failure and became more dedicated to reaching the most challenging populations, not less. This, buttressed by the Maoist medical model, which intermingled extensive government resources with shrewd strategies to motivate local compliance and participation, successfully compensated for many of the problems that haunt elite-run, vertically oriented campaigns.

THE REFORM-ERA CAMPAIGN

Efforts to prevent snail fever and improve rural health did not fare well during the Reform period (1976–present), primarily because they lacked the motivating force of the Maoist medical model. When the government moved toward a free-market system, it dismantled communes, the primary funding source for rural health, and reoriented its goals toward coastal industrial development. As a result, funding, personnel, and top-down pressure on localities to prioritize health all diminished dramatically. As medical care became a patient responsibility, rural people increasingly found health care unaffordable; rural doctors focused on money-making drug prescriptions, rather than primary health care; and unprofitable prevention activities were mostly phased out.[23]

Luckily for the snail fever campaign, major technical advances partially counteracted these larger trends. Praziquantel, a new snail fever medicine developed by Bayer and Merck in Germany, was cheap, nontoxic, very effective, and entailed taking a pill for a day or two. This drug, widely available in China after 1980, allowed individuals to self-medicate and avoid the rapidly eroding rural medical system. Similar advances were made in treatment for cattle. The efficacy of the new medicine transformed the global disease protocol from one that disrupted snail transmission and gave some treatment to one that controlled morbidity by making treatment the primary target of campaign work.[24]

Unlike most places, China continued to make snail elimination a central part of its work in the 1980s and 1990s, perhaps because it was politically challenging to abandon the most important symbol of the campaign. More effective and affordable molluscicides, better snail elimination techniques, and the use of geographical information systems and remote sensing have improved snail eradication. The reassertion of professional expertise at all levels, the ability to disseminate and assimilate scientific knowledge, and better record keeping have also assisted the campaign.[25] However, the dearth of funding has decreased efficacy, particularly in poorer provinces. Thus, with only enough molluscicides and tractors in the late 1970s and 1980s to clear one-seventh of the snail-covered land each year, the infectious area in Jiangxi Province began growing again in the late 1980s.[26]

From 1992 to 2001, the World Bank administered a snail fever project that loaned China US$71 million on the condition that China supply matching funds, prompting a third campaign peak. This peak left more areas under control but did not eliminate the disease everywhere.[27] A few places, such as the area surrounding Jiangxi's Poyang Lake and stretches of the Yangtze River that are snail reservoirs, will probably never eradicate snail fever.

Since the government took sole responsibility for the campaign in 2001, there has been a dramatic increase in disease rates. Today there are close to a million people with the disease, with treatment costs in the many millions of yuan.[28] The explosion of cases includes not only areas where snail fever is endemic, but also places like Shanghai, where the disease had been eliminated. In addition to meager funding, the devastating flood of the Yangtze River in 1998, the Three Gorges Dam basin, and possibly global warming are creating new snail-infested areas without a corresponding degree of increased government support.[29]

The CCP was spurred to dedicate more funding and attention to the health-care system and reconsider the importance of public health because of its initial failings in the 2003 SARS campaign. Thus, in 2004, snail fever was again classified as one of China's most important communicable disease priorities. To signal serious intent, the government tried to resume its place as a global leader of snail fever eradication efforts. Chinese researchers unrolled a new "integrated strategy" for the world's consideration by publishing articles in late 2008 and 2009 in the *Lancet* and *New England Journal of Medicine,* among the world's highest-impact medical journals, and in a high-ranking journal in the field of parasitology, *Tropical Medicine and International Health.* Importantly, the integrated strategy included many of the attributes of the Maoist medical model that actually accounted for its success, while adding preventative strategies to the global focus on treatment, possibly because no campaign symbolizing Chairman Mao could do without them.[30] This new effort employed extensive government human and economic inputs, which appear to be the main factors leading to its notable success. Excellent testing, treatment, and surveillance systems by outside experts, and probable pressure on the community to participate, were also key factors in achieving a precipitous drop in infection rates.[31] In a September 7, 2010, national anti–snail fever meeting, China's vice premier, Li Keqiang, reaffirmed that preventing and controlling snail fever were crucial, signaling that government support and attention were still focused on the problem.[32] However, to effectively clear two villages, government researchers employing the new integrated strategy used over US$263,000 in direct government funding, US$150,000 in subsidies, and close to US$110,000 from villagers.[33] Thus far, the extensive economic and human resources needed to counteract the disease on a broad scale have not been forthcoming. Apparently, even this politically crucial campaign cannot flourish without a return to the Maoist medical model.

THE MAOIST MEDICAL MODEL REJUVENATED: THE CAMPAIGN AGAINST SARS

Most of the rural medical system built under Mao unraveled due to the privatization of health care starting around 1980. However, mass campaigns and the Maoist medical model are being revitalized in China today to deal with major health threats. The campaign against SARS (2002–3) exemplifies this trend. Interestingly, the government narrative explicating the success of the SARS campaign highlighted the same characteristics as the snail fever campaign, namely unitary direction from the top, committed leadership at the bottom, mass mobilization focused on prevention activities, successful health education that spurred popular patriotic participation, and innovative, affordable local solutions. In fact, the SARS campaign replicated many of the unacknowledged strategies that worked so well in the snail fever campaign, reflecting the true way the Maoist medical model operates.

Like the snail fever campaign, the SARS campaign used ideological persuasion and structural coercion to ensure involvement from lower-level leaders and participants. As in the earlier campaign, national leaders designated it a political rather than a health campaign and elevated it via apocalyptic rhetoric, with Premier Wen Jiabao declaring, "The health and security of the people, overall state of reform, development, and stability, and China's national interest and international image are at stake."[34] Next, as was true in the snail campaign, national leaders appropriated the campaign from the Ministry of Public Health and ousted ministry leaders (He Cheng in 1955; Zhang Wenkang in 2003). Over the next months, thousands of lower-level leaders who had not been appropriately responsive were also ousted.[35] These interventions informed lower-level leaders that the campaign was of key political importance and that the government would not let it get bogged down by standard operating procedures or embedded patron-client relationships.[36] Moreover, similar to its behavior in the snail campaign, the government never admitted that MPH had an impossible task due to a dearth of funding, a lack of power to enforce compliance and engagement among citizens, and minimal cooperation from competing government ministries and departments. Instead, after blaming MPH, the government reinstituted the successful organization used in the snail fever campaign to co-opt leaders, establishing a leadership small group called the Anti-SARS Task Force run out of the State Council, led by Vice Premier Wu Yi and with all relevant, previously recalcitrant actors, including the army. This prompted the creation of lower-level LSGs at provincial, city and county levels, each led by a high-level political leader who personally took charge.[37] Once participation became part of political theater, local officials participated with competitive zeal to one-up each other by launching various ostentatious mass campaigns.[38]

The government rallied the whole population to contribute to prevention activities by employing pedagogical strategies, tropes, and themes from prior mass health campaigns. While most of these were no more successful than earlier efforts at education, they served the same purpose: patriotic persuasive strategies that encouraged citizen participation. The SARS campaign was characterized as a citizen's war against invading enemy germs, a fight for survival rather than an effort to manage microorganisms.[39] Between the mass media blasting people with hygiene advice, closed shops and schools, fluttering red banners, and masked neighbors, an all-inclusive environment was created, making it extremely difficult not to participate in the campaign.[40] Because speed, communal effort, and countable accomplishments—such as the number of barricades—came to demonstrate success, campaign activities frequently accomplished little in terms of disease control. For example, eighty million people were marshaled to clean streets and houses in Guangdong.[41] Once the whole population went on a war footing, it became irrelevant whether the work was effective. People developed an esprit de corps, feeling that they would be "letting the people down, and the village committee down," if they let people through blockades. At the same time, it became patriotic, "the responsible thing to do," to spy on one's neighbors.[42] Even though the work was frequently unscientific and ineffective, the militarized, competitive battles gave it a patriotic value that had little to do with health.

Government media emphasized popular engagement in the campaign, but instead of depending solely on the persuasive power of patriotism, the government structurally embedded compliance by restarting the historical household surveillance system, whereby family and neighbors reported on those who were ill. Many rural counties conducted a census of migrants (the potential origin of the disease) and sent health workers and former barefoot doctors daily to take their temperature.[43] Soon, fever paranoia spread to the transport system. Highways and entrances to villages all over China were sprinkled with roadblocks, where drivers had no choice but to stand awaiting laser temperature takers pointed at their heads. Those found feverish were confined until an ambulance arrived to escort them to a clinic.[44] This mass work motivated by a sense of survival, which tried to find every person with fever, while extremely inefficient did compensate for the lack of accurate records for tracing contacts with infected people. In a similar way, during the snail fever campaign, the constant coursing up and down riverbanks facilitated bumping into remnant snails, even without records about prior snail-clearing sites. In the SARS campaign, the Party activated aging neighborhood committees in the cities, a structure created during the Maoist era to observe and control urban dwellers. Committee members went door to door identifying covert fever victims. In some apartment complexes, residents had to report their temperature daily so that their committee could log it.[45] Such tactics replicated the entrenched organizational structures in collectives that made participation required, rather than a choice. The Party also enacted mass quarantines and devised draconian new laws that levied the death penalty for knowingly spreading SARS.[46] Laws forbidding the spread of disease were not a part of the earlier snail fever campaign. However, the Reform-era government employed this new method, not to litigate the many human rights abuses that resulted from the quarantine, but rather to use as a helpful legitimating weapon in addition to the preexisting armamentarium of coercive strategies.

While the SARS campaign supposedly harkened back to the Party's self-reliant roots, it succeeded, like the snail fever campaign, because of extensive government resource allocation. The national government established a 2 billion yuan fund (US$250 million), with an additional 7 billion yuan contribution from local governments to build or reconstruct medical institutions, fever clinics, and an entire hospital system dedicated to this disease, just as it did for snail fever.[47] Once it became clear that some SARS patients were absconding from hospitals midtreatment because they could not afford the cost, treatment was completely subsidized, providing free therapy and increased access for the poorest citizens, as was done for snail fever treatment. The national campaign also made sure that rural places were provided with medicine, medical equipment, and some additional training, particularly in infection control.[48] Importantly, in a strategy reminiscent of sending skilled practitioners to the countryside during the snail campaign, lack of competent personnel was mitigated by posting county health workers and thousands of expert doctors and Chinese medicine practitioners from the civilian, traditional Chinese medicine, and military medical systems to this new medical structure.[49] At designated hospitals in urban areas, complete medical teams were dispatched to take over treatment, and expert surveillance teams circulated to all fever clinics and hospitals to establish who was really ill.[50] The government also sent many members of the People's Liberation Army and millions of reservists and militia to educate rural people and help with quarantine and other prevention measures in cities.[51] Additional funds increased staffing, making it possible for hard-pressed health agencies to complete their tasks.[52] Finally, the Party used the old strategy of site visits by top-level cadres, sending inspection and medical surveillance teams to twenty-six provinces, dispatching local leaders in SARS working groups to increase transparency and accountability, and thus spurring grassroots ardor.[53] Once again, appropriate funding and outside expertise and leadership were crucial components of success.

In the wake of the SARS campaign, some scholars have posited that the government's initial cover-up, combined with radical control measures that trampled human rights, would result in the "internal legitimacy of the regime [being] . . . under greater pressure than at any time since the 1989 Tiananmen Square incident."[54] In fact, the snail fever and other famous Maoist health campaigns normalized extreme measures and reified them as the correct way to address public health emergencies. The result, as surveys in Beijing show, is that the more excessive and coercive the government became during the SARS campaign, the more Chinese citizens gained confidence that the government had the problem well in hand, restoring their faith.[55]

The Maoist primary health-care model has been disseminated around the world. Its popularity is allegedly based on mass education's leading to high participation, low cost methods directed toward prevention, and large numbers of bottom- and midtier medical providers such as barefoot doctors. Evidence from the snail fever campaign, with confirmation from the SARS campaign, suggests that the core attributes of the model lie elsewhere. Mobilization in both campaigns was achieved by structurally entrenching participation. It was made palatable by patriotic and ideological persuasion, rather than by educational efforts that explained why campaign activities were necessary. Small, specialized teams of trained locals were consistently most effective in combatting both snail fever and SARS, while the signature feature of the model, mass prevention campaigns, was most helpful as a compensatory measure for poor record keeping and poor quality control. Finally, although treatment is rarely mentioned in the Maoist medical model, it often accounted for campaign success. Moreover, successful treatment depended on extensive government financial inputs via treatment subsidies. Most importantly, it depended on the professional medical personnel who undertook the more complex medical work while transmitting knowledge and expertise to the barefoot doctors who acted as their helpers. These campaigns were also contingent on newly educated rural youth learning the necessary organizational, medical, and technical skills to take on leadership roles. Together these realities suggest a very successful, but entirely different Maoist primary health-care model, one that if understood could become a real model for improving global public health and addressing the many disease crises the world faces today.

NOTES

INTRODUCTION

1. Joshua Horn, *Away With All Pests: An English Surgeon in People's China, 1954–1969* (New York: Monthly Review Press, 1969), 94–106; "Report of the American Schistosomiasis Delegation to the People's Republic of China," *American Journal of Tropical Medicine and Hygiene* 26.3 (1977): 427–62; F. R. Sandbach, "Farewell to the God of Plague—the Control of Schistosomiasis in China," *Social Science and Medicine* 11 (1977): 27–33; China Health Care Study Group, *Health Care in China, an Introduction: The Report of a Study Group in Hong Kong* (Geneva: Christian Medical Commission, 1974), 60, 67–71.

2. Interest in Maoist medicine is starting to revive. A recent book by Fang Xiaoping explores barefoot doctors, but does not discuss the wider medical model. Fang Xiaoping, *Barefoot Doctors and Western Medicine* (Rochester, NY: University of Rochester Press, 2012).

3. "Parasites—Schistosomiasis," Centers for Disease Control and Prevention, www.cdc.gov/parasites/schistosomiasis (accessed July 26, 2015) (quotation); "Schistosomiasis," World Health Organization, Fact Sheet No. 115, February 2010, www .who.int/mediacentre/factsheets/fs115/en/index.html (accessed October 17, 2013); "Schistosomiasis," World Health Organization, www.who.int/schistosomiasis /en (accessed October 17, 2013).

4. A. Davis, "Schistosomiasis," chapter 80 in *Manson's Tropical Diseases,* 21st ed. ed. Gordon C. Cook and Alimuddin I. Zumla (Philadelphia: Saunders, Elsevier Science, 2003), 1431–69.

5. Davis, "Schistosomiasis," 1436–38, 1442; Wang Ximeng, *Shanghai xiaomie xuexichongbing de huigu* (Shanghai: Shanghai kexue jishu chubanshe, 1988), 61; A. G. Ross et al., "Schistosomiasis in the People's Republic of China: Prospects and Challenges for the 21st Century," *Clinical Microbiology Reviews* 14.2 (2001): 282.

6. Davis, "Schistosomiasis," 1448–52.

7. Cheng Tien-hsi, "Schistosomiasis in Mainland China: A Review of Research and Control Programs since 1949," *American Journal of Tropical Medicine and*

Hygiene 20.1 (January 1971): 26; He Lianyin, "Policy Making and Organization in Managing Tropical Diseases in China," *Chinese Medical Journal* 114.7 (2001): 770; John Harland Reed, "Brass Butterflies of the Thoughts of Mao Tsetung: The Sociology of Schistosomiasis Control in China" (Ph.D. diss., Cornell University, 1979), 37.

8. Wang Ximeng, *Shanghai xiaomie xuexichongbing de huigu,* 1.

9. Fan Xingzhun, "You guan riben zhuxuexichong bing de zhongyi wenxian de chubu tantao," *Zhonghua yixue zazhi* 11 (1954): 862–64.

10. O. T. Logan, "A Case of Dysentery in Hunan Province Caused by the Trematode *Schistosoma japonicum,*" *Chinese Medical Journal* 19 (1905): 243–45; Akira Issii, Miyasu Tsuji, and Isao Tada, "History of Katayama Disease: Schistosomiasis Japonica in Katayama District, Hiroshima, Japan," *Parasitology International* 52 (2003): 313–16; R. T. Leiper and E. L. Atkinson, "Observations on the Spread of Aseatic Schistosomiasis," *Chinese Medical Journal* 29.3 (May 1915): 143–49; Iijima Wataru, "'Farewell to the God of Plague': Anti–*Schistosoma japonicum* Campaign in China and Japanese Colonial Medicine," *Memoirs of the Toyo Bunko* 66 (2008): 56–65.

11. John Farley, *Bilharzia: A History of Imperial Tropical Medicine* (New York: Cambridge University Press, 2003), 93–96; Kan Huai-chieh and Yao Yung-tsung, "Some Notes on the Anti–Schistosomiasis Japonica Campaign in Chih-huai-pan, Kaihua, Chekiang," *Chinese Medical Journal* 48.4 (April 1934): 323; Ka-Che Yip, *Health and National Reconstruction in Nationalist China: The Development of Modern Health Services, 1928–1937* (Ann Arbor, MI: Association for Asian Studies, 1995), 45–49, 57, 105, 110, 111; SHA: 372, 176.

12. "The Henry Lester Institute and Hospital," *Science* 69.1785 (March 15, 1929): 290–91; SMA: U1–16–2651, 1934–1937; SMA: U1–16–2652, 1931–1937; Su De-long and Carl E. Taylor, "The Community Health Teaching Center in China," *American Journal of Public Health* 72.9, suppl. (September 1982): 89.

13. Mao Shou-Pai, "Parasitological Research in Institutes in China," chapter 10 in *Parasitology: A Global Perspective,* ed. Kenneth S. Warren and John Z. Bowers (New York: Springer-Verlag, 1983), 117–25 (quotation p. 119).

14. David M. Lampton, *The Politics of Medicine in China: The Policy Process, 1949–1977* (Boulder, CO: Westview Press, 1977), 59; Yip, *Health and National Reconstruction in Nationalist China,* 159; Szeming Sze, *China's Health Problems* (Washington, D.C.: Chinese Medical Association, 1943), 26–27.

15. Jin Jiqing, ed., *Qingpu xian fangzhi xuexichongbing sanshiwu nian: Tubiao ji* (Shanghai: Shanghai kexue jishu chubanshe, 1986), 159–65; Ma Xuewen, *Qingpu xian zhi* (Shanghai: Shanghai renmin chubanshe, 1990), 600–615.

16. Xu Fuzhou, "Fangbing zhibing zaofu renmin—Qingpu weisheng gongzuo si shinian," in *Qingpu wenshi, di si qi* (Qingpu [Shanghai]: Zhongguo renmin zhengzhi xieshang huiyi Qingpu xian weiyuanhui wenshi ziliao weiyuanhui, 1989), 161–62.

17. YJA: 43, 12/1976.

18. Yu Laixi and Zhonggong Yujiang xianwei xuefang lingdao xiaozu bangongshi, *Jiangxi sheng Yujiang xian xuefang zhi: 1953–1980* (Yujiang: Zhonggong Yujiang xianwei xuefang lingdao xiaozu bangongshi, 1984), 12; YJA: 10, 1–12/1956. By way of

comparison, in 1949 Qingpu already had 290 practitioners, 5.4 times the number Yujiang had after almost a decade under Communist rule. Xu Fuzhou, "Fangbing zhibing," 161; YJA: 38, 1–12/1972.

19. Jin Yimin, Qingpu xian shuiliju, "Shuili xing ze wenming cun—Qingpu xian shuilishi qiantan," in *Qingpu wenshi, di yi qi* (Qingpu [Shanghai]: Zhongguo renmin zhengzhi xieshang huiyi Qingpu xian weiyuanhui wenshi ziliao weiyuanhui 1989), 34–40.

20. Huang Qijing and Luo Zhuliu, "Tongxin xieli song wenshen—qing puxiang xue xi chongbing yiqing ji fangzhi chengguo," in *Qingpu wenshi, di si qi,* 154–58; QPA: 95–1-1, 3/1951.

21. Honggen Chen and Dandan Lin, "The Prevalence and Control of Schisto-somiasis in Poyang Lake Region, China," *Parasitology International* 53.2 (2004): 115–16.

22. Yu Laixi and Zhonggong Yujiang xianwei xuefang lingdao xiaozu bangong-shi, *Jiangxi sheng Yujiang xian xuefang zhi,* 9, 22; Yu Laixi, "Yujiang renmin fangzhi xuexichongbing de weida douzheng," in *Song wenshen jishi,* vol. 43, ed. Liu Yurui and Wan Guohe (Nanchang: Jiangxi sheng zhengxie wenshi ziliao yanjiu weiyuan-hui, 1992), 1; JXA: XIII–02–269, 12/1957.

23. Yu Laixi and Zhonggong Yujiang xianwei xuefang lingdao xiaozu bangong-shi, *Jiangxi sheng Yujiang xian xuefang zhi,* 25; YJA: 13, 1–12/1957; JXA: X035–06–514, 1958; Qian Xinzhong, *Zhonghua renmin gongheguo xuexichongbing dituji, shangce* (Shanghai: Zhonghua dituxue she chuban, 1987), 28.5. According to Zou Huayi, of China's more than three hundred counties with snail fever, Yujiang rated in the bottom third in terms of prevalence rates. Zou Huayi, *Kuayue siwang didai* (Nanchang: Baihuazhou wenyi chubanshe, 1993), 249–50.

24. Quanguo fangzhi wu da jishengchongbing jingyan jiaoliu huiyi, *Renmin shouce 1959 nian* (Beijing: Renmin ribao chubanshe, 1960), 511; Qian Xinzhong, *Zhonghua renmin gongheguo xuexichongbing dituji, shangce,* 22.5.

25. Franz Schurmann, *Ideology and Organization in Communist China* (Berke-ley: University of California Press, 1968), 52, 166, 226, 233, 236; Vivienne Shue, *The Reach of the State: Sketches of the Chinese Body Politic* (Stanford, CA: Stanford Uni-versity Press, 1988), 118–19, 149; Joel Andreas, *Rise of the Red Engineers: The Cultural Revolution and the Origins of China's New Class* (Stanford, CA: Stanford University Press, 2009), 216, 223, 237–39; Susan Greenhalgh, *Just One Child: Science and Policy in Deng's China* (Berkeley: University of California Press, 2008), 5, 19, 76–77, 196; Richard P. Suttmeier, *Science, Technology and China's Drive for Modernization* (Stanford, CA: Hoover Institute Press, 1980), 43.

I. CHAIRMAN MAO WEIGHS IN

1. SMA: C3–1-11, 2/1950.

2. Ibid.; SMA: Q249–1-137, 12/24/1949–4/11/1950; Huang Qijing and Luo Zhuliu, "Tongxin xieli song wenshen—qing puxiang xue xi chongbing yiqing ji

fangzhi chengguo," in *Qingpu wenshi, di si qi* (Qingpu [Shanghai]: Zhongguo renmin zhengzhi xieshang huiyi Qingpu xian weiyuanhui wenshi ziliao weiyuanhui, 1989), 154; Shanghai kexue daxue liuxingbingxue jiaoyanshi, *Su Delong jiaoshou lunwen xuanji* (Tianjin: Tianjin kexue jishu chubanshe, 1985), 1.

3. JSA: 3235, 126, duanqi, 1953–1954; SMA: B242–1-816, 11/1955; JXA: X035–04–802, 1956.

4. Jonathan D. Spence, *The Search for Modern China,* 2nd ed. (New York: W. W. Norton & Company, 1999), 505.

5. John Harland Reed, "Brass Butterflies of the Thoughts of Mao Tsetung: The Sociology of Schistosomiasis Control in China" (Ph.D. diss., Cornell University, 1979), 37–40.

6. Ibid.; Wei Wen-po [Wei Wenbo], "Battle against Schistosomiasis," translated and reprinted from *Hongqi,* no. 2 (1960), *Chinese Medical Journal* 80 (1960): 302. According to current studies, data on decreased productivity are likely exaggerated except for very late-stage patients. However, this was the data available to CCP leadership at the time and it likely influenced their decisions.

7. Zhong Zubiao and Jiangxi sheng jiachu xuexichongbing fangzhi zhan, *Jiangxi sheng jiachu xuefang zhi: 1956–1996* (Nanchang: Jiangxi sheng jiachu xuexichongbing fangzhi zhan, 1989), 16.

8. Croizier believes CCP health work fell on the humanitarian side; this study disagrees, finding that national strength was the primary motivation. Ralph Croizier, "Medicine and Modernization in China: An Historical Overview," in *Medicine in Chinese Cultures,* ed. Arthur M. Kleinman et al. (Washington, D.C.: U.S. Department of Health, Education and Welfare, National Institutes of Health, 1975), 28.

9. YJA: 9, 1–12/1956.

10. JXA: X001–03–079, 1957; JSA: 3119, 1017, duanqi, 4/4/1963–1/12/1964; QPA: 95-1-10, 1956–1958; JSA: 3119, 503, duanqi, 7/3/1958–10/14/1958.

11. Randall M. Packard, "Malaria Dreams: Postwar Visions of Health and Development in the Third World," *Medical Anthropology* 17.3 (1997): 281.

12. "A Study of Physical Education" (April 1917) and "Basic Tactics" (1937), in *Selected Works of Mao Tse-tung,* vol. 6, www.marxists.org/reference/archive/mao /selected-works/index.htm. (accessed April 22, 2010); Edgar Snow, *Red Star over China* (New York: Grove Press, 1994), 92, 280.

13. Snow, *Red Star over China,* 280; "Be Concerned with the Well-Being of the Masses, Pay Attention to Methods of Work" (January 27, 1934), in *Selected Works of Mao Tse-tung,* vol. 1; David M. Lampton, *The Politics of Medicine in China: The Policy Process, 1949–1977* (Boulder, CO: Westview Press, 1977), 13.

14. "Strengthen Party Unity and Carry forward Party Traditions" (August 30, 1956), in *Selected Works of Mao Tse-tung,* vol. 5.

15. JXA: X035–04–802, 1956.

16. SMA: B242–1-814, 1955.

17. Sun Yongjiu, "Gonggu chengguo ying nan er shang; ba xuefang hongqi ju de genggao," in *Song wenshen jishi,* vol. 43, ed. Liu Yurui and Wan Guohe (Nanchang:

Jiangxi sheng zhengxie wenshi ziliao yanjiu weiyuanhui, 1992), 102; JXA: X035–04–802, 1956.

18. SMA: B242–1-815, 11/1955; "Xin Zhongguo zai fangzhi xuexichongbing wentishang suo kaizhan de yi xie yanjiu gongzuo," *Zhonghua yixue zazhi,* 7 (1955): 394. Almost all references to the campaign's international import were in reports from upper-level meetings, suggesting that this line of patriotic propaganda gave value to those guiding the campaign, rather than bolstering the efforts of villagers or grassroots personnel.

19. Stephen Endicott and Edward Hagerman, *The United States and Biological Warfare: Secrets from the Early Cold War and Korea* (Bloomington: Indiana University Press, 1998), 8, 20.

20. Iijima Wataru, "'Farewell to the God of Plague': Anti–*Schistosoma japonicum* Campaign in China and Japanese Colonial Medicine," *Memoirs of the Toyo Bunko* 66 (2008): 61.

21. Sun Yongjiu, "Gonggu chengguo ying nan er shang," 110.

22. Zhang Yi, "Chen yun hui guxiang, diaocha xuexichongbing fangzhi qingkuang," in *Qingpu wenshi, di san qi* (Qingpu [Shanghai]: Zhongguo renmin zhengzhi xieshang huiyi Qingpu xian weiyuanhui wenshi ziliao weiyuanhui, 1989), 105.

23. Reed, "Brass Butterflies," 179; Kenneth S. Warren, "'Farewell the Plague Spirit': Chairman Mao's Crusade against Schistosomiasis," in Science and Medicine in Twentieth-Century China: Research and Education, ed. John Z. Bowers, J. William Hess, and Nathan Sivin (Ann Arbor: Center for Chinese Studies, University of Michigan, 1988), 123–24.

24. "Circular Requesting Opinions on 17 Articles on Agricultural Work" (December 21, 1955) and "Second Preface to *Upsurge of Socialism in China's Countryside*" (December 27, 1955), in *The Writings of Mao Zedong, 1949–1976,* ed. Michael Kau and John Leung, vol. 1 (Armonk, NY: M. E. Sharpe, 1986), 688, 691; "Instructions on Report on Schistosomiasis Prevention Conference" (March 7, 1956), in *The Writings of Mao Zedong, 1949–1976,* ed. Michael Kau and John Leung, vol. 2 (Armonk, NY: M. E. Sharpe, 1992), 31.

25. Wei Wenbo, "Farewell the 'God of Plague,'" in *Mao Zedong: Biography-Assessment-Reminiscences,* comp. Zhong Wenxian (Beijing: Foreign Language Press, 1986), 219–20; H. N. Engle and P. Engle, *Poems of Mao Tse-tung* (New York: Simon and Schuster, 1973), 105–6.

26. JSA: 3119, 486; SMA: B242–1-815, 11/1955.

27. Huang Lanyan, "Sunan xuexichongbing yufang gongzuo," *Jiankang bao,* no. 202, November 8, 1951, 6; Wang Ximeng, *Shanghai xiaomie xuexichongbing de huigu* (Shanghai: Shanghai kexue jishu chubanshe, 1988), 12, 13; Fu Lien-Chang, "An Address to the Members of the Medical Profession among the Delegates to the Peace Conference of the Asian and Pacific Regions," *Chinese Medical Journal* 71 (January–February 1953): 2.

28. Fu, "Address to the Members of the Medical Profession," 6.

29. Fu Lien-Chang, "Summing-Up of the Ninth General Conference of the Chinese Medical Association Held in Peking on December Fourteenth to Seventeenth, 1952," *Chinese Medical Journal* 71 (March–April 1953): 160–61.

30. David M. Lampton, *Health, Conflict, and the Chinese Political System,* Michigan Papers in Chinese Studies No. 18. (Ann Arbor: University of Michigan, 1974), 13, 24–26, 62; Lampton, *Politics of Medicine in China,* 61; Dai Chun, "Pengzi xian fangzhi xuexibing gongzuo weishenme mei gaoqilai?," *Jiangxi ribao,* December 15, 1956, 3.

31. "Some Aspects of Research in the Prevention and Treatment of Schistosomiasis Japonica in New China," *Chinese Medical Journal* 72 (March–April 1955): 100; Boerdeliefu, Zhonghua renmin gongheguo weishengbu sulian zhuanjia zuzhang, "Guanyu xiaomie xuexichong bing cuoshi de jidian yijian," *Jiankang bao,* no. 425, February 17, 1956, 3–4.

32. Ibid. (both sources); "Report of the American Schistosomiasis Delegation to the People's Republic of China," *American Journal of Tropical Medicine and Hygiene* 26.3 (1977): 428.

33. H. F. Hsu and Li S. Y. Hsu, "Schistosomiasis in the Shanghai Area," in *China Medicine as We Saw It,* ed. Joseph R. Quinn and John E. Fogarty International Center, DHEW Publication No. (NIH) 75–684 (Washington, D.C.: U.S. Department of Health, Education, and Welfare, 1974), 348. The Shanghai Institute of Parasitic Diseases was renamed multiple times. Names have included the Shanghai Schistosomiasis Treatment and Prevention Institute, the Shanghai Research Institute of Parasitic Diseases, and currently, the National Institute of Parasitic Diseases. I have chosen to call it the Shanghai Institute of Parasitic Diseases throughout the book.

34. Mao Shou-Pai, "Parasitological Research in Institutes in China," chapter 10 in *Parasitology: A Global Perspective,* ed. Kenneth S. Warren and John Z. Bowers (New York: Springer-Verlag, 1983), 120–21; SMA: B34-2-195, 1954; JXA: XIII–02–269, 12/1957.

35. Ka-Che Yip, *Health and National Reconstruction in Nationalist China: The Development of Modern Health Services, 1928–1937* (Ann Arbor, MI: Association for Asian Studies, 1995), 190.

36. For more information on germ warfare and PPHCs, see Yang Nianqun, "Disease Prevention, Social Mobilization and Spatial Politics: The Anti Germ-Warfare Incident of 1952 and the 'Patriotic Health Campaign,'" *Chinese Historical Review* 11.2 (Fall 2004): 155–82; Ruth Rogaski, "Nature, Annihilation, and Modernity: China's Korean War Germ-Warfare Experience Reconsidered," *Journal of Asian Studies* 61.2 (May 2002), 381–415; QPA: 95-2-2, 10/25/1952.

37. Aaron Shirly, "Community Health," in *Rural Health in the People's Republic of China: Report of a Visit by the Rural Health Systems Delegation, June 1978,* by Committee on Scholarly Communication with the People's Republic of China, NIH Publication No. 81–2124 (Washington, D.C.: U.S. Department of Health and Human Services, Public Health Service, National Institutes of Health, November 1980), 9–15; YJA: 6, 1954.

38. QPA: 95–2-9, 1953.

39. Shanghai kexue, *Su Delong jiaoshou lunwen xuanji,* 1; Ji Shunkang, Qingpu xian fangzhi xuexichongbing sanshiwu nian weiyuanhui, "Qingpu xian xuexi-chongbing fangzhi zhan jianzhan qianhou," in *Qingpu xian fangzhi xuexichongbing sanshiwu nian: Zonglunji* (Shanghai: Shanghai kexue jishu chubanshe), 88–90; Yao Yuanxiang, *Zhonggong Qingpu dangshi dashiji* (Shanghai: Shanghai shehui kexuey-uan chubanshe, 1994), 287–88; SMA: Q244–1-290, 1–7/1952.

40. Cui Yitian, "Dali zhankai huadong nongcun xuexichongbing fangzhi gong-zuo," *Jiefang ribao,* no. 885, November 9, 1951, 3; SMA: B242–1-814, 1955. Cui Yitian was the head of the East China Military Region's public health department as well as Shanghai's Municipal Health Bureau.

41. "17 Articles on Agricultural Work" (December 12, 1955), in *Writings of Mao Zedong,* ed. Kau and Leung, vol. 1, 688.

42. Ka wai Fan and Honkei Lai, "Mao Zedong's Fight against Schistosomiasis," *Perspectives in Biology and Medicine* 51.2 (Spring 2008): 180.

43. Ibid.

44. SMA: B242–1-815, 11/1955.

45. Lampton, *Politics of Medicine in China,* 46.

46. SMA: B242–1-815, 11/1955.

47. Ibid.

48. Maurice Meisner, *Mao's China and After: A History of the People's Republic,* rev. and expanded 1st ed. (New York: Free Press, 1986), 140–43.

49. Lampton, *Health, Conflict, and the Chinese Political System,* 15–16, 71–73.

50. Ibid., 144–49; "We Must Learn to Do Economic Work" (January 10, 1945), in *Selected Works of Mao Tse-tung,* vol. 3.

51. "Second Preface to *Upsurge of Socialism in China's Countryside*" (December 27, 1955), in *Writings of Mao Zedong,* ed. Kau and Leung, vol. 1, 689–92.

52. Spence, *Search for Modern China,* 522–23.

53. Kiangxi, Yü-chiang Hsien, Revolutionary Committee, Culture, Education, Health, and Antischistosomiasis Section with Yü-chiang Antischistosomiasis Sta-tion, "A Great Victory of Mao Zedong's Thought in the Battle against Schistosomia-sis: The 10 Years Since the Eradication of Schistosomiasis in Yukiang County in 1958," *China's Medicine* 10 (October 1968): 592 (quotation); Li Junjiu, "Diyi mian hongqi shi zenyang chashang de," in *Song wenshen jishi,* ed. Liu and Wan, 96; SMA: B242–1-815, 11/1955.

54. "Instruction on Leadership Work of Health Department of Military Com-missions" (April 3, 1953), "Criticism of the Ministry of Public Health" (October 1953), and "Comment on Department of Public Health" (1953), in *Writings of Mao Zedong,* ed. Kau and Leung, vol. 1, 339–40, 425, 441–42 (quotation p. 442). For a broader discussion of Chinese medicine and statecraft, see Ralph C. Croizier, *Tra-ditional Medicine in Modern China: Science, Nationalism, and the Tensions of Cul-tural Change* (Cambridge, MA: Harvard University Press, 1968); Kim Taylor, *Chi-nese Medicine in Early Communist China, 1945–1963: A Medicine of Revolution* (New York: RoutledgeCurzon, 2005).

55. William Y. Chen, "Medicine and Public Health," in *Sciences in Communist China: A Symposium Presented at the New York Meeting of the American Association for the Advancement of Science, December 26–27, 1960*, ed. Sidney H. Gamble (Washington, D.C.: American Association for the Advancement of Science, 1961), 405; JSA: 3235, 41, yongjiu, 3/26/1951–4/18/1957; "Directive on Work in Traditional Chinese Medicine" (July 30, 1954), in *Writings of Mao Zedong*, ed. Kau and Leung, vol. 1, 464–66.

56. "The United Front in Cultural Work" (October 10, 1944), in *Selected Works of Mao Tse-tung*, vol. 3 (quotation); Yip, *Health and National Reconstruction in Nationalist China*, 190.

57. J. Yudkin, "Medicine and Medical Education in the New China," *Journal of Medical Education* 33.7 (July 1958): 519; J. Z. Bowers, "Medicine in Mainland China: Red and Rural," *Current Scene: Developments in Mainland China* 8.12 (June 15, 1970): 1–11.

58. "Directive on Work in Traditional Chinese Medicine" (July 30, 1954) and "Implementing Correct Policy in Dealing with Doctors of Traditional Chinese Medicine" (October 20, 1954), in *Writings of Mao Zedong*, ed. Kau and Leung, vol. 1, 464–66, 488 (quotation).

59. "Implementing Correct Policy" (October 20, 1954), in *Writings of Mao Zedong*, ed. Kau and Leung, vol. 1, 486–91.

60. Ibid.; "Talk with Music Workers" (August 24, 1956), in *Writings of Mao Zedong*, ed. Kau and Leung, vol. 2, 94–98.

61. "On Practice" (July 1937) in *Selected Works of Mao Tse-tung*, vol. 1; "RMRB Editorial on Cultivating Traditional Chinese Medicine" (May 27, 1956), in *Writings of Mao Zedong*, ed. Kau and Leung, vol. 2, 77–79.

62. For a comprehensive discussion of this issue, see Elizabeth Fee, *Disease and Discovery: A History of the Johns Hopkins School of Hygiene and Public Health, 1916–1939* (Baltimore: Johns Hopkins University Press, 1987); F. R. Sandbach, "The History of Schistosomiasis Research and Policy for Its Control," *Medical History* 20.3 (July 1976): 270–73; John Farley, *Bilharzia: A History of Imperial Tropical Medicine* (New York: Cambridge University Press, 2003), 81, 173, 177–81, 194.

63. SMA: B242-1-814, 1955.

64. Ibid. Lampton speculates that one reason the six military regions were dissolved in 1954 was that the Party wanted to "limit the growth of regionally based professional independence." If so, as the Shanghai case shows, this tactic backfired. Lampton, *Health, Conflict, and the Chinese Political System*, 66.

65. Ibid.

66. Ibid.; Lampton, *Politics of Medicine in China*, 46–47.

67. Lampton, *Politics of Medicine in China*, 23, 46–47; "Directive on Work in Traditional Chinese Medicine" (July 30, 1954), in *Writings of Mao Zedong*, ed. Kau and Leung, vol. 1, n466.

68. SMA: B242-1-814, 1955.

69. Iijima, "Farewell to the God of Plague," 61; "Association News: Visit of Japanese Schistosomiasis Specialists," *Chinese Medical Journal* 75.1 (January 1957): 84; "Association News," *Chinese Medical Journal* 76.1 (January 1958): 101.

70. Iijima, "'Farewell to the God of Plague,'" 56–59.

71. Another Japanese schistosomiasis delegation returned to China in October 1981 to assess the work. Iijima, "Farewell to the God of Plague," 61–63, 66, 69; "Report of the American Schistosomiasis Delegation," 429 (quotations); Y. Komiya, "Recommendatory Note for the Control Problem of Schistosomiasis in China," *Japanese Journal of Medical Science and Biology* 10 (1957): 461–71.

72. SMA: B242–1-814, 1955; Shanghai kexue, *Su Delong jiaoshou lunwen xuanji,* 1; Lampton, *Health, Conflict, and the Chinese Political System,* 60. It is unclear whether Dr. Su's agreement was wholly scientifically based, given that almost all of Mao's rural reconstruction measures at the time were slated to be accomplished in seven years.

73. SMA: B242–1-815, 11/1955.

74. JXA: X035–04–802, 1956.

75. SMA: A71–2-375, 5/21/1955–12/24/1955.

76. Shanghai kexue, *Su Delong jiaoshou lunwen xuanji,* 1.

77. Shen Ch'i-chen, "Report on Prevention of Schistosomiasis," in *Speeches Given at the Second Session of the Second National People's Congress, Communist China* (Washington, D.C.: U.S. Joint Publications Research Service, 1961), 3; Warren, "'Farewell to the Plague Spirit,'" 131.

78. Ernest Faust and Henry Meleney, *Studies on Schistosomiasis Japonica,* Monograph Series No. 3. (Baltimore: American Journal of Hygiene, 1924), 263, 265, 266; SMA: Q244–1-290, 1–7/1952.

79. Komiya, "Recommendatory Note," 461–71.

80. Li Zhisui, *The Private Life of Chairman Mao* (New York: Random House, 1994), 215; Meisner, *Mao's China and After,* 285.

81. Li Zhisui, *Private Life of Chairman Mao,* 214–17; Ch'ien Hsin-chung, "Summing Up of Mass Technical Experiences with a View to Expediting Eradication of the Five Major Parasitic Diseases," *Chinese Medical Journal* 77.6 (January 1958): 522; QPA: 95–2-44, 1958.

82. Farley, *Bilharzia,* 269; R. L. Andreano, *More on the God of Plague: Schistosomiasis in Mainland China,* Report No. 7 (Madison, WI: Health Economics Research Center, 1971), 5–10; JXA: X035–05–398, 1963; JSA: 3119, 75, yongjiu, 1964.

83. YJA: 28, 1963.

84. QPA: 95–1-29, 1/3/1962; "The Orientation of the Revolution in Medical Education as seen in the Growth of 'Barefoot Doctors': Report of an Investigation from Shanghai," reprinted from *Hongqi,* no. 3 (1968), *Chinese Medical Journal* 87.10 (1968): 574–75.

85. JSA: 3119, 75, yongjiu, 1964; QPA: 95–2-76, 1961; Wang Ximeng, *Shanghai xiaomie xuexichongbing de huigu,* 7, 39, 117.

86. Roderick MacFarquhar, *The Origins of the Cultural Revolution,* vol. 3, *The Coming of the Cataclysm, 1961–1966* (New York: Columbia University Press, 1997), 3, 91, 95.

87. SMA: B242–1-1624, 5/1963–12/1964.

88. SMA: B257–1-2471, 1–12/1961; SMA: B257–1-3597, 10/1963–12/1964; QPA: 95–2-75, 1961.

89. The section epigraph is quoted from Li, *The Private Life of Chairman Mao,* 420.

90. Yang Nianqun, "Memories of the Barefoot Doctor System," in *Governance of Life in Chinese Moral Experience,* ed. Everett Zhang, Arthur Kleinman, and Tu Weiming (New York: Routledge, 2011), 131.

91. "Directive on Public Health" (June 26, 1965), from *Long Live Mao Tse-tung Thought,* a Red Guard publication, in *Selected Works of Mao Tse-tung,* vol. 9.

92. Everett M. Rogers, "Barefoot Doctors," in *Rural Health in the People's Republic of China,* by Committee on Scholarly Communication with the People's Republic of China, 45.

93. In 1966, Liu Shaoqi was purged for, among other things, his views on public health, placed under house arrest, mistreated, vilified, and denied medical treatment before dying in 1969.

94. Li Zhisui, *Private Life of Chairman Mao,* 413–20; Editor, "The Mao-Liu Controversy over Rural Public Health," *Current Scene* 7.12 (June 15, 1969): 1, 3; "Talk on Health Services" (January 24, 1964), from *Long Live Mao Tse-tung Thought,* a Red Guard publication, in *Selected Works of Mao Tse-tung,* vol. 9.

95. "News and Notes," *Chinese Medical Journal* 85.9 (1966): 633.

96. "Directive on Public Health" (June 26, 1965), in *Selected Works of Mao Tse-tung,* vol. 9 (quotation); Li Zhisui, *Private Life of Chairman Mao,* 413–20; SMA: B242–3-283, 1–8/1972; QPA: 95–2-117, 1965–1966.

97. "Directive on Public Health" (June 26, 1965), in *Selected Works of Mao Tse-tung,* vol. 9.

98. Fang Xiaoping, *Barefoot Doctors and Western Medicine* (Rochester, NY: University of Rochester Press, 2012), 33.

99. Ibid., 47; YJA: 38, 1–12/1972; C. C. Chen, *Medicine in Rural China: A Personal Account* (Berkeley: University of California Press, 1989), 77, 92; SMA: B242–1-1774, 7–10/1966.

100. Roderick MacFarquhar and Michael Schoenhals, *Mao's Last Revolution* (Cambridge, MA: Belknap Press of Harvard University Press, 2006), 339

101. Anita Chan, Richard Madsen, and Jonathan Unger, *Chen Village: The Recent History of a Peasant Community in Mao's China* (Berkeley: University of California Press, 1984), 231.

102. S. M. Hillier and J. A. Jewell, *Health Care and Traditional Medicine in China, 1800–1982* (London: Routledge & Kegan Paul, 1983), 176; "Southern China Launches Antischistosomiasis Campaign," *Chinese Medical Journal* 3.4 (July 1977), 286; Wu Ningkun, *A Single Tear: A Family's Persecution, Love, and Endurance in Communist China* (New York: Atlantic Monthly Press, 1993), 333.

103. SMA: B242–3-283, 1–8/1972; Shanghai shi difangzhi bangongshi, "Diba pian zhuan bing fangzhi, diyi zhang xuexichongbing, disan jie jigou," *Shanghai weishengzhi,* www.shtong.gov.cn/node2/node2245/node67643/node67655/node67719/node67847/userobject1ai65180.html (accessed September 29, 2013).

104. Ibid. (both sources); YJA: 35, 1–12/1970; YJA: 36, 1–12/1971.

105. MacFarquhar and Schoenhals, *Mao's Last Revolution,* 339–42; Hillier and Jewell, *Health Care and Traditional Medicine in China,* 365.

106. "Southern China Launches Antischistosomiasis Campaign," 286–87. The World Bank, with matching funds from the PRC, sponsored a third campaign peak from 1992 to 2001, discussed in the conclusion.

107. Qian Xinzhong, *Zhonghua renmin gongheguo xuexichongbing dituji, shangce* (Shanghai: Zhonghua dituxue she chuban, 1987), 22.5.

108. Interview on September 13, 2007, with personnel of the Shanghai Institute of Parasitic Diseases.

2. DODGING LEADERSHIP IN AN ERA OF DECENTRALIZATION

1. Wang Ximeng, *Shanghai xiaomie xuexichongbing de huigu* (Shanghai: Shanghai kexue jishu chubanshe, 1988), 119.

2. YJA: 20, 1–12/1962.

3. A. Doak Barnett, *Cadres, Bureaucracy, and Political Power in Communist China* (New York: Columbia University Press, 1967), 86, 129, 372, 421; Harry Harding, *Organizing China: The Problem of Bureaucracy, 1949–1976* (Stanford, CA: Stanford University Press, 1981), 348–49.

4. Vivienne Shue, *The Reach of the State: Sketches of the Chinese Body Politic* (Stanford, CA: Stanford University Press, 1988), 56.

5. JXA: X111–02–201, 2/1957, pp. 157–58.

6. QPA: 95-2-44, 1958.

7. Li Guohua, "Chabing, zhibing, de jijian wangshi," in *Song wenshen jishi,* vol. 43, ed. Liu Yurui and Wan Guohe (Nanchang: Jiangxi sheng zhengxie wenshi ziliao yanjiu weiyuanhui, 1992), 136.

8. Deng Shilin, "Bingfang she zai wode jia," in *Song wenshen jishi,* ed. Liu and Wan, 142.

9. YJA: 15, 1957.

10. Zou Huayi, *Kuayue siwang dida* (Nanchang: Baihuazhou wenyi chubanshe, 1993), 88–89.

11. YJA: 9, 1–12/1956.

12. JXA: X111–05–128, 1961.

13. JXA: X111–02–140, 1955; SMA: B34–2–195, 1954.

14. Li Junjiu, "Diyi mian hongqi shi zenyang chashang de," in *Song wenshen jishi,* ed. Liu and Wan, 95.

15. Ibid.

16. SMA: B242–1-816, 11/1955.

17. Lieberthal, *Governing China,* 169.

18. Ibid., 170, 174.

19. David M. Lampton, *The Politics of Medicine in China: The Policy Process, 1949-1977* (Boulder, CO: Westview Press, 1977), 61; Dai Chun, "Pengzi xian

fangzhi xuexibing gongzuo weishenme mei gaoqilai?," *Jiangxi ribao,* December 15, 1956, 3.

20. Kenneth Lieberthal, *Governing China: From Revolution through Reform* (New York: W. W. Norton & Company, 1995), 192–95.

21. Wang Ximeng, *Shanghai xiaomie xuexichongbing de huigu,* 13; SMA: B242–1-816, 11/1955; SMA: A71–2-465, 5/3/1956–12/22/1956; SMA: B242–1-50, 12/16/1955; JSA: 3119, 75, yongjiu, 1964.

22. SMA: B242–1-816, 11/1955; YJA: 3, 1954; QPA: 95–1-11, 1–12/1956; JXA: X009–01–010, 1957.

23. Lampton, *Politics of Medicine in China,* 46–49; David M. Lampton, *Health, Conflict, and the Chinese Political System,* Michigan Papers in Chinese Studies No. 18 (Ann Arbor: University of Michigan, 1974), 62–63.

24. SMA: B242–1-54, 4–12/1956; JSA: 3119, 198, duanqi, 3/1/1956–12/19/1956; JXA: X111–02–269, 12/1957.

25. YJA: 6, 1954.

26. Dai, "Pengze xian," 3 (quotation); JXA: X009–01–010, 1957.

27. JXA: X035–04–484, 1955.

28. QPA: 95–2-45, 1958.

29. JXA: X045–01–017, 1956.

30. Ibid.; JSA: 3119, 75, yongjiu, 1964.

31. SMA: B3–2-68, 1/18/1956–8/18/1956; JXA: X035–02–817, 1/12/1953–10/7/1953. Having more resources made this problem worse. Shanghai created a flurry of constantly changing snail fever organizations with overlapping missions and transferred personnel repeatedly between them. The result was chaos on the ground. SMA: B242–1-907, 6–11/1956.

32. SMA: Q244–1-290, 1–7/1952.

33. SMA: B242–1-815, 11/1955.

34. YJA: 40, 1–12/1973.

35. YJA: 11, 1–12/1956.

36. JXA: X001–01–403, 1–9/1957.

37. QPA: 95–1-12, 1956.

38. JXA: X111–02–201, 2/1957, 261.

39. Shue, *Reach of the State,* 107–8.

40. Harding, *Organizing China,* 348–49.

41. Barnett, *Cadres, Bureaucracy, and Political Power,* 193, 215, 216, 421 (quotation).

42. JXA: X001–01–403, 1–9/1957.

43. QPA: 95–1-10, 1956–1958.

44. JXA: X009–01–010, 1957.

45. JXA: X001–03–079, 1957.

46. JSA: 3119, 322, changqi, 2/10/1957–12/28/1957.

47. JXA: X001–01–403, 1–9/1957; JXA: X111–02–269, 12/1957, 6 (quotation).

48. JXA: X009–01–010, 1957.

49. Ibid.

50. Ibid.

51. JSA: 3119, 198, duanqi, 3/1/1956–12/19/1956.

52. JSA: 3119, 1017, duanqi, 4/4/1963–1/12/1964.

53. JXA: X009–01–010, 1957; JXA: X111–02–269, 12/1957, p. 3 (quotation).

54. SMA: B3–2–68, 1/18/1956–8/18/1956.

55. JXA: X045–01–044, 1957.

56. YJA: 6, 1954; JXA: X111–01–078, 3/19/1957–11/30/1957 (quotation); JSA: 3235, 146, changqi, 1/23/1955–12/1955.

57. JSA: 3119, 418, duanqi, 2/28/1957–12/18/1957.

58. JXA: X001–01–403, 1–9/1957. One mu is one-fifteenth of a hectare.

59. QPA: 95–2-76, 1961.

60. YJA: 27, 1–12/1963.

61. JXA: X111–01–078, 3/19/1957–11/30/1957.

62. JXA: X111–02–087, 1954.

63. Ibid.; JXA: X009–01–010, 1957 (quotation).

64. QPA: 95–1-12, 1956.

65. The snail fever campaign reflected a general problem of all health work. For example, as of 1957 in Jiangxi, "64 percent of county-level [health] department heads didn't manage to stay a year." JXA: X111–01–078, 3/19/1957–11/30/1957.

66. Lü Liang, "Xu," in *Song wenshen jishi,* ed. Liu and Wan, 1; JXA: X111–02–200, 1956.

67. JXA: X009–01–010, 1957.

68. Ibid.

69. Lü Liang, "Xu," 3; SMA: B242–1-816, 11/1955.

70. JXA: X039–03–432, 1/1957–12/1957.

71. Ibid.

72. JXA: X009–01–010, 1957.

73. JXA: X039–01–571, 1959.

74. "Jiangxi sheng xuexichongbing ji," in *Song wenshen jishi,* ed. Liu and Wan, 221.

3. DENYING ECONOMIC RESPONSIBILITY WHILE BRANDISHING AN EMPTY PURSE

1. Luo Chengqing, "Songzou wenshen zhanhongtu—wei min zaofu shi qianqiu—ji Fang Zhichun tongzhi lingdao xiaomie xuexichongbing gongzuo pianduan," in *Song wenshen jishi,* vol. 43, ed. Liu Yurui and Wan Guohe (Nanchang: Jiangxi sheng zhengxie wenshi ziliao yanjiu weiyuanhui, 1992), 10. One mu is one-fifteenth of a hectare.

2. "Resolving the Problem of the 'Five Excesses'" (March 19, 1953), in *The Writings of Mao Zedong, 1949–1976,* ed. Michael Kau and John Leung, vol. 1 (Armonk, NY: M. E. Sharpe, 1986), 337.

3. QPA: 95–2-12, 12/1954.

4. SMA: A71-2-465, 5/3/1956–12/22/1956. Campaign work could most conveniently be done during the slack season. However, because snails hid underground during the winter and summer, they had to be eliminated in the spring or fall in direct competition with production.

5. Zhonggeng Jiangxi sheng weifangzhi xuexichongbing wuxiaozu banggongshi bianxie, *Yujiang xian shi zenyang genzhi xuexichongbing de* (Nanchang: Jiangxi renmin chubanshe, 1958), 20.

6. Wu Zaocun, "Feng zheng jin zu qu wenshen," in *Song wenshen jishi,* ed. Liu and Wan, 125.

7. JSA: 3119, 1017, duanqi, 4/4/1963–1/12/1964; JXA: X111–02–201, 2/1957.

8. QPA: 95-2-85, 1/19/1962.

9. Vivienne Shue, *The Reach of the State: Sketches of the Chinese Body Politic* (Stanford, CA: Stanford University Press, 1988), 67, 107–8.

10. JSA: 3119, 75, yongjiu, 1964.

11. David M. Lampton, *Health, Conflict, and the Chinese Political System,* Michigan Papers in Chinese Studies No. 18 (Ann Arbor: University of Michigan, 1974), 18–19.

12. JSA: 3235, 145, changqi, 7/30/1954–4/16/1957.

13. SMA: B242-1-1090, 11/1957–4/1958.

14. JXA: X001–03–079, 1957.

15. YJA: 8, 1–12/1955.

16. YJA: 28, 1963.

17. JSA: 3119, 231, changqi, 6/23/1956.

18. YJA: 12, 1956.

19. JXA: X035–04–567, 1956; JXA: X111–02–201, 2/1957, 156 (quotation).

20. JXA: X001–01–403, 1–9/1957.

21. JXA: X009–01–010, 1957.

22. QPA: 95-2-76, 1961; YJA: 26, 1–12/1963.

23. SMA: A50-1-12, 1956; SMA: Q243-1-658, 1951.

24. JXA: X001–01–403, 1–9/1957.

25. YJA: 2, 4–11/1953.

26. YJA: 12, 1956.

27. QPA: 95-1-12, 1956; Yu Laixi and Zhonggong Yujiang xianwei xuefang lingdao xiaozu bangongshi, *Jiangxi sheng Yujiang xian xuefang zhi: 1953–1980* (Yujiang: Zhonggong Yujiang xianwei xuefang lingdao xiaozu bangongshi, 1984), 72; QPA: 95-2-108, 1965 (quotation).

28. YJA: 30, 1964; JSA: 3119, 198, duanqi, 3/1/1956–12/19/1956.

29. QPA: 95-1-15, 1957.

30. Ibid.; QPA: 95-2-76, 1961; JXA: X009–01–010, 1957; Yu Laixi and Zhonggong Yujiang xianwei xuefang lingdao xiaozu bangongshi, *Jiangxi sheng Yujiang xian xuefang zhi,* 72 (quotation).

31. YJA: 13, 1–12/1957 (quotation); JXA: X009–01–010, 1957.

32. JXA: X039–04–421, 11/27/1965–12/26/1966; SMA: B242-1-1174, 8–12/1959.

33. Wang Zude, Chen Zhengxuan, Wang Bosheng, and Bianzhuan weiyuanhui bian, *Shanghai nongye zhi* (Shanghai: Shanghai Shehui kexueyuan, 1996), 102; Mao Huiren, Li Guifa, and Jiangxi sheng Yujiang xian xianzhi bianzuan weiyuanhui bianji, *Yujiang xianzhi* (Nanchang: Jiangxi renmin chubanshe, 1993), 660; *Jiangsu sheng nongcun jingji 50 nian* (Beijing: Zhongguo tongji chubanshe, 2000), 115; QPA: 95-2-27, 1956.

34. SMA: B3–2-78, 1/21/1956–12/11/1956.

35. QPA: 95–2-2, 10/25/1952.

36. JSA: 3119, 198, duanqi, 3/1/1956–12/19/1956.

37. JSA: 3119, 231, changqi, 6/23/1956.

38. SMA: B242–1-1011, 1–11/1957; YJA: 25, 1962.

39. JSA: 3119, 231, changqi, 6/23/1956.

40. QPA: 95–1-6, 1954.

41. JXA: X035–03–724, 1957.

42. JSA: 3119, 231, changqi, 6/23/1956.

43. QPA: 95–2-7, 1953.

44. SMA: Q244–1-290, 1–7/1952.

45. SMA: B242–1-1011, 1–11/1957. It is possible that such a directive existed but was not found in the archives.

46. SMA: Q244–1-290, 1–7/1952; QPA: 95–1-2, 1–10/1952.

47. QPA: 95–1-11, 1–12/1956.

48. YJA: 10, 1–12/1956.

49. JXA: X111–02–268, 1957.

50. JSA: 3119, 198, duanqi, 3/1/1956–12/19/1956.

51. JXA: X035–04–567, 1956; JXA: X035–03–440, 1956.

52. United clinics *(lianhe zhensuo)* were composed of previous private practitioners of Chinese medicine forced by the government into cooperative work. During this transitional period, some doctors evaded the clinics and retained a private practice.

53. QPA: 95–2-9, 1953.

54. QPA: 95–2-19, 1955; YJA: 6, 1954.

55. JSA: 3119, 198, duanqi, 3/1/1956–12/19/1956 (quotation); William Y. Chen, "Medicine and Public Health," in *Sciences in Communist China: A Symposium Presented at the New York Meeting of the American Association for the Advancement of Science, December 26–27, 1960*, ed. Sidney H. Gamble (Washington, D.C.: American Association for the Advancement of Science, 1961), 399; QPA: 95–1-15, 1957.

56. JXA: X035–03–440, 1956.

57. JSA: 3119, 231, changqi, 6/23/1956 (quotation); S. M. Hillier and J. A. Jewell, *Health Care and Traditional Medicine in China, 1800–1982* (London: Routledge & Kegan Paul, 1983), 107.

58. Ibid. (both sources).

59. Ibid.

60. JSA: 3119, 232, changqi, 5/25/1956–7/21/1956.

61. "Directive on Work in Traditional Chinese Medicine" (July 30, 1954) and "Implementing the Correct Policy in Dealing with Doctors of Traditional Chinese

Medicine" (October 20, 1954), in *Writings of Mao Zedong,* ed. Kau and Leung, vol. 1, 464–66, 486–91; "RMRB Editorial on Cultivating Traditional Chinese Medicine" (May 27, 1956), in *The Writings of Mao Zedong, 1949–1976,* ed. Michael Kau and John Leung, vol. 2(Armonk, NY: M.E. Sharpe, 1992), 77–79.

62. QPA: 95-2-27, 1956; JXA: X035–04–802, 1956; SMA: B242–1-1017, 4–6/1957.

63. JXA: X035–04–802, 1956.

64. YJA: 6, 1954; SMA: A23-2-499, 4–12/1959; QPA: 95-2-19, 1955; QPA: 95-2-85, 1/19/1962. Some doctors also earned money by providing illegal birth control pills and abortions and false certificates of illness so that people could stay home and work on their private plots. Michael B. Frolic, *Mao's People: Sixteen Portraits of Life in Revolutionary China* (Cambridge, MA: Harvard University Press, 1980), 221.

65. JSA: 3119, 231, changqi, 6/23/1956.

66. Ibid.

67. JSA: 3119, 418, duanqi, 2/28/1957–12/18/1957.

68. QPA: 95-1-10, 1956–1958; JSA: 3119, 231, changqi, 6/23/1956 (quotation).

69. QPA: 95-1-10, 1956–1958; JXA: X009–01–010, 1957.

70. It is unclear when Jiangxi's subsidy started: a November 1957 report suggests one was needed and a June 1958 report listed one in place. JXA: X001–03–079, 1957; JXA: X039–01–571, 1959; JXA: X035–04–802, 1956.

71. JSA: 3119, 525, duanqi, 2/9/1958–1/1959.

72. QPA: 95-2-76, 1961; QPA: 95-1-28, 1962; Mao Zhixiao, "Wo canjia song-wenshen de licheng (Guangfeng)," in *Song wenshen jishi,* ed. Liu and Wan, 38.

73. JSA: 3119, 1017, duanqi, 4/4/1963–1/12/1964.

74. Ibid.

75. JXA: X035–05–539, 1966. To receive reimbursement for supplying free treatment, each medical institution would submit expenses to its own level in the hierarchy (i.e., a county-level institution would submit to the county health department). The first year of the mandate, health departments had these bills covered by their level's general budget office. After that, when areas submitted their general annual budget, they included a request for funds to cover predicted amounts of treatment. This bill would ultimately be paid by the national government. JXA: X039–04–421, 11/27/1965–12/26/1966.

76. SMA: B242-3-72, 1–9/1968.

77. Ibid.

78. JXA: X111–04–052, 1951; Yu Laixi and Zhonggong Yujiang xianwei xuefang lingdao xiaozu bangongshi, *Jiangxi sheng Yujiang xian xuefang zhi,* 22, 41.

79. Li Junjiu, "Diyi mian hongqi shi zenyang chashang de," in *Song wenshen jishi,* ed. Liu and Wan; YJA: 17, 1–12/1959; Yu Laixi and Zhonggong Yujiang xianwei xuefang lingdao xiaozu bangongshi, *Jiangxi sheng Yujiang xian xuefang zhi,* 86, 133.

80. Yu Laixi and Zhonggong Yujiang xianwei xuefang lingdao xiaozu bangongshi, *Jiangxi sheng Yujiang xian xuefang zhi,* 41.

81. Ibid., 41, 52; JXA: X035–06–514, 1958; YJA: 9, 1–12/1956; Li Junjiu, "Diyi mian hongqi shi zenyang chashang de," 97 (quotation); JXA: X111–02–269, 12/1957,

p. 20. Not all of Yujiang's township-level cadres supported the campaign. But because they were forced to attend county-level meetings with the energetic Party secretary monthly, they could not go too far astray. Yu Laixi and Zhonggong Yujiang xianwei xuefang lingdao xiaozu bangongshi, *Jiangxi sheng Yujiang xian xuefang zhi,* 52.

82. Zou Huayi, *Kuayue siwang didai* (Nanchang: Baihuazhou wenyi chubanshe, 1993), 88–89.

83. Yu Laixi and Zhonggong Yujiang xianwei xuefang lingdao xiaozu bangongshi, *Jiangxi sheng Yujiang xian xuefang zhi,* 20; JXA: X111–02–269, 12/1957, 19.

84. While archives from Yujiang and Jiangxi agree on the number of people who became ill, one dates the illnesses to 1953–54, the other to 1954–55. YJA: 7, 1955; JXA: X111–03–089, 1959.

85. YJA: 28, 1963.

86. JXA: X111–03–089, 1959; YJA: 7, 1955; Li Junjiu, "Diyi mian hongqi shi zenyang chashang de," 97.

87. JXA: X111–02–269, 12/1957, 21.

88. Sun Yongjiu, "Gonggu chengguo ying nan er shang; ba xuefang hongqi ju de genggao," in *Song wenshen jishi,* ed. Liu and Wan, 103.

89. Ibid., 110.

90. Ibid., 108.

91. Ibid., 110.

92. YJA: 41, 1–12/1973.

93. As of 1995, 51 percent of Jiangxi's original infectious counties had eliminated the disease, 20 percent had brought it under control, and 29 percent had still not controlled the disease. Zhong Zubiao and Jiangxi sheng jiachu xuexichongbing fangzhi zhan, *Jiangxi sheng jiachu xuefang zhi: 1956–1996* (Nanchang: Jiangxi sheng jiachu xuexichongbing fangzhi zhan, 1989), 82.

4. BUILDING THE NEW SCIENTIFIC SOCIALIST SOCIETY

1. The chapter epigraph is from Wei Wen-po [Wei Wenbo], "The People's Boundless Energy during the Current Leap Forward: New Victories on the Anti-schistosomiasis Front," *Chinese Medical Journal* 77 (1958): 108.

2. For a full discussion of the incorporation of science into China's political philosophy and its transformation into scientism, see D. W. Y. Kwok, *Scientism in Chinese Thought, 1900–1950* (New Haven, CT: Yale University Press, 1965).

3. Maurice Meisner, "Leninism and Maoism: Some Populist Perspective on Marxism-Leninism in China," in *Marxism Maoism and Utopianism: Eight Essays* (Madison: University of Wisconsin Press, 1982), 96. This essay provides a wider discussion of the populist elements in Marxism.

4. "Sixty Points on Working Methods—a Draft Resolution from the Office of the Centre of the CPC" (February 2, 1958), in *Selected Works of Mao Tse-tung,* vol. 8, www.marxists.org/reference/archive/mao/selected-works/index.htm. (accessed April 22, 2010).

5. JSA: 3119, 525, duanqi, 2/9/1958–1/1959.

6. "Methods of Work of Party Committees" (March 13, 1949) and "Sixty Points on Working Methods" (February 2, 1958), in *Selected Works of Mao Tse-tung,* vols. 4, 8; C. H. G. Oldham, "Science and Technology Policies," *Proceedings of the Academy of Political Science* 31.1 (March 1973): 91; Gardel MacArthur Feurtado, "Mao Tse-tung and the Politics of Science in Communist China, 1949–1965" (Ph.D. diss., Stanford University, 1986), 46.

7. QPA: 95-1-2, 1–10/1952; JXA: X035–04–802, 1956. A special bureau to disseminate scientific ideas was developed, but it was more effective in urban areas. Sigrid Schmalzer, *The People's Peking Man: Popular Science and Human Identity in Twentieth-Century China* (Chicago: University of Chicago Press, 2008), 62–66.

8. SMA: Q244–1-290, 1–7/1952.

9. YJA: 5, 1–12/1954; Li Zhenglan, compiled by Ning Haisheng, "Wo canjia xuefang kepu gongzuo," in *Song wenshen jishi,* vol. 43, ed. Liu Yurui and Wan Guohe (Nanchang: Jiangxi sheng zhengxie wenshi ziliao yanjiu weiyuanhui, 1992), 133.

10. Yu Laixi and Zhonggong Yujiang xianwei xuefang lingdao xiaozu bangongshi, *Jiangxi sheng Yujiang xian xuefang zhi: 1953–1980* (Yujiang: Zhonggong Yujiang xianwei xuefang lingdao xiaozu bangongshi, 1984), 44; Li Zhenglan, "Wo canjia xuefang kepu gongzuo," 133; QPA: 95-1-2, 1–10/1952.

11. Zheng Junli, dir., *Kumu feng chun* (Shanghai: Haiyan Film, 1961).

12. QPA: 95-2-20, 1/29/1955; JXA: X009–01–010, 1957; H. F. Hsu and Li S. Y. Hsu, "Schistosomiasis in the Shanghai Area," *China Medicine as We Saw It,* ed. Joseph R. Quinn and John E. Fogarty International Center, DHEW Publication No. (NIH) 75–684 (Washington, D.C.: U.S. Department of Health, Education, and Welfare, 1974), 349.

13. YJA: 16, 1958.

14. YJA: 3, 1954; Li Zhenglan, "Wo canjia xuefang kepu gongzuo," 134; QPA: 95–1-2, 1–10/1952.

15. QPA: 95-2-19, 1955 (quotations); Yu Laixi and Zhonggong Yujiang xianwei xuefang lingdao xiaozu bangongshi, *Jiangxi sheng Yujiang xian xuefang zhi,* 44.

16. SMA: B34–2-195, 1954; QPA: 95-2-4, 1952.

17. YJA: 10, 1–12/1956.

18. Yu Laixi and Zhonggong Yujiang xianwei xuefang lingdao xiaozu bangongshi, *Jiangxi sheng Yujiang xian xuefang zhi,* 44. In some cases, even pictures of exciting new technology were enough to draw attention. For example, an article about Wucheng's snail fever work in Jiangxi prominently displays a movie projector, rather than anything directly related to the campaign, to entice people to read the story. "Wuchengzhen de xuexichongbing fangzhi xiaozu," *Jiangxi ribao,* no. 2341, December 3, 1955, 3.

19. Wang Ximeng, *Shanghai xiaomie xuexichongbing de huigu* (Shanghai: Shanghai kexue jishu chubanshe, 1988), 10.

20. "Boyang xuefang zhan yijia dang san jia: Jiejue xianweijing buzu de kunnan," *Jiangxi ribao,* no. 3221, May 15, 1958.

21. Wang Ximeng, *Shanghai xiaomie xuexichongbing de huigu,* 10; YJA: 6, 1954 (quotation); QPA: 95–1-10, 1956–1958.

22. "On Practice" (July 1937), in *Selected Works of Mao Tse-tung,* vol. 1.

23. Shangrao Prevention Station, "Xiaomie weihai renmin jiankang de xuexichongbing," in *Shangrao shi wenshi ziliao,* vol. 9 (Jiangxi: Zhengxie Shangrao Shi weiyuanhui wenshi ziliao bangongshi, 1989), 171–72.

24. Yu Laixi and Zhonggong Yujiang xianwei xuefang lingdao xiaozu bangongshi, *Jiangxi sheng Yujiang xian xuefang zhi,* 44; Wang Ximeng, *Shanghai xiaomie xuexichongbing de huigu,* 10; QPA: 95–1-10, 1956–1958.

25. Li Zhenglan, "Wo canjia xuefang kepu gongzuo," 133.

26. S.M. Hillier and J.A. Jewell, *Health Care and Traditional Medicine in China, 1800–1982* (London: Routledge & Kegan Paul, 1983), 170.

27. John Harland Reed, "Brass Butterflies of the Thoughts of Mao Tsetung: The Sociology of Schistosomiasis Control in China" (Ph.D. diss., Cornell University, 1979), 173.

28. Yu Laixi and Zhonggong Yujiang xianwei xuefang lingdao xiaozu bangongshi, *Jiangxi sheng Yujiang xian xuefang zhi,* 44; QPA: 95–1-10, 1956–1958.

29. Wang Lun, "Xuefang zhanzhang," *Jiangxi ribao,* October 5, 1957, 3.

30. QPA: 95–1-6, 1954; YJA: 3, 1954.

31. QPA: 95–1-10, 1956–1958.

32. Exhibits with microscopes successfully explained scientific ideas for other diseases too. A Qingpu villager thought his child's death a few days postpartum was due to a lock being moved, a syndrome called *suokou zheng.* After attending a 1954 Qingpu exhibit on midwifery, he realized that the death was due to umbilical tetanus and that his wife needed to use new birthing methods. QPA: 95–2-11, 1954–1955.

33. JSA: 3119, 1017, duanqi, 4/4/1963–1/12/1964.

34. QPA: 95–1-10, 1956–1958.

35. QPA: 95–2-4, 1952.

36. JSA: 3235, 41, yongjiu, 3/26/1951–4/18/1957.

37. SMA: B34-2-195, 1954.

38. QPA: 95–2-4, 1952 (quotation); QPA: 95–1-29, 1/3/1962.

39. QPA: 95–2-7, 1953.

40. Zhonggeng Jiangxi sheng weifangzhi xuexichongbing wuxiaozu banggongshi bianxie, *Yujiang xian shi zenyang genzhi xuexichongbing de* (Nanchang: Jiangxi renmin chubanshe, 1958), 11.

41. C.C. Chen, *Medicine in Rural China: A Personal Account* (Berkeley: University of California Press, 1989), 132.

42. JXA: X035-04-802, 1956 (quotation); Zhonggeng Jiangxi, *Yujiang xian shi zenyang genzhi xuexichongbing de,* 20.

43. YJA: 40, 1-12/1973.

44. H. Kristian Heggenhougen, Veronica Hackethal, and Pramila Vivek, *The Behavioral and Social Aspects of Malaria and Its Control: An Introduction and Annotated Bibliography* (Geneva: World Health Organization, 2003), 44 (quotation);

Deborah L. Helitzer-Allen, Carl Kendall, and Jack J. Wirima, "The Role of Ethnographic Research in Malaria Control: An Example from Malaŵi," *Research in the Sociology of Health Care* 10 (1993): 279–80.

45. Zhonggong zhongyang fangzhi xuexichongbing jiuren xiaozu bangongshi, *Song wenshen* (Shanghai: Shanghai wenyi chubanshe, 1961), 4; Lü Qizuo, "Ganzou wenshen," *Jiankang bao,* no. 695, November 26, 1958, 2; QPA: 95–2-19, 1955 (quotation).

46. For a detailed discussion, see Edwin Joseph Allen Jr., "Disease Control in China: An Investigation into the Ways In Which Public Health Propaganda Effects Changes in Medicine and Hygiene, with Emphasis on Schistosomiasis Control" (master's thesis, Columbia University, 1965), 56–57; Wei Wen-po, "People's Boundless Energy during the Current Leap Forward," 109; Zhonggeng Jiangxi, *Yujiang xian shi zenyang genzhi xuexichongbing de,* 29, 32; JSA: 3119, 231, changqi, 6/23/1956; JSA: 3119, 525, duanqi, 2/9/1958–1/1959.

47. QPA: 95–2-19, 1955. For a wider discussion of Mao's campaigns as wars on nature, see Judith Shapiro, *Mao's War against Nature: Politics and the Environment in Revolutionary China* (Cambridge: Cambridge University Press, 2001).

48. QPA: 95–1-12, 1956 (quotation); SMA: B3–1-16, 1/31/1956–9/25/1956.

49. Shanghai shi aiguo weisheng yundong weiyuanhui bangongshi, *Chu qi hai* (Shanghai: Shaonian ertong chubanshe, 1958); Wang Qingyuan, "Shi xuexichongbing fangzhi gongzuo yu aiguo weisheng yundong jiehe qilai," *Jiankang bao,* no. 412, November 25, 1955, 3.

50. Reed, "Brass Butterflies," 52; Li Junjiu, "Diyi mian hongqi shi zenyang chashang de," in *Song wenshen jishi,* ed. Liu and Wan, 98.

51. The New Culture Movement was a transformative domestic development that encouraged China to embark on broad social, cultural, and political change.

52. JXA: X001–01–403, 1–9/1957; Wei Wen-po, "People's Boundless Energy during the Current Leap Forward," 108.

53. SMA: B242–1-816, 11/1955.

54. JXA: X001–01–403, 1–9/1957.

55. Bu qiu shenxian zhi qiu yi, *Qingpu bao,* no. 9, August 11, 1956, 2 (quotations); QPA: 95–2-12, 12/1954.

56. JSA: 3119, 1017, duanqi, 4/4/1963–1/12/1964.

57. JXA: X009–01–010, 1957; Wang Ximeng, *Shanghai xiaomie xuexichongbing de huigu,* 11; JSA: 3119, 525, duanqi, 2/9/1958–1/1959.

58. Hubei sheng weisheng ting, *Xuexichong bing fangzhi zhishi jianghua* (Wuhan: Hubei sheng weisheng ting, 1966), 7. One jin is 1.1 pounds.

59. QPA: 95–2-85, 1/19/1962.

60. JXA: X111–05–345, 1963.

61. QPA: 95–1-10, 1956–1958.

62. QPA: 95–1-12, 1956.

63. JSA: 3119, 231, changqi, 6/23/1956 (quotation); QPA: 95–2-21, 12/1955.

64. QPA: 95–2-108, 1965. Eventually, the campaign established statistical benchmarks that were quality based, making this tool more helpful.

65. SMA: B3–1-16, 1/31/1956–9/25/1956.

66. "Qingpu xian xiaomie xuexichongbing jiangli banfa (caoan)," *Qingpu bao,* no. 207, August 7, 1958, 3; Schmalzer, *People's Peking Man,* 127; "Quanguo gedi honghong lielie daban kexue shiye," *Qingpu bao,* no. 188, June 26, 1958, 4. Qingpu's model workers, who had to be "people who create inventions," received a gold-tipped fountain pen, an enamel cup, a commemorative diary, and a certificate of merit. "Qingpu xian xiaomie xuexichongbing jiangli banfa (caoan)," *Qingpu bao,* no. 207, August 7, 1958, 3.

67. Wang Ximeng, *Shanghai xiaomie xuexichongbing de huigu,* 10 (quotation); Zou Huayi, *Kuayue siwang didai* (Nanchang: Baihuazhou wenyi chubanshe, 1993), 66.

68. SMA: A71-2-465, 5/3/1956–12/22/1956; Reed, "Brass Butterflies," 145.

69. Yu Laixi, "Yi fenguan laoren Wan Fengxin," in *Song wenshen jishi,* ed. Liu and Wan, 121–24.

70. JXA: X035–06–689, 1959 (quotation); Reed, "Brass Butterflies," 154.

71. YJA: 16, 1958 (quotation); YJA: 3, 1954.

72. SMA: Q243–1-658, 1951 (quotation); *Xue xianjin gan xianjin xianjin geng xianjin chu sihai, xiaomie xuexichongbing jingyan* (Nanchang: Jiangxi renmin chubanshe, 1958), 19.

73. QPA: 95–1-6, 1954.

74. QPA: 95–1-12, 1956.

75. Joshua Horn, *Away With All Pests: An English Surgeon in People's China, 1954–1969* (New York: Monthly Review Press, 1969), 98–99.

76. JXA: X111–02–269, 12/1957.

77. Mao Zhixiao, "Wo canjia songwenshen de licheng (Guangfeng)," in *Song wenshen jishi,* ed. Liu and Wan, 34.

78. QPA: 95–2-2, 10/25/1952; QPA: 95–1-4, 1953; JXA: X111–04–052, 1951; Mao Zhixiao, "Xuefang Jishi," in *Guangfeng xian wenshi ziliao,* vol. 3 (Guangfeng xian: Zhongguo renmin zhengzhi xieshang huiyi Jiangxi sheng Guangfeng xian wenshi ziliao yanjiu weiyuanhui, 1989), 17. Military framing in health campaigns was probably also due to many grassroots cadres' pre-1949 background in the Red Army. Franz Schurmann, *Ideology and Organization in Communist China* (Berkeley: University of California Press, 1968), 237.

79. SMA: B242–1-816, 11/1955; Yang Daozheng, "Qumo you dang yizhi jian yin chu pikai xin tiandi (Fengxin)," in *Song wenshen jishi,* ed. Liu and Wan, 17 (quotations).

80. Chekiang, Chia-shan Hsien, Anti-epidemic Station Revolutionary Leading Group, "As Chairman Mao Directs, We Follow: How Schistosomiasis in Jiashan County Was Wiped Out by 'People's War,'" *China's Medicine* 10 (October 1968): 607 ("annihilation" quotation); Mao Zhixiao, "Wo canjia songwenshen de licheng (Guangfeng)," 37 (other quotations).

81. Li Junjiu, "Diyi mian hongqi shi zenyang chashang de," 101 ("combat" quotation); Yang Daozheng, "Qumo you dang yizhi jian yin chu pikai xin tiandi (Fengxin)," 18 (other quotations).

82. Yang Daozheng, "Qumo you dang yizhi jian yin chu pikai xin tiandi (Fengxin)," 18.

83. Mao Zhixiao, "Wo canjia songwenshen de licheng (Guangfeng)," 37–38; Yu Laixi, "Yujiang renmin fangzhi xuexichongbing de weida douzheng," in *Song wenshen jishi,* ed. Liu and Wan, 4 (quotation). Susan Greenhalgh notes that birth planning was also framed militarily as threat control, which was a way to transfer "military values and institutions into the civilian sector." Susan Greenhalgh, *Just One Child: Science and Policy in Deng's China* (Berkeley: University of California Press, 2008), 332.

84. Kenneth Lieberthal, *Governing China: From Revolution through Reform* (New York: W. W. Norton & Company, 1995), 68–70; Gordon Bennett, *Yundong: Mass Campaigns in Chinese Communist Leadership,* China Research Monograph No. 12 (Berkeley: Center for Chinese Studies, University of California, 1976), 43–44; Anita Chan, Richard Madsen, and Jonathan Unger, *Chen Village: The Recent History of a Peasant Community in Mao's China* (Berkeley: University of California Press, 1984), 41–64.

85. YJA: 31, 1965; YJA: 29, 1–12/1964. Perhaps this is another reason why pictures of germs and diseases during this era portray them as evil people.

86. JXA: X009–01–010, 1957.

87. QPA: 95–1-6, 1954.

88. SMA: A71–2-465, 5/3/1956–12/22/1956.

89. JXA: X009–01–010, 1957; YJA: 13, 1–12/1957; YJA: 14, 1–12/1957; Yu Laixi and Zhonggong Yujiang xianwei xuefang lingdao xiaozu bangongshi, *Jiangxi sheng Yujiang xian xuefang zhi,* 56.

90. QPA: 95–2-44, 1958.

91. Over many decades and increasing education levels, the community consensus about appropriate habits changed. While the snail fever campaign contributed to this evolution, in the 1950s and 1960s a new consensus had yet to emerge.

92. QPA: 95–2-4, 1952.

93. QPA: 95–1-2, 1–10/1952; Li Junjiu, "Diyi mian hongqi shi zenyang chashang de," 100 (quotation); Sun Yongjiu, "Gonggu chengguo ying nan er shang; ba xuefang hongqi ju de genggao," in *Song wenshen jishi,* ed. Liu and Wan, 104–5.

94. Y. Komiya, "Recommendatory Note for the Control Problem of Schistosomiasis in China," *Japanese Journal of Medical Science and Biology* 10.6 (1957): 465.

95. Once revolutionary spirit ebbed in the early 1960s, some places gave a monetary award. In 1964, Yujiang gave people three to five yuan for every snail. This strategy was only possible in places with few snails and an impressive campaign budget. YJA: 31, 1965; YJA: 29, 1–12/1964.

96. Bennett, *Yundong,* 79.

97. JXA: X035–06–689, 1959. For a fuller discussion, see Chalmers Johnson, "Chinese Communist Leadership and Mass Response: The Yenan Period and the Socialist Education Period," in *China in Crisis: China's Heritage and the Communist Political System,* ed. Ping-ti Ho and Tang Tsou (Chicago: University of Chicago Press, 1968), 397–437; Bennett, *Yundong.*

1. JXA: X111–02–200, 1956 (first quotation); JXA: X035–04–800, 1956 (second quotation).

2. Joshua Horn, *Away With All Pests: An English Surgeon in People's China, 1954–1969* (New York: Monthly Review Press, 1969), 94–106; Victor W. Sidel and Ruth Sidel, *Serve the People: Observations on Medicine in the People's Republic of China* (Boston: Beacon Press, 1974), 103–6; David M. Lampton, *Health, Conflict, and the Chinese Political System,* Michigan Papers in Chinese Studies No. 18 (Ann Arbor: University of Michigan, 1974); David M. Lampton, *The Politics of Medicine in China: The Policy Process, 1949–1977* (Boulder, CO: Westview Press, 1977); "Report of the American Schistosomiasis Delegation to the People's Republic of China," *American Journal of Tropical Medicine and Hygiene* 26.3 (1977): 431; China Health Care Study Group, *Health Care in China, an Introduction: The Report of a Study Group in Hong Kong* (Geneva: Christian Medical Commission, 1974), 60, 67–71; F. R. Sandbach, "Farewell to the God of Plague—the Control of Schistosomiasis in China," *Social Science and Medicine* 11 (1977): 27–33; Iijima Wataru, "'Farewell to the God of Plague': Anti-*Schistosoma japonicum* Campaign in China and Japanese Colonial Medicine," *Memoirs of the Toyo Bunko* 66 (2008): 67.

3. SMA: Q244-1-290, 1–7/1952.

4. QPA: 95–1-6, 1954.

5. QPA: 95–1-1, 3/1951; JXA: X009–01–010, 1957; YJA: 40, 1–12/1973.

6. Li Zhisui, *The Private Life of Chairman Mao* (New York: Random House, 1994), 158 (quotation); Yu Laixi and Zhonggong Yujiang xianwei xuefang lingdao xiaozu bangongshi, *Jiangxi sheng Yujiang xian xuefang zhi: 1953–1980* (Yujiang: Zhonggong Yujiang xianwei xuefang lingdao xiaozu bangongshi, 1984), 49.

7. SMA: C1–2-2716, 1/10/1958–8/19/1958. The belief that feces was a natural part of the environment also meant that populations with little snail fever saw no reason to stop washing out commodes in the drinking water. QPA: 95–2-117, 1965–1966.

8. Friedrich Engels, "The Part Played by Labour in the Transition from Ape to Man," in *Dialectics of Nature,* trans. and ed. Clemens Dutt (New York: International Publishers, 1940), 279.

9. YJA: 6, 1954; YJA: 40, 1–12/1973.

10. Yu Laixi and Zhonggong Yujiang xianwei xuefang lingdao xiaozu bangongshi, *Jiangxi sheng Yujiang xian xuefang zhi,* 71.

11. QPA: 95–2-13, 12/1954.

12. QPA: 95–1-1, 3/1951.

13. SMA: Q249–1-138, 12/31/1951–4/8/1952; JXA: X035–04–802, 1956 (quotation).

14. QPA: 95–1-1, 3/1951.

15. YJA: 40, 1–12/1973. Disinterest in the sanitation-oriented Patriotic Public Health Campaigns was a province-wide phenomenon. Jiangxi Province's 1956 annual PPHC report stated that in the prior year "the provincial Patriotic Public Health Committee has not met once. They have not communicated or summarized

their experience nor given enough concrete guidance. Some of the lower-level committees exist in form only, with nobody to take an interest in the work." JXA: X009–01–010, 1957.

16. YJA: 4, 1954; Yu Laixi and Zhonggong Yujiang xianwei xuefang lingdao xiaozu bangongshi, *Jiangxi sheng Yujiang xian xuefang zhi,* 49 (quotation).

17. JXA: X111–02–201, 2/1957, 262.

18. Yu Laixi and Zhonggong Yujiang xianwei xuefang lingdao xiaozu bangongshi, *Jiangxi sheng Yujiang xian xuefang zhi,* 49.

19. YJA: 38, 1–12/1972.

20. YJA: 1, 1953.

21. SMA: C1–2-2716, 1/10/1958–8/19/1958; YJA: 6, 1954.

22. QPA: 95–2-6, 12/1953; JXA: X111–02–200, 1956.

23. JXA: X111–02–200, 1956.

24. QPA: 95–2-6, 12/1953.

25. YJA: 23, 1–12/1962; JXA: X111–02–201, 2/1957, 261; Zhonggeng Jiangxi sheng weifangzhi xuexichongbing wuxiaozu banggongshi bianxie, *Yujiang xian shi zenyang genzhi xuexichongbing de* (Nanchang: Jiangxi renmin chubanshe, 1958), 21.

26. SMA: B242–1-815, 11/1955.

27. YJA: 44, p. 84.

28. SMA: Q249–1-138, 12/31/1951–4/8/1952.

29. QPA: 95–2-4, 1952; SMA: Q249–1-138, 12/31/1951–4/8/1952.

30. QPA: 95–2-4, 1952. In 1955, the new currency was exchanged with the old using a 10,000:1 ratio.

31. Ibid.

32. Zou Huayi, *Kuayue siwang didai* (Nanchang: Baihuazhou wenyi chubanshe, 1993), 120–23 (quotation p. 122).

33. Sun Yongjiu, "Gonggu chengguo ying nan er shang; ba xuefang hongqi ju de genggao," in *Song wenshen jishi,* vol. 43, ed. Liu Yurui and Wan Guohe (Nanchang: Jiangxi sheng zhengxie wenshi ziliao yanjiu weiyuanhui, 1992), 109–10.

34. Yu Laixi and Zhonggong Yujiang xianwei xuefang lingdao xiaozu bangongshi, *Jiangxi sheng Yujiang xian xuefang zhi,* 123.

35. Sun Yongjiu, "Gonggu chengguo ying nan er shang," 109–10.

36. The epigraph is from Yu Laixi and Zhonggong Yujiang xianwei xuefang lingdao xiaozu bangongshi, *Jiangxi sheng Yujiang xian xuefang zhi,* 71.

37. SMA: C31–2-532, 3/3/1957–12/12/1957.

38. Ibid.

39. QPA: 95–1-1, 3/1951. While evidence is sparse, densely packed villages in the Shanghai region, familiar with commodes cleaned daily, tended to list dirt as the factor keeping them from the public toilets; scattered villages in Jiangxi, accustomed to filthy private pit toilets, tended to list distance as the reason for avoiding public toilets. YJA: 10, 1–12/1956; JXA: X111–02–201, 2/1957, 262; QPA: 95–2-12, 12/1954.

40. It is unknown whether many places in China had this job or whether proximity to Shanghai—where many people worked full-time processing households'

commodes—had sparked the idea in its suburbs. As the national test site, Qingpu was able to disseminate this idea. QPA: 95–1-2, 1–10/1952.

41. QPA: 95–1-15, 1957.

42. YJA: 1, 1953; QPA: 95–2-117, 1965–1966; YJA: 9, 1–12/1956.

43. Ernest Faust and Henry Meleney, *Studies on Schistosomiasis Japonica,* Monograph Series No. 3 (Baltimore: American Journal of Hygiene, 1924), 257.

44. YJA: 29, 1–12/1964; QPA: 95–1-12, 1956; JSA: 3119, 231, changqi, 6/23/1956.

45. JSA: 3119, 231, changqi, 6/23/1956.

46. SMA: C31–2-532, 3/3/1957–12/12/1957.

47. QPA: 95–2-75, 1961.

48. QPA: 95–1-15, 1957; QPA: 95–1-12, 1956.

49. YJA: 1, 1953; YJA: 10, 1–12/1956; Yu Laixi and Zhonggong Yujiang xianwei xuefang lingdao xiaozu bangongshi, *Jiangxi sheng Yujiang xian xuefang zhi,* 110–111.

50. QPA: 95–1-6, 1954.

51. Wang Ximeng, *Shanghai xiaomie xuexichongbing de huigu* (Shanghai: Shanghai kexue jishu chubanshe, 1988), 75; QPA: 95–1-11, 1–12/1956 (quotation).

52. QPA: 95–1-6, 1954; QPA: 95–1-15, 1957; QPA: 95–2-20, 1/29/1955. Similar patterns have been observed for treated bed nets, a core part of the global campaign against malaria. African people use the nets for many tasks and purposes, including fishing, which seem more compelling than the nets' putative use against mosquitoes. Sonia Shah, *The Fever: How Malaria Has Ruled Humankind for 500,000 Years* (New York: Sarah Crichton Books, 2010), 226.

53. QPA: 95–1-6, 1954.

54. Wang Ximeng, *Shanghai xiaomie xuexichongbing de huigu,* 6.

55. Ibid., 75.

56. QPA: 95–1-11, 1–12/1956.

57. Ibid.; QPA: 95–1-29, 1/3/1962.

58. YJA: 13, 1–12/1957; YJA: 18, 1–12/1961. Yujiang's sole effort toward fisherfolk recommended following Qingpu's example, but seems to have mandated boat-based commodes without providing funding or monitoring. YJA: 12, 1956.

59. QPA: 95–2-4, 1952.

60. JSA: 3119, 231, changqi, 6/23/1956.

61. JXA: X111–02–201, 2/1957, 262.

62. JXA: X009–01–010, 1957.

63. Ibid.

64. JXA: X035–04–800, 1956; JSA: 3119, 1017, duanqi, 4/4/1963–1/12/1964.

65. For example, see Shanghai Zhongyi xueyuan deng bian, *"Chijiao yisheng" shouce* (Shanghai: Shanghai shi chuban geming zu, 1970), 1–13; William L. Parish and Martin King Whyte, *Village and Family in Contemporary China* (Chicago: University of Chicago Press, 1978), 93.

66. F. R. Sandbach, "The History of Schistosomiasis Research and Policy for Its Control," *Medical History* 20.3 (July 1976): 271, 274.

67. He Lianyin, "Policy Making and Organization in Managing Tropical Diseases in China," *Chinese Medical Journal* 114.7 (2001): 770; H. F. Hsu and Li S. Y.

Hsu, "Schistosomiasis in the Shanghai Area," in *China Medicine as We Saw It,* ed. Joseph R. Quinn and John E. Fogarty International Center, DHEW Publication No. (NIH) 75–684 (Washington, D.C.: U.S. Department of Health, Education, and Welfare, 1974), 356; National Schistosomiasis Research Committee, "Studies on Schistosomiasis Japonica in New China," *Chinese Medical Journal* 78.4 (1959): 371–72.

68. John Farley, *Bilharzia: A History of Imperial Tropical Medicine* (New York: Cambridge University Press, 2003), 269; John Harland Reed, "Brass Butterflies of the Thoughts of Mao Tsetung: The Sociology of Schistosomiasis Control in China" (Ph.D. diss., Cornell University, 1979), 44–49.

69. Farley, *Bilharzia,* 121–22; R.L. Andreano, *"Farewell to the God of Plague":* *The Economic Impact of Parasitic Disease (Schistosomiasis) in Mainland China,* Report No. 3 (Madison, WI: Health Economics Research Center, 1971), 4, 21–22; R.L. Andreano, *More on the God of Plague: Schistosomiasis in Mainland China,* Report No. 7 (Madison, WI: Health Economics Research Center, 1971), 5–7; David Shankman and Qiaoli Liang, "Landscape Changes and Increasing Flood Frequency in China's Poyang Lake Region," *Professional Geographer* 55.4 (2003): 434–45.

70. QPA: 95-1-1, 3/1951; QPA: 95-1-11, 1–12/1956.

71. Yu Laixi and Zhonggong Yujiang xianwei xuefang lingdao xiaozu bangong-shi, *Jiangxi sheng Yujiang xian xuefang zhi,* 48.

72. Shangrao Prevention Station, "Xiaomie weihai renmin jiankang de xuexi-chongbing," in *Shangrao shi wenshi ziliao,* vol. 9 (Jiangxi: Zhengxie Shangrao Shi weiyuanhui wenshi ziliao bangongshi, 1989), 172.

73. SMA: B242-1-816, 11/1955.

74. Proximity to and control over factories also meant that the Shanghai government could assign them to mass-produce specialty items solely for the city's use (such as urea, which sped up egg eradication in fertilizer). SMA: B242-1-816, 11/1955; Hsu and Hsu, "Schistosomiasis in the Shanghai Area," 357.

75. Luo Chengqing, "Songzou wenshen zhanhongtu—wei min zaofu shi qian-qiu—ji Fang Zhichun tongzhi lingdao xiaomie xuexichongbing gongzuo pianduan," in *Song wenshen jishi,* ed. Liu and Wan, 10; Zhonggeng Jiangxi, *Yujiang xian shi zenyang genzhi xuexichongbing de,* 27–28.

76. QPA: 95-1-15, 1957; Wang Ximeng, *Shanghai xiaomie xuexichongbing de huigu,* 69–70.

77. Mao Zhixiao, "Wo canjia songwenshen de licheng (Guangfeng)," *Song wen-shen jishi,* ed. Liu and Wan, 38 (quotation); JXA: X009-01-010, 1957.

78. QPA: 95-1-15, 1957; JSA: 3119, 198, duanqi, 3/1/1956–12/19/1956.

79. JXA: X111-02-201, 2/1957, 113.

80. "First County to Wipe Out Schistosomiasis," *China Reconstructs* (July 17, 1968): 15.

81. QPA: 95-1-15, 1957.

82. Shu Xiangmao, oral history compiled by Lei Yu, "Shouzhan Magang," in *Song wenshen jishi,* ed. Liu and Wan, 115–18.

83. Ibid.

84. Ibid.

85. JXA: X009–01–010, 1957.

86. SMA: A23–2–639, 11/1959–9/1960.

87. Wang Ximeng, *Shanghai xiaomie xuexichongbing de huigu,* 72; QPA: 95–1-12, 1956.

88. JSA: 3119, 418, duanqi, 2/28/1957–12/18/1957.

89. SMA: A71–2–465, 5/3/1956–12/22/1956. This had one unintended consequence. Because urbanites had no prior immunity and were working in infectious zones, many came down with acute disease. Wang Ximeng, *Shanghai xiaomie xuexichongbing de huigu,* 49.

90. JSA: 3119, 231, changqi, 6/23/1956; QPA: 95–1-15, 1957 (quotation).

91. Shangrao Prevention Station, "Xiaomie weihai renmin jiankang de xuexichongbing," 173.

92. Reed, "Brass Butterflies," 45–46; Wei Wen-po [Wei Wenbo], "Battle against Schistosomiasis," translated and reprinted from *Hongqi,* 2 (1960), *Chinese Medical Journal* 80 (1960): 303.

93. JSA: 3119, 75, yongjiu, 1964.

94. QPA: 95–1-29, 1/3/1962; QPA: 95–1-28, 1962; "The Orientation of the Revolution in Medical Education as seen in the Growth of 'Barefoot Doctors': Report of an Investigation from Shanghai," reprinted from *Hongqi,* 3 (1968), *Chinese Medical Journal* 87.10 (1968): 574–75.

95. Qingpu xian fangzhi xuexichongbing sanshiwu nian weiyuanhui, *Qingpu xian fangzhi xuexichongbing sanshiwu nian: Zonglunji* (Shanghai: Shanghai kexue jishu chubanshe, 1987), 48.

96. QPA: 95–2-76, 1961.

97. YJA: 31, 1965.

98. As discussed in the next chapter, acute snail fever broke out because the Great Leap treatment campaign was much more successful than prevention work. As irrigation systems built during the Great Leap spread the disease, newly infectiously naïve individuals encountered the disease and contracted acute snail fever. In Yujiang, reasons why work had to continue postelimination ranged from the biological (we have eliminated the disease, but others have not and the disease is coming from them) to the political ("we still have a strata of enemies and they could intentionally harm society"). YJA: 36, 1–12/1971.

99. YJA: 24, 1–12/1962.

100. YJA: 31, 1965.

101. YJA: 24, 1–12/1962.

102. SMA: B242–1-1315, 9–11/1961.

103. Ibid.

104. JSA: 3119, 1017, duanqi, 4/4/1963–1/12/1964.

105. Shah, *Fever,* 125–27 (quotation); Deborah L. Helitzer-Allen, Carl Kendall, and Jack J. Wirima, "The Role of Ethnographic Research in Malaria Control: An Example from Malaŵi," *Research in the Sociology of Health Care* 10 (1993): 277.

106. Gordon Harrison, *Mosquitoes, Malaria and Man: A History of the Hostilities since 1880* (New York: E. P. Dutton, 1978), 244.

107. Wang Ximeng, *Shanghai xiaomie xuexichongbing de huigu*, 35.

108. Reed, "Brass Butterflies," 60–61 (quotation); JXA: X035–06–689, 1959.

109. YJA: 18, 1–12/1961; QPA: 95-2-75, 1961.

110. Wang Ximeng, *Shanghai xiaomie xuexichongbing de huigu*, 10, 60–63; QPA: 95-2-85, 1/19/1962. Shanghai made similar refinements in methods for processing cattle manure. Researchers discovered that adding pig urine to manure cut the fermentation process from 180 days to 120. Wang Ximeng, *Shanghai xiaomie xuexichongbing de huigu*, 93.

111. Lü Liang, "Xu," in *Song wenshen jishi*, ed. Liu and Wan, 1.

112. JXA: X035–04–802, 1956. This tendency was reinforced by barefoot doctor propaganda books that emphasized the danger of incorporating medically competent people from the landlord class into the new barefoot doctor program. Yang Hsiao, *The Making of a Peasant Doctor* (Peking: Foreign Language Press, 1976), 36.

113. QPA: 95-1-12, 1956.

114. JXA: X009–01–010, 1957 (quotation); JXA: X035–06–514, 1958; YJA: 35, 1–12/1970.

115. Li Junjiu, "Diyi mian hongqi shi zenyang chashang de," in *Song wenshen jishi*, ed. Liu and Wan, 96, 101; Li Zhenglan, "Wo canjia xuefang kepu gongzuo," in *Song wenshen jishi*, ed. Liu and Wan, 133–34.

116. QPA: 95-2-108, 1965.

117. YJA: 40, 1–12/1973.

118. Revolutionary Jiangxi foisted detested prevention activities on those with a bad class background long before the Cultural Revolution. In 1954, according to a snail fever campaign report from Magang Township, Yujiang's test site, because the township was "lacking in labor power," it decided to dispatch all of its landlords and rich peasants to go build toilets. Landlords each labored five days, while rich peasants worked three. YJA: 4, 1954.

119. The "mass line" is supposedly the consensus of mass opinion, gathered, clarified, and enacted by the Party.

120. YJA: 36, 1–12/1971.

121. Reed, "Brass Butterflies," 164–65.

122. Liansheng People's Commune, Qingpu County, Shanghai, "Struggle against Schistosomiasis," *Chinese Medical Journal* 87.11 (1968): 671.

123. Anting People's Commune, Jiading County, Shanghai, "Drive Away the God of Plague with Gleaming Mattocks and Mighty Arms," *Chinese Medical Journal* 87.11 (1968): 668.

124. Ibid., 663, 668; Liansheng People's Commune, "Struggle against Schistosomiasis," 672; "News and Notes," *Chinese Medical Journal* 87.11 (1968): 683–84. Speculatively, the limited experience of the Red Guard and urban sent-down youth with the first snail fever campaign likely made them more willing to try the same ineffective campaign tactics.

125. Zhong Zubiao and Jiangxi sheng jiachu xuexichongbing fangzhi zhan, *Jiangxi sheng jiachu xuefang zhi: 1956–1996* (Nanchang: Jiangxi sheng jiachu xuexichongbing fangzhi zhan, 1989), 69; Wang Ximeng, *Shanghai xiaomie xuexichongbing de huigu,* 64, 66, 72.

126. SMA: B34-2-195, 1954.

127. JXA: XIII–02–269, 12/1957, 19; JXA: XIII–03–089, 1959; JSA: 3119, 525, duanqi, 2/9/1958–1/1959; JSA: 3119, 75, yongjiu, 1964.

128. YJA: 10, 1–12/1956; YJA: 29, 1–12/1964; Wang Ximeng, *Shanghai xiaomie xuexichongbing de huigu,* 84.

129. SMA: A71-2-465, 5/3/1956–12/22/1956; YJA: 15, 1957; JXA: X001–01–403, 1–9/1957; JXA: X035–04–802, 1956.

130. There is indeed some evidence that the enormous weight of water in the dam basin triggered the earthquake centuries before it would likely have happened. Richard A. Kerr and Richard Stone, "A Human Trigger for the Great Quake of Sichuan?" *Science* 323.5912 (January 16, 2009): 322. For a discussion of the resurgence of feng shui postcommunization, see Ole Bruun, "The Fengshui Resurgence in China: Conflicting Cosmologies between State and Peasantry," *China Journal* 36 (July 1996): 47–65.

6. THE CHALLENGES OF TREATMENT

1. Yu Laixi and Zhonggong Yujiang xianwei xuefang lingdao xiaozu bangongshi, *Jiangxi sheng Yujiang xian xuefang zhi: 1953–1980* (Yujiang: Zhonggong Yujiang xianwei xuefang lingdao xiaozu bangongshi, 1984), 47.

2. QPA: 95–2-6, 12/1953; YJA: 1, 1953 (quotation).

3. YJA: 1, 1953.

4. H. Kristian Heggenhougen, Veronica Hackethal, and Pramila Vivek, *The Behavioral and Social Aspects of Malaria and Its Control: An Introduction and Annotated Bibliography* (Geneva: World Health Organization, 2003), 9.

5. YJA: 7, 1955 (quotation); YJA: 3, 1954. The Qing dynasty (1644–1911) constructed China's most comprehensive system of disaster-relief granaries, eventually building a granary each for all thirteen hundred counties. Gaps in the system were filled by additional community granaries. Robert B. Marks, *Tigers, Rice, Silk, and Silt: Environment and Economy in Late Imperial South China* (New York: Cambridge University Press, 1998), 226–29.

6. Fang Xiaoping, *Barefoot Doctors and Western Medicine* (Rochester, NY: University of Rochester Press, 2012), 28.

7. YJA: 39, 12/1972; YJA: 16, 1958; SMA: B242–1-815, 11/1955. The global malaria campaign faced similar problems. Microscopy was the best way to identify parasites, but most sites lacked personnel with enough time, skill, and appropriate reagents to effectively employ this seemingly accessible testing method. Kenneth J. Arrow, Claire Panosian, and Hellen Gelband, eds., *Saving Lives, Buying Time: Economics*

of Malaria Drugs in and Age of Resistance (Washington, D.C.: National Academies Press, 2004), 220.

8. SMA: Q244–1–290, 1–7/1952.

9. Yu Laixi and Zhonggong Yujiang xianwei xuefang lingdao xiaozu bangong-shi, *Jiangxi sheng Yujiang xian xuefang zhi,* 105; Li Guohua, "Chabing, zhibing, de jijian wangshi," in *Song wenshen jishi,* vol. 43, ed. Liu Yurui and Wan Guohe (Nan-chang: Jiangxi sheng zhengxie wenshi ziliao yanjiu weiyuanhui, 1992), 137; QPA: 95–2–12, 12/1954; QPA: 95–1–6, 1954. To add insult to injury, at least through 1956 Jiangsu actually charged people for the honor of handing in a stool sample. There is no indication that Jiangxi had similar fees. JSA: 3119, 231, changqi, 6/23/1956.

10. Ibid. (all sources).

11. Yu Laixi and Zhonggong Yujiang xianwei xuefang lingdao xiaozu bangong-shi, *Jiangxi sheng Yujiang xian xuefang zhi,* 47; JXA: X009–01–010, 1957; SMA: C31–2–532, 3/3/1957–12/12/1957.

12. E. L. Munson, "Cholera Carriers in Relation to Cholera Control," *Philippine Journal of Science* 10B (January 1915): 4–5.

13. John Farley, *Bilharzia: A History of Imperial Tropical Medicine* (New York: Cambridge University Press, 2003), 106.

14. JXA: X111–02–087, 1954.

15. SMA: C31–2–532, 3/3/1957–12/12/1957; YJA: 31, 1965 (quotations); YJA: 29, 1–12/1964; JXA: X009–01–010, 1957; Fang, *Barefoot Doctors,* 28.

16. Yu Laixi and Zhonggong Yujiang xianwei xuefang lingdao xiaozu bangong-shi, *Jiangxi sheng Yujiang xian xuefang zhi,* 47.

17. Wang Ximeng, *Shanghai xiaomie xuexichongbing de huigu* (Shanghai: Shanghai kexue jishu chubanshe, 1988), 42–44; Hou Tsung-Ch'ang, Chung Huei-Lan, Ho Lien-Yin, and Weng Hsin-Chih, "Achievements in the Fight against Para-sitic Diseases in New China," *Chinese Medical Journal* 79 (December 1959): 502–3.

18. SMA: C31–2–532, 3/3/1957–12/12/1957.

19. Wang Ximeng, *Shanghai xiaomie xuexichongbing de huigu,* 43.

20. The first section epigraph is from SMA: Q249–1–138, 12/31/1951–4/8/1952; the second is from JXA: X001–01–403, 1–9/1957.

21. YJA: 10, 1–12/1956.

22. QPA: 95–1–15, 1957; SMA: C31–2–532, 3/3/1957–12/12/1957; Mobo Gao, *Gao Village: Rural Life in Modern China* (Honolulu: University of Hawai'i Press, 1999), 74; JSA: 3119, 1017, duanqi, 4/4/1963–1/12/1964 (quotation). The global malaria campaign faced the opposite problem, but it resulted in similar rationales for resist-ance. In Africa, many people associated malaria with only the mild form of the disease, so trivial that treatment was unnecessary. Severe malaria must be another disease, making malaria treatment equally illogical. Arrow, *Saving Lives,* 58; Debo-rah L. Helitzer-Allen, Carl Kendall, and Jack J. Wirima, "The Role of Ethnographic Research in Malaria Control: An Example from Malawi," *Research in the Sociology of Health Care* 10 (1993): 272–76.

23. Yu Laixi and Zhonggong Yujiang xianwei xuefang lingdao xiaozu bangong-shi, *Jiangxi sheng Yujiang xian xuefang zhi,* 81; QPA: 95–2–12, 12/1954.

24. YJA: 23, 1–12/1962 (quotation); YJA: 44, 81, 83.

25. Tong Xianghan, "Shiziyan," in *Song wenshen jishi,* ed. Liu and Wan, 73–75; Yu Laixi and Zhonggong Yujiang xianwei xuefang lingdao xiaozu bangongshi, *Jiangxi sheng Yujiang xian xuefang zhi,* 17.

26. Gao, *Gao Village,* 74.

27. Joshua Horn, *Away With All Pests: An English Surgeon in People's China, 1954–1969* (New York: Monthly Review Press, 1969), 124.

28. JXA: X111–01–030, 3/2/1955–12/27/1955; Horn, *Away With All Pests,* 124.

29. For a few of many examples of fictional stories about quacks, see Zhang Yufeng, Bai Gengsheng, and Qiao Mingxian, eds., *Zhongguo minjian gushi quanshu: Henan, nanzhao juan* (Beijing: Zhishi chanquan chubanshe, 2011); Ou Risheng and Li Baojia, eds., *Zhongguo jindai guanchang xiaoshuo xuan,* vol. 2, *Guanchang xianxing jixia* (Hohhot: Neimenggu renmin chubanshe, 2003); Cao Xueqin, *Honglou meng* (1791; Beijing: Renmin wenxue chubanshe, Xinhua shudian faxing, 1996); YJA: 15, 1957; Zhang Jiwan, oral history compiled by Xiong Yangsheng, "Jianmiao baifo xinqiancheng wanminan miao bu anmin—wanminan jiangcun duanrenyan zao huimie qinjian qinli ji," in *Song wenshen jishi,* ed. Liu and Wan, 60–62; Zhou Fukai, oral history compiled by Xiong Yangsheng, "Yongyi mocai, jifu sangming," in *Song wenshen jishi,* ed. Liu and Wan, 69–72; Horn, *Away With All Pests,* 104–6.

30. YJA: 15, 1957.

31. JXA: X111–01–030, 3/2/1955–12/27/1955.

32. SMA: Q244–1-290, 1–7/1952 (quotation); YJA: 6, 1954.

33. SMA: Q249–1-138, 12/31/1951–4/8/1952.

34. YJA: 1, 1953 (Yujiang quotation); QPA: 95–2-5, 10/1953–9/1955 (Qingpu quotation).

35. JXA: X009–01–010, 1957.

36. Ibid.; JXA: X035–04–800, 1956; JXA: X111–04–423, 1956 (quotations). The unhappy doctors described here were conscripted into the schistosomiasis campaign and predate the large number of physicians sent to the countryside during the Great Leap Forward.

37. JXA: X009–01–010, 1957.

38. QPA: 95–2-6, 12/1953.

39. YJA: 22, 1–12/1962.

40. SMA: Q243–1-658, 1951.

41. YJA: 10, 1–12/1956.

42. YJA: 16, 1958; SMA: Q243–1-658, 1951; SMA: C31-2-532, 3/3/1957–12/12/1957.

43. YJA: 16, 1958; "Medical Activities in New China," *Chinese Medical Journal* 76.5 (1958): 105–6; Kiangxi, Yü-chiang Hsien, Revolutionary Committee, Culture, Education, Health, and Antischistosomiasis Section of Revolutionary Committee of Yukiang County and Yukiang Antischistosomiasis Station, "A Great Victory of Mao Tse-tung's Thought in the Battle against Schistosomiasis: The 10 Years Since the Eradication of Schistosomiasis in Yukiang County in 1958," *China's Medicine* 10

(October 1968): 592. The older an urban doctor, the more likely he or she would be labeled a rightist and dispatched to the countryside during the Great Leap Forward or Cultural Revolution. The interesting result was that rightist doctors often had more immediate credibility and respect than barefoot doctors simply because of their age. Arthur W. Chung, *Of Rats, Sparrows and Flies . . .: A Lifetime in China* (Stockton, CA: Heritage West Books, 1995), 205.

44. QPA: 95-2-27, 1956; Edward Friedman, Paul G. Pickowicz, and Mark Selden, *Revolution, Resistance, and Reform in Village China* (New Haven, CT: Yale University Press, 2005), 216–17 (quotations). In March 1953, Qingpu residents had already assimilated the correct procedure for giving shots and insisted on every step being followed, since it was unclear which part made the sequence work. When one team ran out of supplies, "many patients were angry because no gauze was used after the shot." QPA: 95-2-7, 1953.

45. Ch'ien Hsin-chung, "Summing Up of Mass Technical Experiences with a View to Expediting Eradication of the Five Major Parasitic Diseases," *Chinese Medical Journal* 77.6 (December 1958): 522. See also A. Davis, "Schistosomiasis," chapter 80 in *Manson's Tropical Diseases,* 21st ed., ed. Gordon C. Cook and Alimuddin I. Zumla (Philadelphia: Saunders, Elsevier Science, 2003), 1431–69; George T. Tootell, "Tartar Emetic in Schistosomiasis Japonica," *Chinese Medical Journal* 38.4 (April 1924): 276–77.

46. Arthur Kleinman, "Traditional Doctors," in *Rural Health in the People's Republic of China: Report of a Visit by the Rural Health Systems Delegation, June 1978,* by Committee on Scholarly Communication with the People's Republic of China, NIH Publication No. 81–2124 (Washington, D.C.: U.S. Department of Health and Human Services, Public Health Service, National Institutes of Health, November 1980), 67–69; Ernest Faust and Henry Meleney, *Studies on Schistosomiasis Japonica,* Monograph Series No. 3 (Baltimore: American Journal of Hygiene, 1924), 238; SMA: Q244–1-290, 1–7/1952; SMA: B242–1-815, 11/1955; QPA: 95-2-9, 1953. Such doctors also tended to mix shots with Chinese herbs without any knowledge of possible drug interactions. Kleinman, "Traditional Doctors," 67–69.

47. Li Guohua, "Chabing, zhibing, de jijian wangshi," 138; Kan Huai-chieh and Yao Yung-tsung, "Some Notes on the Anti–Schistosomiasis Japonica Campaign in Chih-huai-pan, Kaihua, Chekiang," *Chinese Medical Journal* 48.4 (April 1934): 328; SMA: Q244–1-290, 1–7/1952 (quotation); SMA: Q243–1-658, 1951; SMA: B34–2-195, 1954.

48. JSA: 3119, 198, duanqi, 3/1/1956–12/19/1956 (quotation); Edward Friedman, Paul G. Pickowicz, and Mark Selden, *Chinese Village, Socialist State* (New Haven, CT: Yale University Press, 1991), 207–8; JXA: X035–04–567, 1956; JXA: X009–01–010, 1957.

49. QPA: 95-1-12, 1956; Zhonggeng Jiangxi sheng weifangzhi xuexichongbing wuxiaozu banggongshi bianxie, *Yujiang xian shi zenyang genzhi xuexichongbing de* (Nanchang: Jiangxi renmin chubanshe, 1958), 21 (quotation).

50. "First County to Wipe Out Schistosomiasis," *China Reconstructs* (July 17, 1968): 15; YJA: 10, 1–12/1956; JXA: X111–02–266, 1957; Xiong Peikang, "Zhenma

qiepi, Zhansheng wenshen (Boyang xian)," in *Song wenshen jishi,* ed. Liu and Wan, 27–30; Li Guohua, "Chabing, zhibing, de jijian wangshi," 138.

51. SMA: Q249-1-138, 12/31/1951–4/8/1952.

52. YJA: 43, 12/1976.

53. JXA: X009-01-010, 1957 (first quotation); SMA: C31-2-532, 3/3/1957–12/12/1957 (second quotation).

54. SMA: B242-1-815, 11/1955; Huang Qijing and Luo Zhuliu, "Tongxin xieli song wenshen—qing puxiang xue xi chongbing yiqing ji fangzhi chengguo," in *Qingpu wenshi, di si qi* (Qingpu [Shanghai]: Zhongguo renmin zhengzhi xieshang huiyi Qingpu xian weiyuanhui wenshi ziliao weiyuanhui, 1989), 157; Ye Songling, "Xuexichongbing fangzhi gongzuo de huigu (De'an)," in *Song wenshen jishi,* ed. Liu and Wan, 25.

55. Withholding work points was a very effective strategy but mainly happened only in model areas where cadres were very dedicated to the campaign. YJA: 10, 1–12/1956; SMA: C31-2-532, 3/3/1957–12/12/1957; SMA: A71-2-465, 5/3/1956–12/22/1956 (quotation); SMA: Q243-1-658, 1951.

56. Deng Shilin, oral history compiled by Shu Mingliang, "Bingfang she zai wode jia," in *Song wenshen jishi,* ed. Liu and Wan, 143; QPA: 95-1-6, 1954 (quotation).

57. Families tended to have one set of bedding that stayed with the family at home.

58. Deng, "Bingfang she zai wode jia," 141; SMA: Q243-1-658, 1951; QPA: 95-1-2, 1–10/1952; Mao Zhixiao, "Wo canjia songwenshen de licheng (Guangfeng)," in *Song wenshen jishi,* ed. Liu and Wan, 33; SMA: Q249-1-138, 12/31/1951–4/8/1952.

59. JXA: X111-02-087, 1954; Mao Zhixiao, "Wo canjia songwenshen de lichen (Guangfeng)," 32 (quotations).

60. QPA: 95-2-45, 1958; QPA: 95-2-18, 1–12/1954; QPA: 95-1-6, 1954. Some villagers assessed the conditions on the rural wards and instead of viewing them as convenient, asked to be sent to the snail fever station or a hospital where they could be assured of better care. Yu Laixi and Zhonggong Yujiang xianwei xuefang lingdao xiaozu bangongshi, *Jiangxi sheng Yujiang xian xuefang zhi,* 65.

61. Similar antagonistic undercurrents occurred during colonial health campaigns. In an American campaign against cholera in the Philippines, a disease that is also initially asymptomatic, Filipino villagers were disturbed that "the search [for sick people] was made among persons apparently healthy to themselves and others who could scarcely fall even within the class of suspects." Once forcibly quarantined or corralled into wards, they were "subjected to all the inconveniences of isolation, separation from family, loss of earning capacity, etc." Munson, "Cholera Carriers in Relation to Cholera Control," 4–5. Like Chinese villagers, many ran away due to the "severity of the drug reactions" and economic barriers, since a "day in the annex was a day without wages." Farley, *Bilharzia,* 99 ("annex" quotation), 106, 197 ("severity" quotation).

62. SMA: B34-2-195, 1954; SMA: Q243-1-658, 1951; SMA: Q249-1-138, 12/31/1951–4/8/1952; QPA: 95-2-6, 12/1953; QPA: 95-2-9, 1953; QPA: 95-2-12, 12/1954.

63. SMA: Q243–1-658, 1951.

64. SMA: Q249–1-138, 12/31/1951–4/8/1952; SMA: Q243–1-658, 1951; QPA: 95–1-6, 1954.

65. Ibid. (all sources).

66. Zhonggeng Jiangxi, *Yujiang xian shi zenyang genzhi xuexichongbing de,* 19, 21; *Health Statistics Information in China, 1949–88* (Beijing: Ministry of Public Health, 1989), cited in William C. L. Hsiao, "The Chinese Health Care System: Lessons for Other Nations," *Social Science and Medicine* 41.8 (1995): 1047; YJA: 24, 1–12/1962 (quotation).

67. QPA: 95–1-10, 1956–1958.

68. SMA: B34–2-195, 1954; SMA: C31–2-532, 3/3/1957–12/12/1957; QPA: 95–2-23, 1956.

69. Zhonggeng Jiangxi, *Yujiang xian shi zenyang genzhi xuexichongbing de,* 21.

70. SMA: Q243–1-658, 1951.

71. Even after the famine when people received small private plots, the commune system still made a difference. For example, a December 1961 report from Yujiang advises, "If when getting treated the person has nobody to look after his own fields, then the production team should find people to look after it for him." Women's work was not so easily delegated. YJA: 20, 1–12/1962.

72. SMA: C31–2-532, 3/3/1957–12/12/1957; Li Guohua, "Chabing, zhibing, de jijian wangshi," 136.

73. Li Zhenglan, "Wo canjia xuefang kepu gongzuo," in *Song wenshen jishi,* ed. Liu and Wan, 133; SMA: Q243–1-658, 1951; SMA: C31–2-532, 3/3/1957–12/12/1957; Zhonggeng Jiangxi, *Yujiang xian shi zenyang genzhi xuexichongbing de,* 19, 36, 37. Observing the problematic disease-based family dynamics, sometimes young women's own mothers would intervene by announcing that their daughters were getting treated and then personally escorting them to the hospital. Prior to the start of high-level cooperatives, members of medical teams would also occasionally try to cover a patient's household duties. Li Zhenglan, "Wo canjia xuefang kepu gongzuo," 133; SMA: Q243–1-658, 1951.

74. Li Guohua, "Chabing, zhibing, de jijian wangshi," 136; Zhonggeng Jiangxi, *Yujiang xian shi zenyang genzhi xuexichongbing de,* 21; SMA: C31–2-532, 3/3/1957–12/12/1957.

75. Yang Ruidong, "Wo canjia xuefang gongzuo de pianduan huiyi," *Jingjiang wenshi ziliao* (Jiangsu, 7, 1987): 186; Li Guohua, "Chabing, zhibing, de jijian wangshi," 137; QPA: 95–1-1, 3/1951.

76. SMA: C31–2-532, 3/3/1957–12/12/1957.

77. QPA: 95–2-27, 1956; QPA: 95–2-26, 1956; QPA: 95–2-32, 1–12/1957; QPA: 95–1-2, 1–10/1952; QPA: 95–2-12, 12/1954.

78. QPA: 95–1-12, 1956. According to Roderick MacFarquhar, in 1958 ten billion work days, or one-third of the time normally employed for grain production, were lost to backyard steel production. Roderick MacFarquhar, *The Origins of the Cultural Revolution,* vol. 2, *The Great Leap Forward, 1958–1960* (New York: Columbia University Press, 1983), 103, 119, 198.

79. Li Guohua, "Chabing, zhibing, de jijian wangshi," 136; SMA: C31-2-532, 3/3/1957–12/12/1957; QPA: 95–1-12, 1956. The Jiangxi provincial Party secretary Fang Zhichun suggested that cadres go to women's houses and work with neighbors to apportion work so that treatment would be possible. Zou Huayi, *Kuayue siwang didai* (Nanchang: Baihuazhou wenyi chubanshe, 1993), 98–100.

80. The Party attempted to alter work and eating patterns through communal labor and dining halls, pregnancy through new family planning regimes, and movement via the rural residency permit.

81. JSA: 3119, 1017, duanqi, 4/4/1963–1/12/1964;; Zou Huayi, *Kuayue siwang dida*, 249–50. Even in Shanghai, there was significant downsizing, including closing one of the main hospitals (Xujiahui) that had two hundred beds dedicated to snail fever. Due to decreased government subsidies, other Shanghai hospitals started to refuse treatment to people with insurance, because policies awarded less money than those who paid out of pocket. Since most people were unable to pay without assistance, this decision decreased patient access. SMA: B242-1-1299, 5/1960–8/1961; SMA: B242-1-1315, 9–11/1961.

82. JXA: X035-05-398, 1963; JSA: 3119, 75, yongjiu, 1964. During the famine the national government planned to mandate that other counties learn from Yujiang. However, Yujiang had no feces or water management system and had such a high rate of snail fever that it could not be used as an example. Zou Huayi, *Kuayue siwang didai,* 249–50.

83. JXA: X035-06-689, 1959.

84. When treatment left patients with a permanent disability, assessment of treatment changed from useless to actively harmful, making it harder to mobilize people. QPA: 95–1-12, 1956; YJA: 31, 1965; JXA: X009–01–010, 1957 (quotations).

85. SMA: B242-3-15, 7/21/1967–9/1967; Wang Ximeng, *Shanghai xiaomie xuexichongbing de huigu,* 47.

86. Xiong, "Zhenma qiepi, Zhansheng wenshen (Boyang xian)," 27–30.

87. "News and Notes," *Chinese Medical Journal* 85.4 (1966): 275–76; A. G. Ross et al., "Schistosomiasis in the People's Republic of China: Prospects and Challenges for the 21st Century," *Clinical Microbiology Reviews* 14.2 (2001): 284.

88. Shanghai, the center of the regional cattle market, also had to deal with infusions of sick cattle from surrounding areas that were less avid in their animal treatment programs. To address its inability to track animals' health and location, Shanghai instituted a cattle residency permit *(hukou).* Wang Ximeng, *Shanghai xiaomie xuexichongbing de huigu,* 85–93 (quotation in chapter pp. 90–91).

89. Ibid.; SMA: B45-5-13, 3–12/1967; Zhonggong zhongyang nanfang shisan sheng, shi, qu xuefang lingdao xiaozu bangongshi, *Song wenshen: Huace* (Beijing: Zhonggong zhongyang nanfang shisan sheng, shi, qu xuefang lingdao xiaozu bangongshi, 1978), 77, 80, 84.

90. Late-stage patients, palliative care for drug reactions, and treatment of many preexisting diseases that impeded curing snail fever were also made free. SMA: B242-1-1774, 7–10/1966; SMA: B242-3-77, 1–12/1968.

91. QPA: 95-1-2, 1–10/1952 (first quotation); QPA: 95-1-15, 1957 (second quotation). Medical students and some doctors had come to Qingpu earlier in circulating teams over Spring Festival and to run test site activities. However, only the later large number of expert doctors' staying for extended periods due to the Anti-Rightist Campaign made it possible to treat late-stage patients.

92. SMA: B242-1-816, 11/1955; JSA: 3119, 1017, duanqi, 4/4/1963–1/12/1964. Postfamine, Jiangsu struggled not only from people and communes unable to pay for treatment but also from the extraordinary drop in campaign personnel from twenty-eight hundred in 1955 to five hundred in 1961. Few of the remaining medical personnel were knowledgeable enough to safely treat late-stage patients. JSA: 3119, 75, yongjiu, 1964.

93. Fu Lien-Chang, "Summing-Up of the Ninth General Conference of the Chinese Medical Association Held in Peking on December Fourteenth to Seventeenth, 1952." *Chinese Medical Journal* 71 (March–April 1953): 6; YJA: 28, 1963.

94. Gao, *Gao Village*, 86–87; Kiangxi, Yü-chiang Hsien, "Great Victory," 596.

95. Wang Ximeng, *Shanghai xiaomie xuexichongbing de huigu*, 46.

96. It may be that Red Guards' limited experience with the first campaign peak also made them more willing to believe in the efficacy of campaign tactics.

97. Wang Ximeng, *Shanghai xiaomie xuexichongbing de huigu*, 17, 39–44, 46.

98. These numbers are unlikely to be totally accurate, but the aim was to have a minimum of one-third of the urban medical establishment in the countryside at any given time. According to Pi-chao Chen, by 1973, 100,000 medical workers lived permanently in the countryside and the number of workers in mobile teams had grown to 800,000. Pi-chao Chen, *Population and Health Policy in the People's Republic of China,* Occasional Monograph Series No. 9 (Washington, D.C.: Interdisciplinary Communications Program, Smithsonian Institution, December 1976), 52, 54–55. See also "Directive on Public Health" (June 26, 1965), from *Long Live Mao Tse-tung Thought,* a Red Guard publication, in *Selected Works of Mao Tse-tung,* vol. 9, www.marxists.org/reference/archive/mao/selected-works/index.htm. (accessed April 22, 2010); "Weishengbu mianli xinnian qu nongcun de yiyao weisheng renyuan nuli zuodao," *Renmin ribao,* December 31, 1965; "Health Work Serving the Peasants," *Chinese Medical Journal* 85.3 (March 1966): 145–47; Volker Scheid, *Chinese Medicine in Contemporary China: Plurality and Synthesis* (Durham, NC: Duke University Press, 2002), 78; J. Bonner, "Medicine and Public Health," *China Science Notes* 3.1 (January 1972): 6.

99. "Nong mu relie huanying Mao zhuxi pailai de yiliaodui," *Renmin ribao,* October 6, 1965; SMA: B242-2-206, 4–11/1972 (quotation).

100. "Zunzhao Mao zhuxi guanyu 'yingdang jiji de yufang he yiliao renmin de jibing' de jiaodao," *Renmin ribao,* June 26, 1973.

101. Chen, *Population and Health Policy,* 53. While the impact of the mass transfer of urban medical personnel to the countryside is clear, more research is needed to know whether permanent, institutionally based medical linkages also had a large effect on rural medical knowledge.

102. YJA: 38, 1–12/1972.

103. Ibid. (quotations); Chung, *Of Rats, Sparrows and Flies,* 204.

104. Many urban youth were interested in becoming barefoot doctors and had higher education levels than rural youth. However, not only were there strong ideological barriers to access, but also few urban youth had the social networks needed to acquire this plum job. Yang Nianqun, "Memories of the Barefoot Doctor System," in *Governance of Life in Chinese Moral Experience,* ed. Everett Zhang, Arthur Kleinman, and Tu Weiming (New York: Routledge, 2011), 139; Chen Zhengyan, "Wo shi dangnian de chijiaoyisheng," *Wenshi bolan* 4 (2014): 46–48; Marilyn M. Rosenthal and Jay R. Greiner, "The Barefoot Doctors of China: From Political Creation to Professionalization," *Human Organization* 4.4 (1982): 330.

105. David Mechanic and Arthur Kleinman, "Ambulatory Care," and Everett M. Rogers, "Barefoot Doctors," both in *Rural Health in the People's Republic of China,* by Committee on Scholarly Communication with the People's Republic of China, 31, 61 (respectively).

106. Chung, *Of Rats, Sparrows and Flies,* 207.

107. Mao Zhixiao, "Wo canjia songwenshen de lichen (Guangfeng)," 31, 34; QPA: 95-2-117, 1965–1966 (Qingpu quotation).

108. Aaron Shirly, "Community Health," in *Rural Health in the People's Republic of China,* by Committee on Scholarly Communication with the People's Republic of China, 13. A 1975 documentary on barefoot doctors observed the same phenomenon. It also noted the key role that professional doctors played in supplying barefoot doctors' initial training. *The Barefoot Doctors of Rural China, 1975,* National Archives and Records Administration, Washington, D.C., ARC: 46549.. See also Gao, *Gao Village,* 86; Kiangxi, Yü-chiang Hsien, "Great Victory," 601; "Directive on Public Health" (June 26, 1965), in *Selected Works of Mao Tse-tung,* vol. 9; YJA: 37, 1–12/1972; YJA: 38, 1–12/1972.

109. Prompted by the discovery of an exceptional single-dose medicine, praziquantel, in the late 1970s international snail fever control work also shifted to a primary focus on treatment of people and animals, rather than on eliminating snails. Farley, *Bilharzia,* 285–89, 303, 304.

110. SMA: B242–3-283, 1–8/1972; Shanghai shi difangzhi bangongshi, "Diba pian zhuan bing fangzhi, diyi zhang xuexichongbing, disan jie jigou," *Shanghai weishengzhi,* www.shtong.gov.cn/node2/node2245/node67643/node67655 /node67719/node67847/userobject1ai65180.html (accessed September 29, 2013).

111. Cheng Tien-hsi, "Schistosomiasis in Mainland China: A Review of Research and Control Programs since 1949," *American Journal of Tropical Medicine and Hygiene* 20.1 (January 1971): 26; Wang Ximeng, *Shanghai xiaomie xuexichongbing de huigu,* 48; Ross et al., "Schistosomiasis in the People's Republic of China," 282; Quanguo fangzhi wu da jishengchongbing jingyan jiaoliu huiyi, *Renmin shouce 1959 nian* (Beijing: Renmin ribao chubanshe, 1960), 511; Qian Xinzhong, *Zhonghua renmin gongheguo xuexichongbing dituji, shangce* (Shanghai: Zhonghua dituxue she chuban, 1987), 22.5.

112. "Biopower" is a term coined by Michel Foucault to describe a key management strategy of the modern state, which is "an explosion of numerous and diverse

techniques for achieving the subjugations of bodies and the control of populations." Ideally, such bodily disciplines will be normalized so that citizens will police themselves into correct behavior without the use of overt force. Michel Foucault, *The History of Sexuality,* vol. 1 (New York: Vintage, 1990), 140 (quotation); Michel Foucault, *Discipline and Punish: The Birth of the Prison* (New York: Vintage, 1979), 26–27, 295, 308.

7. DOING THE UNTHINKABLE

1. The chapter epigraph is from Zhonggeng Jiangxi sheng weifangzhi xuexichongbing wuxiaozu banggongshi bianxie, *Yujiang xian shi zenyang genzhi xuexichongbing de* (Nanchang: Jiangxi renmin chubanshe, 1958), 24.

2. Maurice Meisner, *Mao's China and After: A History of the People's Republic,* rev. and expanded 1st ed. (New York: Free Press, 1986), 140–48.

3. Jessica Ching-Sze Wang, *John Dewey in China: To Teach and to Learn* (New York: SUNY Press, 2008), 15–16.

4. Friedrich Engels, "The Part Played by Labour in the Transition from Ape to Man," in *Dialectics of Nature,* trans. and ed. Clemens Dutt (New York: International Publishers, 1940); Friedrich Engels, *Ludwig Feuerbach and the Outcome of Classical German Philosophy* (London: M. Lawrence, 1934); Carolyn Fluehr-Lobban, "Frederick Engels and Leslie White: The Symbol versus the Role of Labor in the Origin of Humanity," *Dialectical Anthropology* 11.1 (1986): 119–26.

5. "Implementing Correct Policy in Dealing with Doctors of Traditional Chinese Medicine" (October 20, 1954), in *The Writings of Mao Zedong,* ed. Michael Kau and John Leung, vol. 1 (Armonk, NY: M. E. Sharpe, 1986), 487.

6. Wei Wen-po [Wei Wenbo], "The People's Boundless Energy during the Current Leap Forward: New Victories on the Anti-schistosomiasis Front," *Chinese Medical Journal* 77 (1958): 108–9, 111.

7. JSA: 3119, 525, duanqi, 2/9/1958–1/1959.

8. Ibid. (quotation); "Yishi dapo mixin, xiaxiang shuxue qiangjiu bingren," *Qingpu bao,* no. 193, July 9, 1958, 3.

9. QPA: 95-2-108, 1965.

10. For a fuller discussion of the transformation of the meaning of superstition, see Sigrid Schmalzer, *The People's Peking Man: Popular Science and Human Identity in Twentieth-Century China* (Chicago: University of Chicago Press, 2008), 120–21.

11. "On the Ten Great Relationships" (April 25, 1956), in *The Writings of Mao Zedong,* ed. Michael Kau and John Leung, vol. 2 (Armonk, NY: M. E. Sharpe, 1992), 61.

12. Meisner, *Mao's China and After,* 316.

13. JXA: X035-04-802, 1956.

14. SMA: A50-1-12, 1956.

15. SMA: A71-2-465, 5/3/1956–12/22/1956.

16. QPA: 95–1-4, 1953. Chairman Mao also believed that sickness and superstition were connected. Watt argues that this was one reason he strongly promoted health care. John R. Watt, *Saving Lives in Wartime China: How Medical Reformers Built Modern Healthcare Systems amid War and Epidemics, 1928–1945* (Leiden: Brill, 2014), 256–58.

17. Bailey K. Ashford and Pedro Gutiérrez Igaravidez, *Uncinariasis (Hookworm disease) in Porto Rico: A Medical and Economic Problem* (Washington D.C.: Government Printing Office, 1911), 89–90.

18. JXA: X035–04–802, 1956.

19. Ibid.; Li Junjiu, "Diyi mian hongqi shi zenyang chashang de," in *Song wenshen jishi,* vol. 43, ed. Liu Yurui and Wan Guohe (Nanchang: Jiangxi sheng zhengxie wenshi ziliao yanjiu weiyuanhui, 1992), 94 (quotation).

20. JXA: X035–06–689, 1959 (quotation); SMA: B242–1-816, 11/1955.

21. Susan Greenhalgh, *Just One Child: Science and Policy in Deng's China* (Berkeley: University of California Press, 2008), 8.

22. Attacks on temples long predated the Party. In the late Qing dynasty (1890s), priests were ousted from temples so that they could be used for schools. The Nationalists (1911–49) continued assaults on traditional culture for many of the same reasons as the Communists. Sally Borthwick, *Education and Social Change in China: The Beginnings of the Modern Era* (Stanford, CA: Hoover Institution Press, 1983), 47, 63–64, 81, 97–103.

23. QPA: 95–1-1, 3/1951.

24. YJA: 3, 1954.

25. Ye Songling, "Xuexichongbing fangzhi gongzuo de huigu (De'an)," in *Song wenshen jishi,* ed. Liu and Wan, 25–26.

26. YJA: 6, 1954; JSA: 3119, 198, duanqi, 3/1/1956–12/19/1956; QPA: 95–2-2, 10/25/1952. The idea of subverting holidays by making them cleanup days predates the PRC. Chairman Mao was already repurposing Spring Festival in 1944, while at Yan'an. Watt, *Saving Lives,* 292.

27. Gordon Bennett, *Yundong: Mass Campaigns in Chinese Communist Leadership,* China Research Monograph No. 12 (Berkeley: Center for Chinese Studies, University of California, 1976), 41–42.

28. Joshua Horn, *Away With All Pests: An English Surgeon in People's China, 1954–1969* (New York: Monthly Review Press, 1969), 97.

29. Sun Yongjiu, "Gonggu chengguo ying nan er shang; ba xuefang hongqi ju de genggao," in *Song wenshen jishi,* ed. Liu and Wan, 105.

30. JXA: X111–02–269, 12/1957, 14, 21; QPA: 95–2-2, 10/25/1952. In Yujiang, youth's symbolic position as societal leaders was built into the mass mobilization campaigns. They were organized "as the front line to set the example." Women's caretaking role was also reemphasized by giving them the job of bringing water and tea to workers. *Xue xianjin gan xianjin xianjin geng xianjin chu sihai, xiaomie xuexichongbing jingyan* (Nanchang: Jiangxi renmin chubanshe, 1958), 17–18, 22 (quotation p. 18).

31. As discussed in the next chapter, many male educated youth in the Youth League participated as backbone elements, but not as activists.

32. JSA: 3119, 1017, duanqi, 4/4/1963–1/12/1964; YJA: 9, 1–12/1956; QPA: 95-1-15, 1957.

33. YJA: 9, 1–12/1956; JXA: X001–01–403, 1–9/1957; John Harland Reed, "Brass Butterflies of the Thoughts of Mao Tsetung: The Sociology of Schistosomiasis Control in China" (Ph.D. diss., Cornell University, 1979), 154; SMA: B242–1-813, 11/1954–11/1955.

34. Yu Laixi, "Yi fenguan laoren Wan Fengxin," in *Song wenshen jishi*, ed. Liu and Wan, 121–24; QPA: 95-2-21, 12/1955. Women were equally happy when other women took over the commode-cleaning task. However, unlike with men, their appreciation was based on not having to do the task themselves, rather than on gratitude toward the night soil worker.

35. QPA: 95-2-12, 12/1954.

36. QPA: 95-2-21, 12/1955; Horn, *Away With All Pests,* 98–99; Reed, "Brass Butterflies," 176; QPA: 95-1-11, 1–12/1956.

37. QPA: 95–1-12, 1956.

38. Li Guohua, "Chabing, zhibing, de jijian wangshi," in *Song wenshen jishi,* ed. Liu and Wan, 138; SMA: B34-2-195, 1954; QPA: 95-1-6, 1954.

39. SMA: B34-2-195, 1954.

40. QPA: 95–1-10, 1956–1958.

41. Ibid.

42. The broad-scale free treatment starting in 1966 likely caused a surge in loyal activists that may have helped rally popular participation in the Cultural Revolution.

43. QPA: 95–2-108, 1965 (quotation); Huang Qijing and Luo Zhuliu, "Tongxin xieli song wenshen—qing puxiang xue xi chongbing yiqing ji fangzhi chengguo," in *Qingpu wenshi, di si qi* (Qingpu [Shanghai]: Zhongguo renmin zhengzhi xieshang huiyi Qingpu xian weiyuanhui wenshi ziliao weiyuanhui, 1989), 155.

44. SMA: B34-2-195, 1954.

45. SMA: B242–1-816, 11/1955.

46. SMA: B34-2-195, 1954.

47. QPA: 95–1-6, 1954.

48. While poor and landless peasants who did not have enough land welcomed the new system, middle and rich peasants and landlords saw few advantages and tried their best to resist.

49. Other coercive strategies include increasing taxes, withholding access to irrigation, and soldiers' materializing to "aid agriculture," among others. G. William Skinner and Edwin A. Winckler, "Compliance Succession in Rural Communist China: A Cyclical Theory," in *A Sociological Reader on Complex Organizations,* 2nd ed., ed. Amitai Etzioni (New York: Holt, Rinehart and Winston, 1969), 430.

50. "Second Preface to *Upsurge of Socialism in China's Countryside*" (December 27, 1955), in *Writings of Mao Zedong,* ed. Kau and Leung, vol. 1, 691.

51. SMA: B242–1-815, 11/1955.

52. SMA: B242-1-816, 11/1955.

53. Sun, "Gonggu chengguo ying nan er shang," 108; JXA: X039–04–421, 11/27/1965–12/26/1966.

54. The impact of sanitation campaigns' joint snail eradication and irrigation-channel reconstruction projects on moving people to APCs needs further study. In the process of digging channels, fields' old boundary stones were moved and newly dug waterways reconfigured the agricultural space, transforming the topography. It was difficult to establish exactly where one's old fields used to be, which perhaps made it easier to accept the new status quo. Yu Laixi and Zhonggong Yujiang xian-wei xuefang lingdao xiaozu bangongshi, *Jiangxi sheng Yujiang xian xuefang zhi: 1953–1980* (Yujiang: Zhonggong Yujiang xianwei xuefang lingdao xiaozu bangong-shi,, 1984), 54; Kiangxi, Yü-chiang Hsien, Revolutionary Committee, Culture, Education, Health, and Antischistosomiasis Section, with Yü-chiang Antischisto-somiasis Station, "A Great Victory of Mao Zedong's Thought in the Battle against Schistosomiasis: The 10 Years Since the Eradication of Schistosomiasis in Yukiang County in 1958," *China's Medicine,* 10 (October 1968): 596.

55. Yu Laixi and Zhonggong Yujiang xianwei xuefang lingdao xiaozu bangong-shi, *Jiangxi sheng Yujiang xian xuefang zhi,* 71.

56. QPA: 95–1-2, 1–10/1952.

57. SMA: B242-1-877, 1–4/1956; Andrew Morris, "'Fight for Fertilizer!': Excre-ment, Public Health, and Mobilization in New China," *Journal of Unconventional History* 6.3 (Spring 1995): 64.

58. SMA: B242-1-877, 1–4/1956.

59. Ibid.

60. SMA: B242-1-816, 11/1955 (quotation); QPA: 95–2-6, 12/1953.

61. Zhonggeng Jiangxi, *Yujiang xian shi zenyang genzhi xuexichongbing de,* 21.

62. YJA: 10, 1–12/1956.

63. Chen Qilin, "Dengfuzhen chujian fenguan de huiyi," in *Song wenshen jishi,* ed. Liu and Wan, 120.

64. QPA: 95–1-15, 1957.

65. JXA: X035–04–802, 1956 (quotation); SMA: B242-1-816, 11/1955.

66. QPA: 95–1-12, 1956.

67. Wang Ximeng, *Shanghai xiaomie xuexichongbing de huigu* (Shanghai: Shanghai kexue jishu chubanshe, 1988), 76 (quotation); SMA: B242-1-816, 11/1955.

68. QPA: 95–1-15, 1957.

69. JXA: X035–04–802, 1956. In the Shanghai area, some people put part of their fields in the collective and kept part for private use. They had the same problem as sole proprietors with extracting fertilizer from the co-op. Shanghai co-ops gave people a monthly ticket to submit when they came to collect. But since no actual records were kept, the injunction that "the amount used should not exceed the amount originally handed in" seems unlikely to have worked. SMA: B242-1-1090, 11/1957–4/1958.

70. Yu Laixi and Zhonggong Yujiang xianwei xuefang lingdao xiaozu bangong-shi, *Jiangxi sheng Yujiang xian xuefang zhi,* 110–11; Sun, "Gonggu chengguo ying nan er shang," 103–5.

71. QPA: 95-2-75, 1961; YJA: 19, 1–12/1961 (quotation).

72. More research is needed to determine if science served a similarly helpful consolidation function in urban settings.

8. SCIENTIFIC CONSOLIDATION IN THE LATE 1960S AND 1970S

1. Franz Schurmann, *Ideology and Organization in Communist China* (Berkeley: University of California Press, 1968), 52, 166, 226, 233, 236; Vivienne Shue, *The Reach of the State: Sketches of the Chinese Body Politic* (Stanford, CA: Stanford University Press, 1988), 118–19, 149; Joel Andreas, *Rise of the Red Engineers: The Cultural Revolution and the Origins of China's New Class* (Stanford, CA: Stanford University Press, 2009), 216, 223, 237–39; Susan Greenhalgh, *Just One Child: Science and Policy in Deng's China* (Berkeley: University of California Press, 2008), 5, 19, 76–77, 196; Richard P. Suttmeier, *Science, Technology and China's Drive for Modernization* (Stanford, CA: Hoover Institute Press, 1980), 43.

2. For one of many examples, see "Twenty Manifestations of Bureaucracy" (February 1970), in *Selected Works of Mao Tse-tung,* vol. 9, www.marxists.org/reference /archive/mao/selected-works/index.htm. (accessed April 22, 2010), where bureaucracy is called truculent, authoritarian, brainless, dishonest, irresponsible, stupid, and useless.

3. Understandings of science also varied in the Party. Because Chairman Mao was the leading voice through most of this era (1949–76), his idiosyncratic use of science is explored here.

4. Gordon Bennett, *Yundong: Mass Campaigns in Chinese Communist Leadership* (China Research Monograph No. 12 (Berkeley: Center for Chinese Studies, University of California, 1976); Charles P. Cell, *Revolution at Work: Mobilization Campaigns in China* (New York: Academic Press, 1977).

5. A. Doak Barnett, *Cadres, Bureaucracy, and Political Power in Communist China* (New York: Columbia University Press, 1967); Schurmann, *Ideology and Organization;* Harry Harding, *Organizing China: The Problem of Bureaucracy, 1949–1976* (Stanford, CA: Stanford University Press, 1981); Shue, *Reach of the State;* Kenneth Lieberthal, *Governing China: From Revolution through Reform* (New York: W. W. Norton & Company, 1995); Roderick MacFarquhar, *The Origins of the Cultural Revolution,* vols. 1–3 (New York: Columbia University Press, 1974–97); Roderick MacFarquhar and Michael Schoenhals, *Mao's Last Revolution* (Cambridge, MA: Belknap Press of Harvard University Press, 2006).

6. Yeh Wen-hsin, *Shanghai Splendor: Economic Sentiments and the Making of Modern China, 1843–1949* (Berkeley: University of California Press, 2007), 30–50; Frederick Winslow Taylor, *The Principles of Scientific Management* (1911; New York: W. W. Norton and Company, 1967).

7. Jessica Ching-Sze Wang, *John Dewey in China: To Teach and to Learn* (New York: SUNY Press, 2008), 15–16; John Dewey, *Lectures in China, 1919–1920,* ed. and

trans. Robert Clopton and Tsuin-chen Ou (Honolulu: University of Hawai'i, 1973), 127, cited in ibid., 15.

8. Editor's introduction, "The Founding and Progress of the 'Strengthen Learning Society'" (July 21, 1919), and "Letter to Li Jinxi" (June 7, 1920), in *Mao's Road to Power: Revolutionary Writings, 1912–1949*, vol. 1, *The Pre-Marxist Period, 1912–1920*, ed. Stuart R. Schram, (Armonk, NY: M. E. Sharpe, 1992), xxxvi, 376 (quotations), 519.

9. Roger R. Thompson, trans., *Mao Zedong: Report from Xunwu* (Stanford, CA: Stanford University Press, 1990), 23–24; "Oppose Bookism" (May 1930), in *Mao's Road to Power: Revolutionary Writings, 1912–1949*, vol. 3, *From the Jinggangshan to Establishment of the Jiangxi Soviet, July 1927–December 1930*, ed. Stuart R. Schram (Armonk, NY: M. E. Sharpe, 1995), 419 (quotation).

10. V. I. Lenin, "The Taylor System—Man's Enslavement by the Machine" (1914), in *Collected Works,* vol. 20 (Moscow: Foreign Languages Publishing House, 1964), 154; Thomas Parke Hughes, *American Genesis: A Century of Invention and Technological Enthusiasm, 1870–1970* (Chicago: University of Chicago Press, 2004), 254–57, 269–70 (Trotsky quotations p. 256).

11. Susan Greenhalgh makes this point about the role of science in public policy. Greenhalgh, *Just One Child,* 8.

12. Originally, scientific management did not contain this contradiction. Each group was supposed to specialize in what it did best: workers labored efficiently; managers ensured a standardized work process; and scientists, engineers, and academics developed innovative or efficient ways of doing the work. It was because Chairman Mao insisted that the tools of science, technology, and scientific management be placed in the hands of the people that these inconsistencies were created.

13. "Resolving the Problem of the 'Five Excesses'" (March 19, 1953) and editors' notes on *Upsurge of Socialism in China's Countryside* (December 27, 1955), in *The Writings of Mao Zedong, 1949–1976*, vol. 1, ed. Michael Kau and John Leung (Armonk, NY: M. E. Sharpe, 1986), 335–36, 711–14; "Methods of Work of Party Committees" (March 13, 1949) and "Sixty Points on Working Methods—a Draft Resolution from the Office of the Centre of the CPC" (February 2, 1958), in *Selected Works of Mao Tse-tung*, vols. 4, 8.

14. "Methods of Work of Party Committees" (March 13, 1949), "Sixty Points on Working Methods" (February 2, 1958), in *Selected Works of Mao Tse-tung*, vols. 4, 8.

15. "Sixty Points on Working Methods" (February 2, 1958), in *Selected Works of Mao Tse-tung*, vol. 8; "Conversation with Security Guards" (mid-July 1955), in *Writings of Mao Zedong*, vol. 1, ed. Kau and Leung, 613.

16. Harding, *Organizing China,* 348–49. Franz Schurmann notes that during the Great Leap rural areas implemented a "rational work organization" (i.e., a stringent division of labor), where communes "were being administered like a factory," which resulted in a vast increase in productivity rates, a reality that he feels was the Great Leap's real revolution. Once the coercive policies of the Great Leap were over, communes jettisoned these more efficient work patterns and returned to traditional patterns of labor. Despite these findings, Schurmann still concludes that revolutionary periods were incompatible with technical organization. Schurmann, *Ideology*

and *Organization,* 464–72, 498. See also Barnett, *Cadres, Bureaucracy, and Political Power,* 174–76.

17. Barnett, *Cadres, Bureaucracy, and Political Power,* 179; Schurmann, *Ideology and Organization,* 572.

18. According to Harry Harding, in the 1960s the earlier gap in administrative knowledge was offset by sent-down urban and rural educated youth. Harding, *Organizing China,* 348–49.

19. Robert Weller, *Discovering Nature: Globalization and Environmental Culture in China and Taiwan* (New York: Cambridge University Press, 2006), 40.

20. "Methods of Work of Party Committees" (March 13, 1949), in *Selected Works of Mao Tse-tung,* vol. 4.

21. JXA: X111–02–140, 1955 (quotation); Yu Laixi and Zhonggong Yujiang xianwei xuefang lingdao xiaozu bangongshi, *Jiangxi sheng Yujiang xian xuefang zhi: 1953–1980* (Yujiang: Zhonggong Yujiang xianwei xuefang lingdao xiaozu bangongshi, 1984), 45; YJA: 3, 1954.

22. JXA: X001–01–403, 1–9/1957.

23. Wang Ximeng, *Shanghai xiaomie xuexichongbing de huigu* (Shanghai: Shanghai kexue jishu chubanshe, 1988), 61; YJA: 7, 1955.

24. QPA: 95–1-1, 3/1951; JXA: X035–04–800, 1956 (quotation). The same problem of testing biased samples haunted the global campaign against malaria: "And so along with a high level of underreporting, there is a high level of overreporting. Nevertheless, statistics are duly gathered." Sonia Shah, *The Fever: How Malaria Has Ruled Humankind for 500,000 Years* (New York: Sarah Crichton Books, 2010), 133 (quotation), 210–11; H. Kristian Heggenhougen, Veronica Hackethal, and Pramila Vivek, *The Behavioral and Social Aspects of Malaria and Its Control: An Introduction and Annotated Bibliography* (Geneva: World Health Organization, 2003), 91–92.

25. JXA: X111–02–201, 2/1957, 114; Wang Ximeng, *Shanghai xiaomie xuexichongbing de huigu,* 62.

26. Analogous problems impeded the global malaria campaign. When surveillance teams could not survey their whole assigned territory, got bored, or began to doubt campaign efficacy, they would typically neglect the work and falsify data, including taking "extra blood samples from more accessible residents." Shah, *Fever,* 210–11 (quotation); Gordon Harrison, *Mosquitoes, Malaria and Man: A History of the Hostilities since 1880* (New York: E. P. Dutton, 1978), 244–46.

27. Similarly, the World Health Organization and the Joint United Nations Programme on HIV/AIDS (UNAIDS) sometimes collected skewed statistics in order to maximize funding. Shah, *Fever,* 134; Craig Timberg and Daniel Halperin, *Tinderbox: How the West Sparked the AIDS Epidemic and How the World Can Finally Overcome It* (New York: Penguin, 2013), 140–42.

28. QPA: 95–1-10, 1956–1958; QPA: 95–1-15, 1957; "Di yici quanguo renkou pucha," posted at the National Bureau of Statistics, June 25, 2002, www.stats.gov.cn (accessed May 6, 2008).

29. SMA: Q243–1-658, 1951.

30. QPA: 95–2-21, 12/1955 (quotation); YJA: 6, 1954. Qingpu was one of the few places that placed a heavy emphasis on forms, even in nonmodel areas. Yet even there, forms were "filled out wrong, or they lost them, or in every way messed them up!" QPA: 95–2-21, 12/1955.

31. SMA: A71–2-465, 5/3/1956–12/22/1956.

32. Professional doctors conducting Shanghai's campaign in 1952 greatly mitigated this problem by posting each person's correct dosage above his or her bedside. But this innovation was never mentioned in any other report, and the frequent comments about incorrect dosage indicates that most places found no replacement for patient charts. SMA: Q243–1-658, 1951.

33. QPA: 95–1-6, 1954 (quotation); SMA: A71–2-465, 5/3/1956–12/22/1956.

34. JSA: 3119, 198, duanqi, 3/1/1956–12/19/1956.

35. As described later in the chapter, mass mobilization campaigns, which reached their apogee at the same moment as administration was under attack, partially compensated for the drop in record keeping by endlessly retesting people and repeatedly rehunting for snails.

36. QPA: 95–2-44, 1958 (quotation); John Harland Reed, "Brass Butterflies of the Thoughts of Mao Tsetung: The Sociology of Schistosomiasis Control in China" (Ph.D. diss., Cornell University, 1979), 150.

37. Qingpu xian xiaomie xuexichongbing jiangli banfa (caoan), *Qingpu bao,* no. 207, August 7, 1958, 3; JXA: X035–06–689, 1959.

38. QPA: 95–2-75, 1961.

39. SMA: B242–3-283, 1–8/1972. Even midlevel medical institutions had not grasped why records were necessary. A U.S. delegation visiting China in the late 1970s observed that neither communes nor county hospitals kept a medical record library. Doctors wrote down patient information on small scraps of paper and handed them to the patients, after which these pieces of paper were rarely seen again. Richard C. Reynolds, "Hospital Care," *Rural Health in the People's Republic of China: Report of a Visit by the Rural Health Systems Delegation, June 1978,* by Committee on Scholarly Communication with the People's Republic of China, NIH Publication No. 81–2124 (Washington, D.C.: U.S. Department of Health and Human Services, Public Health Service, National Institutes of Health, November 1980), 38–39.

40. Wang Ximeng, *Shanghai xiaomie xuexichongbing de huigu,* 40, 54; Sun Yongjiu, "Gonggu chengguo ying nan er shang; ba xuefang hongqi ju de genggao," in *Song wenshen jishi,* vol. 43, ed. Liu Yurui and Wan Guohe (Nanchang: Jiangxi sheng zhengxie wenshi ziliao yanjiu weiyuanhui, 1992), 108.

41. Even campaign activities that potentially had an impact on production, such as changing paddy fields to dry crops, generally were not evaluated unless they occurred in test sites. As a 1956 Jiangxi report noted, "When paddy fields are changed to dry fields there's no preparation or survey work done, and afterward there's no check on the results." JXA: X111–02–200, 1956.

42. Anting People's Commune, Jiading County, Shanghai, "Drive Away the God of Plague with Gleaming Mattocks and Mighty Arms," *Chinese Medical Journal* 87.11 (1968): 668.

43. SMA: Q249–1-138, 12/31/1951–4/8/1952; YJA: 1, 1953 (quotation).

44. QPA: 95–2-21, 12/1955.

45. Wang Ximeng, *Shanghai xiaomie xuexichongbing de huigu,* 62.

46. QPA: 95–1-1, 3/1951; QPA: 95–1-8, 3/1955; QPA: 95–2-23, 1956.

47. QPA: 95–1-12, 1956.

48. QPA: 95–2-75, 1961. Speculatively, rather than an ineffective medicine, researchers' problem may have been their testing method, since stool tests miss up to half of the cases.

49. JSA: 3119, 322, changqi, 2/10/1957–12/28/1957; JXA: X111–04–604, 1958; JXA: X039–01–571, 1959; SMA: B242–1-938, 1–6/1956. Funding for research started as early as 1956, the official beginning of the broader campaign. SMA: B242–1-938, 1–6/1956.

50. "22: Methods of Thinking and Methods of Work" (February, 5, 1940; originally from "On Practice," July 1937) and "Sixty Points on Working Methods" (February 2, 1958), in *Selected Works of Mao Tse-tung, Red Book* and vol. 8.

51. Anting, "Drive Away the God of Plague," 665–66; Liansheng People's Commune, Qingpu County, Shanghai, "Struggle against Schistosomiasis," *Chinese Medical Journal* 87.11 (1968): 670; "Quanguo gedi honghong lielie daban kexue shiye," *Qingpu bao,* no. 188, June 26, 1958, 4.

52. QPA: 95–1-15, 1957. By the Cultural Revolution, scientific performances seem to have crept into grassroots work of all types. For example, A. Doak Barnett notes that after receiving general instructions, counties would try their own limited experiments, disseminate the "results of the experiment" to subordinate units, and then carry out the directive as mandated. Barnett, *Cadres, Bureaucracy, and Political Power,* 140.

53. SMA: B242–1-815, 11/1955.

54. Jiangsu sheng xuexichongbing fangzhi yanjiusuo, *Youguan zhiliao xuexichongbing de ziliao* (Nanjing: Jiangsu sheng xuexichongbing fangzhi yanjiusuo, 1965); Jiangxi sheng xuexichongbing yanjiu weiyuanhui, *Xuexichongbing yanjiu, 1956–1985* (Nanchang: Jiangxi sheng xuexichongbing yanjiu weiyuanhui, [198?]).

55. Yu Laixi and Zhonggong Yujiang xianwei xuefang lingdao xiaozu bangongshi, *Jiangxi sheng Yujiang xian xuefang zhi,* 48; YJA: 14, 1–12/1957.

56. YJA: 3, 1954; Wu Zaocun, "Feng zheng jin zu qu wenshen," in *Song wenshen jishi,* ed. Liu and Wan, 126–27; *Xue xianjin gan xianjin xianjin geng xianjin chu sihai, xiaomie xuexichongbing jingyan* (Nanchang: Jiangxi renmin chubanshe, 1958), 16.

57. Wang Ximeng, *Shanghai xiaomie xuexichongbing de huigu,* 93.

58. Yang Daozheng, "Qumo you dang yizhi jian yin chu pikai xin tiandi (Fengxin)," in *Song wenshen jishi,* ed. Liu and Wan, 17; SMA: C31–2–532, 3/3/1957–12/12/1957.

59. There was a strong connection between this sort of grassroots science and achieving model status. For example, in her book on science in the context of the one-child policy, Susan Greenhalgh notes that "some grassroots localities began to develop innovative methods of mass data gathering [for birth planning] that won them model status." Greenhalgh, *Just One Child,* 63.

60. QPA: 95–1–28, 1962.

61. Qian Xinzhong, *Zhonghua renmin gongheguo xuexichongbing dituji, shangce* (Shanghai: Zhonghua dituxue she chuban, 1987), 22.5.

62. Wang Ximeng, *Shanghai xiaomie xuexichongbing de huigu,* 63–64.

63. Qingpu xian fangzhi xuexichongbing sanshiwu nian weiyuanhui, *Qingpu xian fangzhi xuexichongbing sanshiwu nian: Dashiji ji* (Shanghai: Shanghai kexue jishu chubanshe, 1988), 8–9; QPA: 95–1–2, 1–10/1952.

64. SMA: B242–1–816, 11/1955; SMA: B242–1–937, 1–3/1956; Qingpu xian, *Sanshiwu nian: Dashiji ji,* 8–26.

65. Ibid. (all sources).

66. SMA: A71–2–465, 5/3/1956–12/22/1956.

67. QPA: 95–1–12, 1956.

68. JSA: 3119, 198, duanqi, 3/1/1956–12/19/1956; SMA: B3–1–16, 1/31/1956–9/25/1956.

69. Wang Ximeng, *Shanghai xiaomie xuexichongbing de huigu,* 116–17.

70. "The Orientation of the Revolution in Medical Education as Seen in the Growth of 'Barefoot Doctors': Report of an Investigation from Shanghai," reprinted from *Hongqi,* no. 3 (1968), *Chinese Medical Journal* 87.10 (1968): 574–75.

71. Wang Ximeng, *Shanghai xiaomie xuexichongbing de huigu,* 63–64; Mao Zhixiao, "Wo canjia songwenshen de licheng (Guangfeng)," in *Song wenshen jishi,* ed. Liu and Wan, 37 (quotation).

72. Joshua Horn, *Away With All Pests: An English Surgeon in People's China, 1954–1969* (New York: Monthly Review Press, 1969), 101.

73. SMA: B242–1–816, 11/1955; SMA: A71–2–465, 5/3/1956–12/22/1956; Yu Laixi and Zhonggong Yujiang xianwei xuefang lingdao xiaozu bangongshi, *Jiangxi sheng Yujiang xian xuefang zhi,* 52; *Xue xianjin gan xianjin xianjin geng xianjin,* 22.

74. JXA: X009–01–010, 1957; JSA: 3119, 198, duanqi, 3/1/1956–12/19/1956; Li Junjiu, "Diyi mian hongqi shi zenyang chashang de," in *Song wenshen jishi,* ed. Liu and Wan, 98.

75. Bennett, *Yundong,* 39, 50.

76. "Sixty Points on Working Methods" (February 2, 1958), in *Selected Works of Mao Tse-tung,* vol. 8.

77. YJA: 28, 1963; QPA: 95–1–10, 1956–1958. For example, in early December 1958, eighty-one Jiangxi cadres were dragged to a Xingzi County model to study its snail fever work in cattle, a previously neglected part of the campaign. After this, a "high tide in cattle work" ensued. By late December that year, 97,538 head of cattle were tested and 4,089 were treated. Zhong Zubiao and Jiangxi sheng jiachu xuexichongbing fangzhi zhan, *Jiangxi sheng jiachu xuefang zhi: 1956–1996* (Nanchang: Jiangxi sheng jiachu xuexichongbing fangzhi zhan, 1989), 176.

78. Zhonggeng Jiangxi sheng weifangzhi xuexichongbing wuxiaozu banggongshi bianxie, *Yujiang xian shi zenyang genzhi xuexichongbing de* (Nanchang: Jiangxi renmin chubanshe, 1958), 25 (first quotation); QPA: 95–1–10, 1956–1958 (second quotation). In Anting People's Commune, a model campaign site in Jiading County on the periphery of Shanghai, campaign workers reversed the normal process by

going to errant areas, disseminating proper procedures, and then acting as unobtrusive peer supervision by directly participating in snail eradication work for a month. Anting, "Drive Away the God of Plague," 665–66.

79. JSA: 3119, 1017, duanqi, 4/4/1963–1/12/1964; JSA: 3119, 418, duanqi, 2/28 /1957–12/18/1957 (quotation).

80. JSA: 3119, 525, duanqi, 2/9/1958–1/1959; Yu Laixi and Zhonggong Yujiang xianwei xuefang lingdao xiaozu bangongshi, *Jiangxi sheng Yujiang xian xuefang zhi*, 110.

81. Wang Ximeng, *Shanghai xiaomie xuexichongbing de huigu*, 131.

82. Mara Hvistendahl, "The Numbers Game," *Science* 340 (May 31, 2013): 1037–38.

CONCLUSION

1. William C.L. Hsiao, "The Chinese Health Care System: Lessons for Other Nations," *Social Science and Medicine* 41.8 (1995): 1047; Judith Banister, "Population, Public Health and the Environment in China," *China Quarterly* 156 (December 1998): 986; Ansley J. Coale, "Rapid Population Change in China, 1952–1982," *Committee on Population and Demography,* Committee on Population and Demography Report No. 27 (Washington, D.C.: National Academy Press, 1984): 12; Qian Xinzhong, *Zhonghua renmin gongheguo xuexichongbing dituji, shangce* (Shanghai: Zhonghua dituxue she chuban, 1987), 22.5; China Health Care Study Group, *Health Care in China, an Introduction: The Report of a Study Group in Hong Kong* (Geneva: Christian Medical Commission, 1974), 58.

2. When the Chinese government was criticized for its handling of SARS, *Time of Disasters* was filmed in 2004, depicting the unity and strength of the masses in overcoming natural disasters, one of which was schistosomiasis. "China Produces First Documentary on Disasters," www.china.org.cn/english/culture/96762.htm (accessed March 10, 2006).

3. The following discussion is largely inspired by Sonia Shah, *The Fever: How Malaria Has Ruled Humankind for 500,000 Years* (New York: Sarah Crichton Books, 2010); Marcel Tanner and Don de Savigny, "Malaria Eradication Back on the Table," *Bulletin of the World Health Organization* 86.2 (February 2008): 82.

4. Randall M. Packard, "Malaria Dreams: Postwar Visions of Health and Development in the Third World," *Medical Anthropology* 17.3 (1997): 279–96.

5. Peter J. Brown, "Malaria, Miseria, and Underpopulation in Sardinia: The 'Malaria Blocks Development' Cultural Model," *Medical Anthropology* 17.3 (1997): 250.

6. Packard, "Malaria Dreams," 289; Brown, "Malaria," 245, 252.

7. Laurie Garrett, *The Coming Plague: Newly Emerging Diseases in a World out of Balance* (New York: Penguin, 1994), 48 (quotation); Shah, *Fever,* 197–98.

8. L.W. Hackett, *Malaria in Europe: An Ecological Study* (London: Oxford University Press, 1937), 266.

9. J. A. Najera, "Malaria and the Work of WHO," *Bulletin of the World Health Organization* 67.3 (1989): 233–35.

10. Packard, "Malaria Dreams," 290.

11. Najera, "Malaria and the Work of WHO," 233.

12. Ibid., 240; Shah, *Fever,* 51; Garrett, *Coming Plague,* 51.

13. WHO Technical Report Series 38:46 (1951), quoted in M. J. Dobson, M. Malowany, and R. W. Snow, "Malaria Control in East Africa: The Kampala Conference and the Pare-Taveta Scheme: A Meeting of Common and High Ground," *Parassitologia* 42 (2000): 150; Packard, "Malaria Dreams," 290

14. Joshua Blu Buhs, *The Fire Ant Wars: Nature, Science, and Public Policy in Twentieth-Century America* (Chicago: University of Chicago Press, 2004), 66.

15. Dobson, "Malaria Control in East Africa," 151, 157, 158.

16. Afr/Mal/Conf/25: 97–98, quoted in Dobson, "Malaria Control in East Africa," 159.

17. James Whorton, *Before Silent Spring: Pesticides and Public Health in Pre-DDT America,* (Princeton, NJ: Princeton University Press, 1974), 249; Buhs, *Fire Ant Wars,* 68; Edmund P. Russell III, "'Speaking of Annihilation': Mobilizing for War against Human and Insect Enemies, 1914–1945," *Journal of American History* 82.4 (March 1996): 1505–29.

18. Buhs, *Fire Ant Wars,* 66, 68, 73; Russell, "Speaking of Annihilation," 1505–29.

19. Najera, "Malaria and the Work of WHO," 235, 240; Packard, "Malaria Dreams," 286, 287.

20. H. Kristian Heggenhougen, Veronica Hackethal, and Pramila Vivek, *The Behavioral and Social Aspects of Malaria and Its Control: An Introduction and Annotated Bibliography* (Geneva: World Health Organization, 2003), 87–102, 150; Dobson, "Malaria Control in East Africa," 165; Jeffrey Gettleman, "Meant to Keep Malaria Out, Mosquito Nets Are Used to Haul Fish In," *New York Times,* January 24, 2015.

21. Donald G. McNeil Jr., "Gate Foundation's Influence Criticized," *New York Times,* February 16, 2008.

22. Dobson, "Malaria Control in East Africa," 159, 164;

23. David Blumenthal and William Hsiao, "Privatization and Its Discontents—the Evolving Chinese Health Care System," *New England Journal of Medicine* 353.11 (September 15, 2005): 1165–70; Mobo C. F. Gao, *Gao Village: A Portrait of Rural Life in Modern China* (Honolulu: University of Hawai'i Press, 1999), 87.

24. Jürg Utzinger et al., "Conquering Schistosomiasis in China: The Long March," *Acta Tropica* 96 (2005): 74, 81.

25. Ibid., 86; Wang Ximeng, *Shanghai xiaomie xuexichongbing de huigu* (Shanghai: Shanghai kexue jishu chubanshe, 1988), 21, 22, 43, 44, 54; Zhou Xiaonong et al., "Application of Geographic Information Systems and Remote Sensing to Schistosomiasis Control in China," *Acta Tropica* 79.1 (2001): 97–106.

26. Zhong Zubiao and Jiangxi sheng jiachu xuexichongbing fangzhi zhan, *Jiangxi sheng jiachu xuefang zhi: 1956–1996* (Nanchang: Jiangxi sheng jiachu xuexichongbing fangzhi zhan, 1989), 69.

27. Chen Xianyi et al., "Schistosomiasis Control in China: The Impact of a 10-Year World Bank Loan Project (1992–2001)," *Bulletin of the World Health Organization* 83 (2005): 44–45.

28. Zhong and Jiangxi sheng jiachu xuexichongbing fangzhi zhan, *Jiangxi sheng jiachu xuefang zhi,* 82, 159, 160; Utzinger et al., "Conquering Schistosomiasis in China," 69, 70, 73; Dongbao Yu et al., "Cost-Effectiveness Analysis of the Impact on Infection and Morbidity Attributable to Three Chemotherapy Schemes against *Schistosoma japonicum* in Hyperendemic Areas of the Dongting Lake Region, China," *Southeast Asian Journal of Tropical Medicine Public Health* 33.3 (September 2002): 441.

29. Vincent Lee, "Snail Scare," *Shanghai Star,* June 24, 2004; Utzinger et al., "Conquering Schistosomiasis in China," 70.

30. L.D. Wang, J. Utzinger, and X.N. Zhou, "Schistosomiasis Control: Experiences and Lessons," *Lancet* 372.9652 (November 2008): 1793–95; L.D. Wang, H.G. Chen, et al., "A Strategy to Control Transmission of *Schistosoma japonicum* in China," *New England Journal of Medicine* 360.2 (January 8, 2009): 121–28; L.D., Wang, J.G. Guo, et al., "China's New Strategy to Block *Schistosoma japonicum* Transmission: Experience and Impact beyond Schistosomiasis," *Tropical Medicine and International Health* 14.12 (December 2009): 1475–83.

31. Wang, Utzinger, and Zhou, "Schistosomiasis Control," 126.

32. Utzinger et al., "Conquering Schistosomiasis in China," 76; Li Keqiang, "National Schistosomiasis Treatment and Prevention Working Conference—Li Keqiang's Attendance and Speech" (September 6, 2010), www.gov.cn/ldhd/2010–09/06/content_1697124.htm (accessed October 15, 2010).

33. Wang, Utzinger, and Zhou, "Schistosomiasis Control," 126.

34. Zhongguo xinwen wang, April 13, 2003, http://news.sina.com.cn/o/2003–09–23/0934803130s.shtml, cited in Yanzhong Huang, "The SARS Epidemic and Its Aftermath in China: A Political Perspective," in *Learning from SARS: Preparing for the Next Disease Outbreak; Workshop Summary,* ed. Stacey Knobler, Adel Mahmoud, Stanley Lemon, Alison Mack, Laura Sivitz, and Katherine Oberholtzer(Washington, D.C.: National Academies Press, 2004), 116–17 (quotation); Phillip P. Pan, "Village by Village, China Fights Virus; SARS Battle Shows Party Can Still Mobilize the Masses," *New York Times,* June 8, 2003; Joan Kaufman, "SARS and China's Health-Care Response: Better to Be Both Red and Expert!," in *SARS in China: Prelude to Pandemic?,* ed. Arthur Kleinman and James L. Watson (Stanford, CA: Stanford University Press, 2006), 65.

35. Lai Hongyi, "Local Management of SARS in China: Guangdong and Beijing," in *The SARS Epidemic: Challenges to China's Crisis Management,* ed. John Wong and Zheng Yongnian (Singapore: World Scientific Publishing Company, 2004), 91.

36. Christopher A. McNally, "Baptism by Storm: The SARS Crisis' Imprint on China's New Leadership," in *The New Global Threat: SARS and Its Impacts,* ed. Tommy Koh, Aileen Plant, and Eng Hin Lee (Singapore: World Scientific Publishing Company, 2003), 78; Zheng Yongnian and Lye Liang Fook, "SARS and China's

Political System," in *SARS Epidemic,* ed. Wong and Zheng, 64; Kaufman, "SARS and China's Health-Care Response," 65.

37. Mangai Balasegaram and Alan Schnur, "China: From Denial to Mass Mobilization," *SARS: How a Global Epidemic Was Stopped* (Geneva: World Health Organization, Western Pacific Region, 2006), 80; Yanzhong Huang, "SARS Epidemic," 125; Qin Zhu, "SARS in Beijing: An Urban Response," in *SARS from East to West,* ed. Eva Karin Olsson and Lan Xue (Lanham, MD: Lexington Books, 2012), 62; Lai, "Local Management of SARS," 91–94. The army sequestered most SARS cases in its separate medical system, making it almost impossible for the health ministry to act effectively. Tony Saich, "Is SARS China's Chernobyl or Much Ado about Nothing?," in *SARS in China,* ed. Kleinman and Watson, 80–82.

38. Yanzhong Huang, "SARS Epidemic," 125.

39. Marta Hanson, "The Art of Medicine: Maoist Public-Health Campaigns, Chinese Medicine, and SARS," *Lancet* 372 (October 25, 2008): 1457–58; Balasegaram and Schnur, "China: From Denial to Mass Mobilization," 81–84; Lynn T. White III, "SARS, Anti-populism, and Elite Lies: Temporary Disorders in China," in *New Global Threat,* ed. Koh, Plant, and Lee, 38–40. The government also manufactured a new set of human enemies, supposedly undermining the campaign, in case the war against pathogens was not enough. However, instead of landlords and rightists, the new targets were migrants who complained about the Three Gorges Dam resettlement program and members of the Falun Gong accused of having "evil intentions of anti-mankind, anti-science, and anti-society." Saich, "Is SARS China's Chernobyl?," 89.

40. Pan, "Village by Village"; McNally, "Baptism by Storm," 73; Balasegaram and Schnur, "China: From Denial to Mass Mobilization," 81–84.

41. Yanzhong Huang, "SARS Epidemic," 125; Balasegaram and Schnur, "China: From Denial to Mass Mobilization," 81–84.

42. Pan, "Village by Village."

43. Kaufman, "SARS and China's Health-Care Response," 63; Balasegaram and Schnur, "China: From Denial to Mass Mobilization," 81–84.

44. Pan, "Village by Village"; Yanzhong Huang, "SARS Epidemic," 129; Balasegaram and Schnur, "China: From Denial to Mass Mobilization," 81–84.

45. McNally, "Baptism by Storm," 73; Tim Brookes, *Behind the Mask: How the World Survived SARS, the First Epidemic of the 21st Century* (Washington, D.C.: American Public Health Association, 2005), 204; Balasegaram and Schnur, "China: From Denial to Mass Mobilization," 81–84.

46. Balasegaram and Schnur, "China: From Denial to Mass Mobilization," 81–84; McNally, "Baptism by Storm," 77; Brookes, *Behind the Mask,* 197–98; Zou Keyuan, "SARS and the Rule of Law in China," in *SARS Epidemic,* ed. Wong and Zheng, 114.

47. Yanzhong Huang, "SARS Epidemic," 125, 128; Brookes, *Behind the Mask,* 197; Kaufman, "SARS and China's Health-Care Response," 63–64.

48. Ibid. (all sources); Zheng and Lye, "SARS and China's Political System," 65; Brookes, *Behind the Mask,* 204.

49. Kaufman, "SARS and China's Health-Care Response," 64; Saich, "Is SARS China's Chernobyl?," 86; Liu Wei, "Hunan Province Takes Measures to Prevent Spread of SARS," *China Radio International,* April 22, 2003, http://english.cri .cn/144/2003-4-23/14@10764.htm (accessed January 31, 2015); *SARS: Clinical Trials on Treatment Using a Combination of Traditional Chinese Medicine and Western Medicine* (Geneva: World Health Organization, 2004), 1.

50. Brookes, *Behind the Mask,* 200, 204; Zheng and Lye, "SARS and China's Political System," 64.

51. McNally, "Baptism by Storm," 77.

52. Pan, "Village by Village."

53. Yanzhong Huang, "SARS Epidemic," 124–25, 130; Lai, "Local Management of SARS," 91–94; McNally, "Baptism by Storm," 81.

54. McNally, "Baptism by Storm," 86.

55. Zhu, "SARS in Beijing," 66; Zheng and Lye, "SARS and China's Political System," 64.

BIBLIOGRAPHY

The notes and bibliography contain the following abbreviations:

Second Historical Archive	SHA
Shanghai Municipal Archive	SMA
Jiangsu Provincial Archive	JSA
Jiangxi Provincial Archive	JXA
Qingpu Area Archive	QPA
Yujiang County Archive at the Commemorative Museum	YJA

ARCHIVES

Second Historical Archive

SHA: 372, 176. Zhe weishengchu Hainan tequ gongshu qing bao fangzhi xuexi-chongbing jingfei redaibing yaopin de jihua kou youguan jiguan laiwang wenshu [Official correspondences between Zhejiang Health Agency, Hainan Special Administrative Government Office, and related departments on the proposal of applying for funding to prevent schistosomiasis and purchasing tropical diseases medicines].

Shanghai Municipal Archive

SMA: A23–2-499, 4–12/1959. Zhonggong Shanghai shiwei jiaoyu weisheng gong-zuobu guanyu nongcun weisheng gongzuo de tongzhi, qingkuang huibao, huiyi jilu [Announcements, reports, and meeting memos on health work in rural areas from the education and health agencies of Shanghai Municipal Committee of CCP].

SMA: A23–2-639, 11/1959–9/1960. Shanghai shi weishengju, shi aiguo weisheng yundong weiyuanhui youguan aiguo weisheng yundong de baogao [Shanghai Health Bureau and Municipal Patriotic Health Campaign Committee's reports on the Patriotic Health Campaign].

SMA: A50–1-12, 1956. Zhonggong Shanghai shi di er qinggongye weiyuanhui guanyu kaizhan chu "sihai" yundong de tongbao, tongzhi [Reports and announcements of the Second Light Industry Committee of Shanghai Municipal Committee of CCP on launching the Campaign against Four-Pests].

SMA: A71–2-375, 5/21/1955–12/24/1955. Zhonggong shanghai shiwei jiaoqu gong-zuo weiyuanhui guanyu jiaqiang zhongxiaoxue gongzuo yu xuefang, gongzhai, bingyi gongzuo de qingkuang baogao [Reports and proposals of the Rural Area Work Committee of Shanghai Municipal Committee of CCP on strengthening the work on elementary and secondary education, prevention of schistosomiasis, public bonds, and military service].

SMA: A71–2-465, 5/3/1956–12/22/1956. Zhonggong Shanghai shiwei jiaoqu gong-zuo weiyuanhui, xijiao quwei guanyu shengchan, shengzhu siliao, fangzhi bing-chong, xixuechong wenti tongzhi yu baogao [Announcements and reports of the West Rural Area Committee of the Rural Area Work Committee of Shanghai Municipal Committee of CCP on production, pig feed, pest control, and preven-tion of schistosomiasis].

SMA: B3–1-16, 1/31/1956–9/25/1956. Shanghai shi renwei, weishengju, chusihai ban-gongshi deng guanyu chusihai gongzuo de jihua, zongjie, guihua, jueding ji tongzhi [Proposals, summaries, plans, decisions, and announcements of People's Committee of Shanghai, Health Bureau, and Office of Eliminating Four-Pests on the work against four-pests].

SMA: B3–2-68, 1/18/1956–8/18/1956. Shanghai shi weishengju guanyu xuexichong-bing fangzhizhan, suo weiyuanhui zuzhi lingdao de baogao [Shanghai Health Bureau's report on organizing and directing schistosomiasis prevention and treat-ment stations].

SMA: B3–2-78, 1/21/1956–12/11/1956. Weishengbu, Shanghai shi weishengju guanyu bingren yiyao shoufei, yujiaofei, jianmian deng de guiding [Ministry of Health and Shanghai Health Bureau's regulations on medical charges, prepayment, and fee remission].

SMA: B34–2-195, 1954. Shanghai shi weishengju guanyu xuexichong, changchuan-ran, naoyan, Tianhua fangzhi qingkuang jihua, baogao [Proposals and reports of Shanghai Health Bureau on prevention and treatment of schistosomiasis, gas-trointestinal infectious disease, and smallpox].

SMA: B45–5-13, 3–12/1967. Shanghai shi nongyeju ji ge xianju zhiding de youguan gengniu xuefang, yang niu fangmian de jigou, baogao tongzhi [Reports and announcements of Shanghai Bureau of Agriculture and other county depart-ments on aspects of schistosomiasis prevention of draft oxen and for raising cattle].

SMA: B242–1-50, 12/16/1955. Zhonggong Shanghaishi weishengju dangzu guanyu zucheng Shanghaishi xuexichongbing qi ren xiaozu di pishi [Memo from the leading group of the Party Shanghai Health Bureau regarding the composition of Shanghai's seven-person schistosomiasis small group].

SMA: B242-1-54, 4-12/1956. Zhonggong Shanghai shiwei guanyu Shanghai shi weishengju ganbu renmian, diaodong ji Shanghai shi weishengju dangwei qiyong xinyin de tongzhi, pifu [Announcements and replies of Shanghai Municipal Committee of CCP on the appointments, dismissals, and transfers of cadres of Shanghai Health Bureau and the Party Committee of the Health Bureau's use of a new seal].

SMA: B242-1-813, 11/1954-11/1955. Shanghai shi weishengju guanyu xuexichongbing liuxing qingkuang ji fangzhi banfa de chubu yijian ji zai liuxingqu jianli fangzhizhan, zu de yijian [Shanghai Health Bureau's preliminary proposal on the situation of the prevalence of schistosomiasis and its prevention and treatment, and proposal on establishing prevention and treatment stations and groups in endemic areas].

SMA: B242-1-814, 1955. Shanghaishi weishengju juzhang zai rendaihui ji guangbo diantai guanyu fangzhi xuexichongbing gongzuo de fayangao [Speech of the director of Shanghai Health Bureau on prevention and treatment of schistosomiasis at People's Congress and on broadcasting stations].

SMA: B242-1-815, 11/1955. Weishengbu guanyu zhaokai quanguo fangzhi xuexichongbing huiyi jianbao ji zongjie baogao, Wang juzhang fayangao [Ministry of Health's news bulletin on holding a national conference on prevention and treatment of schistosomiasis and final report, and speech of Director Wang].

SMA: B242-1-816, 11/1955. Zhonggong zhongyang guanyu xiaomie xuexichong binghai zhishi ji Shanghai sanniannei xiaomie gaibing de fangzhi jihua, jiaoqu fangzhi gongzuo baogao he jianbao [Central Committee of CCP's directives on eliminating schistosomiasis and prevention and treatment proposals of eliminating this disease in Shanghai within three years, work report and news bulletins of prevention and treatment work in the rural areas].

SMA: B242-1-877, 1-4/1956. Shanghai shiwei pizhuan Shanghai shi weishengju dangzu guanyu xiaomie xuexichongbing liangnian guihua he jinyibu kaizhan chunji aiguo weisheng yundong ji jiamin lai hu qu hong hunluan qingkuang de baogao [Shanghai Municipal Committee's approval of the Party organization of Health Bureau's two-year proposal of eliminating schistosomiasis and further carrying out the spring Patriotic Public Health Campaign and the report on the chaotic situation of peasants coming to Shanghai for warmth].

SMA: B242-1-907, 6-11/1956. Shanghai shi weishengju dui xuexichong fangzhisuo de lingdao guanxi, zuzhi bianzhi wenti tichu yijian de baogao yu youguan laihan [Report and related letters of Shanghai Health Bureau on administrative and organizational establishment issues of the Schistosomiasis Prevention and Treatment Agency].

SMA: B242-1-937, 1-3/1956. Shanghai shi weishengju guanyu fangzhi xuexichongbing de banfa guiding gongzuo yaodian ji 1956 nian Shanghai shi jiaoqu xuexichongbing zhiliao gongzuo jihua [Main points of Shanghai Health Bureau's regulations on the prevention and treatment of schistosomiasis, and 1956 work proposal of prevention and treatment of schistosomiasis in Shanghai rural areas].

SMA: B242-1-938, 1–6/1956. Weishengbu, Shanghai shi weishengju guanyu xuexichongbing fangzhi jingfei wenti de tongzhi [Announcements from Ministry of Health and Shanghai Health Bureau on funding for prevention and treatment of schistosomiasis].

SMA: B242-1-1011, 1–11/1957. Shanghai shi weishengju dui gongli yiliao jigou shoufei biaozhun de buchong guiding ji geshu youguan tiaozheng shoufei biaozhun de baogao yu pifu [Shanghai Health Bureau's additional regulations on public medical organizations' fee standard and the reports and replies regarding fee adjustment].

SMA: B242-1-1017, 4–6/1957. Zhongyang zhonggong youguan fangzhi xuexichongbing gongzuo de zhishi [Central Committee of CCP's directives on prevention and treatment of schistosomiasis].

SMA: B242-1-1090, 11/1957–4/1958. Shanghai shi weishengju guanyu Shanghai shi fangzhi jishengchongbing gongzuo de jihua zongjie ji jiti zhiliao shoufei banfa [Shanghai Health Bureau's proposal summary on prevention and treatment of parasitic diseases in Shanghai and on fee collection measures for collective treatment].

SMA: B242-1-1174, 8–12/1959. Shanghai shi weishengju guanyu niding "xiaxiang zhiyuan nongcun chusihai miebing gongzuo zhong youguan gongyong feiyong baoxiao de guiding" ji xiuding "Shanghai shi yiyuan zhuyuan bingren yufufei de guiding" [Shanghai Health Bureau's proposal on "reimbursement of public expenses for helping rural areas eliminate pests and prevent diseases" and "revised regulations on hospital patients' prepayment in Shanghai"].

SMA: B242-1-1299, 5/1960–8/1961. Shanghai shi weishengju guanyu xiongke, Xujiahui yiyuan, Shanghai shi weixiao, rurou guanlisuo, jingmi yiliao qixie chang, ertong yiyuan tiaozheng zuzhi bianzhi de pifu ji chengli zhongyao gongying zhan jiejue renyuan wenti de yijian [Shanghai Health Bureau's replies to Chest Hospital, Xuhui Hospital, Shanghai Health School, Milk and Meat Management Agency, Medical Device Factory, and Children's Hospital regarding adjusting organizational establishment, and suggestions on the establishment of Chinese herbal medicine supply stations and resolving personnel issues].

SMA: B242-1-1315, 9–11/1961. Shanghai shi weishengju guanyu fangzhi nueji he xuexichongbing gongzuo de yijian ji youguan danwei de baogao [Proposal of Shanghai Health Bureau on prevention and treatment of malaria and schistosomiasis and reports from related agencies].

SMA: B242-1-1624, 5/1963–12/1964. Weishengbu, Shanghai shi weishengju guanyu jiaqiang Shanghai shi xuefang gongzuo de zhishi ji Shanghai shi xuefang suo genggai suoming, jianli xianchang shiyan jidi de qingshi baogao [Ministry of Health and Shanghai Health Bureau's directives on strengthening the work of schistosomiasis prevention in Shanghai and proposals of changing the name of Shanghai Schistosomiasis Prevention Agency and establishing laboratory and experimental base].

SMA: B242-1-1774, 7–10/1966. Weishengbu ji Shanghai shi weishengju guanyu xuexichongbing jiancha zhiliao shixing mianfei de tongzhi [Announcements of

Ministry of Health and Shanghai Health Bureau regarding providing free services on checking and treating schistosomiasis].

SMA: B242-2-206, 4–11/1972. Shanghai shi weishengju guanyu si ge yixue yanjiusuo lingdao tizhi gaige yu chengli tiaozheng keyan xiezuo zu ji jiyansuobu zai chengdan Hunan, Yunnan yiliaodui renwu de baogao, tongzhi [Proposal and announcement of Shanghai Health Bureau on guiding the structural reform of four medical research institutes and establishing restructured scientific research cooperative groups, as well as the Parasitic Disease Institute's personnel again being sent as medical teams to Hunan and Yunnan].

SMA: B242-3-15, 7/21/1967–9/1967. Shanghai shi aiguo weisheng zhihuibu, Shanghai shi xuefangsuo guanyu jinyibu kaizhan xuexichong fangzhi gongzuo de baogao [Reports of Shanghai Patriotic Health Headquarters and Shanghai Schistosomiasis Prevention Institute on further carrying out the work of prevention and treatment of schistosomiasis].

SMA: B242-3-72, 1–9/1968. Shanghai shi aiguo weisheng zhihuibu guanyu xiaomie xuexichong guihua ji fangzhi gongzuo jingfei, renyuan daiyu de qingshi, han [Proposal letters of Shanghai Patriotic Health Headquarters regarding the plan of eliminating schistosomiasis, funding for treatment, and personnel benefits].

SMA: B242-3-77, 1–12/1968. Shanghai shi geweihui, Shanghai shi weishengju guanyu jiaqiang mafeng bingren de zhiliao he guanli, xuexichongbing zhiliao shixing mianfei yijian, gongfei yiliao guanli ji zhizhi chongza yiyuan de qingshi, tongzhi [Shanghai Revolution Committee and Shanghai Health Bureau's proposals on enhancing treatment and management of leprosy patients and free treatment for schistosomiasis, reports and announcements on public health service management and stopping attacking hospitals].

SMA: B242-3-143, 2–12/1969. Shanghai shi weishengju guanyu xuefang jihua, diaocha baogao, qingkuang huibao ji shilingdao zai xuefang gongzuo huiyi shang de jianghua [Proposals and reports of Shanghai Health Bureau on prevention of schistosomiasis and municipal leaders' speeches at schistosomiasis prevention conferences].

SMA: B242-3-283, 1–8/1972. Shanghai shi weishengju guanyu xuefangsuo dangan xiaohui baogao ji zhiding wenjian, dangan guanli, huiyi, jingfei baoxiao guiding yijian, yongjun gongyue [Shanghai Health Bureau's reports on destroyed archives of Schistosomiasis Prevention Agency and proposals on creating files, archival management, conferences, and reimbursement, and pledge of supporting the army].

SMA: B257-1-2471, 1–12/1961. Zhongguo kexueyuan Shanghai fenyuan guanyu keji daxue, kexue yiqichang, jishengchongbing yanjiusuo guanyu shiyan dalou, gongchang, fanting, sushe deng jianshe yongdi yu Shanghai shi chengshi jiansheju de laiwang wenshu [Correspondences between the Shanghai Branch of the Chinese Academy of Sciences and Shanghai City Development Bureau regarding land use for constructing laboratory buildings, factories, canteens, and staff quarters of University of Science and Technology, Scientific Device Factory, and Institute of Parasitic Diseases].

SMA: B257–1-3597, 10/1963–12/1964. Zhongkeyuan kexue yiqichang, guangjisuo, yejinsuo, lixuesuo, tianwentai deng danwei jianshe yongdi, chaiqian gongzuo yu Shanghai shi chenshi jiansheju de laiwang wenshu [Correspondences between Shanghai City Development Bureau and Chinese Academy of Sciences on land use, construction, and demolition for Scientific Device Factory, Institute of Optical Precision Machinery, Institute of Metallurgy, Institute of Mechanics, and Observatory].

SMA: C1–2-2716, 1/10/1958–8/19/1958. Shanghai shi gonglian shenghuo zhuzhaibu 1958 nian gongzuo guihua ji lühua yu chu qihai gongzuo de dasuan, tongbao [Proposals of Shanghai Labor Union Quarters on 1958 work planning and proposals and reports on landscaping and seven-pests elimination projects].

SMA: C3–1-11, 2/1950. 1949–1950 nian Shanghai shi yiwu gongzuozhe gonghui chuanda rendaihui huibao, lüxing jiuhu gongzuo zongjie, zhigong canjia jiaoqu zhujun xuefang gongzuo gongchen shiji cailiao, weiwenxin deng [1949–1950 Shanghai medical workers reporting to the People's Congress, summaries of medical emergency work, reports of good deeds of staff attending schistosomiasis prevention work in rural areas, and letters of encouragement, etc.].

SMA: C31–2-532, 3/3/1957–12/12/1957. Shanghai shi fulian nongcun gongzuobu guanyu Shanghai jiaoqu fangzhi xuexichongbing, baohu funü, laodongli yu ertong deng gongzuo baogao ji youguan wenshu [Reports and related documents of Rural Work Department of Shanghai Women Federation on prevention and treatment of schistosomiasis in Shanghai rural areas, protecting women, laborers, and children].

SMA: Q243–1-658, 1951. Shengyuehan daxue yixueyuan xuexichong fangzhi dadui gongzuo baogao he zongjie [Report and summary of schistosomiasis prevention and treatment group from medical school of St. John's University].

SMA: Q244–1-290, 1–7/1952. Zhengdan daxue guanyu yixueyuan zhiliao xuexichongbing juan [Aurora University's report on medical school's treatment of schistosomiasis].

SMA: Q249–1-137, 12/24/1949–4/11/1950. Tongde yixueyuan yu xiaxiang jiefangjun zhi xuexichongbing yanjiu tiaoji yingyang tongxue, jiaoyuan laiwang wenjian ji Shanghai jiaoqu Riben xuexichongbing fangzhi weiyuanhui de jianbao [Correspondences between Tongde Medical School and nutritionist students and instructors of People's Liberation Army in the countryside on study of treatment of schistosomiasis, and report on Japanese Schistosomiasis Prevention and Treatment Committee in Shanghai rural areas].

SMA: Q249–1-138, 12/31/1951–4/8/1952. Huadong jiaoyubu, weishengbu zhifa guanyu dongyuan ge yixueyuan shisheng yu 1951 nian hanjia qijian xiaxiang zhiliao xuexichongbing banfa deng tongzhi ji fangzhi gongzuo jihua caoan, zhiliao xuexi, di fangzhi tongxun deng he benyuan wei zuzhi zhiliaodui yu youguan yiliao danwei jiaoshou laiwang hanjian [East China Ministry of Education and Ministry of Health's announcements and proposals on mobilizing medical school students and instructors to go to the countryside to prevent and treat schistosomiasis during winter break in 1951, Local Schistosomiasis Prevention and Treatment Bulletin, and correspondences between the medical school and related professors in medical agencies regarding organizing medical treatment groups].

SMA: U1-16-2651, 1934-1937. Shanghai gonggongzujie gongbuju weishengchu guanyu xuexichongbing de chuanran ji zhiliao deng wenjian [Documents of Health Office of Shanghai Municipal Council on the spread and treatment of schistosomiasis].

SMA: U1-16-2652, 1931-1937. Shanghai gonggongzujie gongbuju weishengchu youguan xuexichongbing diaocha wenjian [Documents of Health Office of Shanghai Municipal Council on study of schistosomiasis].

Jiangsu Provincial Archive

JSA: 3119, 75, yongjiu, 1964. Zhonggong Jiangsu shengwei, chuwuhai aiguo weisheng yundong, lingdao xiaozu bangongshi, bensheng linian xuexichongbing fangzhi gongzuo baogao, (1961 zhi 1964 nian) [Work reports on prevention and treatment of schistosomiasis in Jiangsu Province from 1961 to 1964, by the Leadership Small Group Office of Eliminating Five-Pests Patriotic Health Campaign of Jiangsu Provincial Committee of CCP].

JSA: 3119, 198, duanqi, 3/1/1956-12/19/1956. Jiangsu sheng weishengting. dangzu, shengwei guanyu fangzhi xuexichongbing, nügongbing bing de zhishi ji ting dang zu guanyu nügongbing bing de diaocha he lianhe zhensuo qianfei chuli de baogao [Jiangsu Provincial Department of Health, Party Unit, Party Provincial Committee's directives on prevention and treatment of schistosomiasis, female workers' diseases, and Party unit of Provincial Health Department's reports on the study of female workers' diseases and funding for joint treatment clinics].

JSA: 3119, 231, changqi, 6/23/1956. Zhonggong Jiangsu shengwei, chuwuhai aiguo weisheng yundong, lingdao xiaozu bangongshi, wo shi xuefang gongzuo jiahua, diaochabaogao, tongzhi [Proposals, study reports, and announcements of the Leadership Small Group Office of Eliminating Five-Pests Patriotic Health Campaign of Jiangsu Provincial Committee of CCP on prevention of schistosomiasis].

JSA: 3119, 232, changqi, 5/25/1956-7/21/1956. Jiangsu sheng weishengting, jihua caiwuchu, xuexichongbing zhiliao gongzuo qingkuang de huibao ji ben ting ni fa de gongyong jingfei kaizhi biaozhun [Reports of Jiangsu Provincial Department of Health and Financial Planning Department on treatment of schistosomiasis and department's directives on public expenditure standard].

JSA: 3119, 322, changqi, 2/10/1957-12/28/1957. Jiangsu weishengting, bangongshi, bensheng xuefang, fangyi he yaozheng gongzuo zongjie ji xuefang gongzuo guihua, Hongshizihui gongzuo baogao [Reports of Jiangsu Provincial Department of Health and Office on prevention of schistosomiasis, epidemic prevention, and drug administration, and proposal on prevention of schistosomiasis, and Red Corss work report].

JSA: 3119, 418, duanqi, 2/28/1957-12/18/1957. Zhonggong Jiangsu shengwei, chuwuhai aiguo weisheng yundong, lingdao xiaozu bangongshi, Wo shi dui xuefang wenjian zhuanfa, niandu gongzuo yijian, dianxing ziliao diaocha [Annual evaluation and study report of the Leadership Small Group Office of Eliminating Five-Pests Patriotic Health Campaign, Jiangsu Provincial Committee of CCP, on prevention of schistosomiasis].

JSA: 3119, 486. Wei Wenbo tongzhi zai Jiangsu sheng xuexichongbing huiyi shang de fayan [Speech of Comrade Wei Wenbo at Jiangsu Schistosomiasis Conference].

JSA: 3119, 503, duanqi, 7/3/1958–10/14/1958. Jiangsu weishengting, zhongyichu, benting guanyu kaizhan zhiliao wanqi Riben xuexichongbing de zhishi, baogao [Directives and reports of Chinese Medicine Office of Jiangsu Provincial Department of Health on treatment of advanced Japanese schistosomiasis].

JSA: 3119, 525, duanqi, 2/9/1958–1/1959. Zhonggong Jiangsu shengwei, chuwuhai aiguo weisheng yundong, lingdao xiaozu bangongshi, benshi dui wo sheng wuba nian xuefang gongzuo qingkuang, gongzuoyijian, pizhuan wenjian, youguan wenti baogao [Suggestions, transmitted documents, and related reports of the Leadership Small Group Office of Eliminating Five-Pests Patriotic Health Campaign, Jiangsu Provincial Committee of CCP, on the work of prevention of schistosomiasis in 1958].

JSA: 3119, 1017, duanqi, 4/4/1963–1/12/1964. Zhonggong Jiangsu shengwei, chuwuhai aiguoweisheng yundong, lingdao xiaozu bangongshi, wo shi dui xuefang gongzuo tongzhi, niandu, shidian, jixing chuanran zhongdian shi xian gongzuo zongjie [Announcements of the Leadership Small Group Office of Eliminating Five-Pests Patriotic Health Campaign, Jiangsu Provincial Committee of CCP, on prevention of schistosomiasis, and annual work summary on experimental units, and cities and counties affected by acute infectious diseases].

JSA: 3235, 41, yongjiu, 3/26/1951–4/18/1957. Jiangsu sheng Songjiang zhuanyuan gongshu, weishengke, guanyu chengli zhuanqu bingchong fangzhizhan ji 1952–1956 nian xuexichongbing fangzhi gongzuo de zongjie baogao, fu: Qingpu xian meiqi huoshao mieluo qingkuang baogao [Summary reports of Health Office of Jiangsu Songjiang Commissioner Office on establishing prefectural pest prevention and treatment station, and on prevention and treatment of schistosomiasis from 1952 to 1956, with attached report on Qingpu County eliminating oncomelania by burning with gas].

JSA: 3235, 126, duanqi, 1953–1954. Jiangsu sheng Songjiang zhuanyu gongshu, weishengke, 1953 nian zhongyi jinxiuban zongjie 1954 xuefang gongzuo qingkuang ji jihua caoan [Summary report of Health Office of Jiangsu Songjiang Commissioner Office on 1953 Chinese medicine training class, and 1954 report and proposal on prevention of schistosomiasis].

JSA: 3235, 145, changqi, 7/30/1954–4/16/1957. Jiangsu sheng Songjiang zhuanyuan gongshu, weishengke, zhuanqu xuefangsuo guanyu zhengdun xuexichongbing fangzhi duiwu zongjie baogao ji 1957 nian fangzhi xuexichongbing keyan jihua [Summary report of Schistosomiasis Prevention Center, Health Office of Jiangsu Songjiang Commissioner Office on consolidating schistosomiasis prevention personnel, and 1957 research proposal on prevention and treatment of schistosomiasis].

JSA: 3235, 146, changqi, 1/23/1955–12/1955. Jiangsu sheng Songjiang zhuanyuan gongshu, weishengke, benke guanyu xuexichongbing fangzhi gongzuo jihuan ji weisheng gongzuo wei nongye shengchan fuwu de yijian. [Proposal by the Health Office of Jiangsu Songjiang Commissioner Office on schistosomiasis treatment and prevention work plans and on health work to assist agricultural production].

Jiangxi Provincial Archive

JXA: X001–01–403, 1–9/1957. Zhongguo gongchandang Jiangxi sheng weiyuanhui (bangongting) shengwei guanyu wenhua jiaoyu kexue biyesheng laodong, shengxue wenti de chuli de pishi, tongzhi, pishi [Directives, announcements and instructions of Jiangxi Provincial Committee (General Office) of CCP on employment and further education of the graduates from education and science fields].

JXA: X001–03–079, 1957. Zhonggong zhongyang, xuanchuanbu guanyu guoji, chenei xuanchuan gongzuo de zhishi, baogao, tongzhi he pizhuan quanguo fangzhi xuexichongbing de zhishi shengwei bangongting [Directives, reports, and announcements of Propaganda Department of Central Committee of CCP on international and domestic propaganda work, and directives to provincial general offices on prevention and treatment of schistosomiasis in the country].

JXA: X009–01–010, 1957. Zhonggong zhongyang, shengwei, Nanchang diwei, fangzhi xuexichongbing jiuren xiaozu, wuren xiaozu he sheng aiguo weisheng yundong weiyuanhui guanyu fangzhi xuexichongbing gongzuo de baogao, zongjie, yijian [Reports, summaries, and suggestions of Central Committee of CCP, Provincial Committee, Nanchang City Committee, Schistosomiasis Prevention and Treatment Nine-Person Small Group, Five-Person Small Group, and Provincial Patriotic Health Campaign Committee on prevention of schistosomiasis].

JXA: X035–02–817, 1/12/1953–10/7/1953. Sheng renmin zhengfu zhonggong zhonggong shengwei xuanchuanbu guanyu 1953 nian ganbu xunlian jihua choudiao ge zhuanye zaizhi ganbu xunlian xueyuan de zhishi tongzhi he 1953 nian sheng zhi jiguan tiba ganbu jihua [Directives and announcements of Provincial Government and Department of Propaganda of Provincial Committee of CCP on cadres training plan in 1953 and selecting professional cadres in active services to train students, and 1953 proposal of promoting cadres in the provincial offices].

JXA: X035–03–440, 1956. Sheng renwei guanyu weisheng gongzuo yu Gannan xingshu zhuanshu Lushan guanliju, geshi he waishengshi ge jiguan de laiwang wenshu [Correspondences between Provincial People's Committee and Lushan Administration Bureau of South Jiangxi Administrative Office, various cities, and cities in other provinces on health work].

JXA: X035–03–724, 1957. Shangrao, Ji an, Jiujiang, Fuzhou zhuanshu, Nanchang, Ji an shi, Xinfeng, Ningdu, Fengcheng, Yichun, Shanggao Geyang, Xingan, De'an, Ruichang, Lushan guanliju guanyu weisheng yiliao gongzuo de qingshi baogao he benhui de pifu [Reports of Shangrao, Jian, Jiujiang, Fuzhou Administrative Office, Nanachang, Jian City, Xifeng, Ningdu, Fengcheng, Yichun, Shanggao, Geyang, Xingan, De'an, Ruichang, Lushan Administration Bureau on health and medical work asking for instruction and the committee's reply].

JXA: X035-04-484, 1955. Quansheng wenjiao gongzuo huiyi wenjian [Documents of the Province's Culture and Education Conference].

JXA: X035-04-567, 1956. Jiangxi sheng renmin weiyuanhui bangongting, mishuke, Jiangxi sheng diyijie quansheng renmin daibiao dahui diwuci huiyi daibiao fanyin yijian huibian [Collection of proposals of representatives of the Fifth Session of the First People's Congress of Jiangxi Province, compiled by Secretary Section of General Office of Jiangxi Provincial People's Committee].

JXA: X035-04-800, 1956. Sheng renwei guanyu weisheng, jiuban kexue yuchan he xiezhu kexue jingji dili diaocha gongzuo de tongzhi tonggao [Announcement and reports of Provincial People's Committee on health, scientific reproduction, and assisting scientific, economic, and geographical research].

JXA: X035-04-802, 1956. Gannan xingshu, zhuanshu, Lushan guanliju, xianshi guanyu weisheng gongzuo de jihua, baogao, Nanchang shi shiqu cesuo ji fenbian guanli banfa he Nanchang shi tiyu yundong weiyuanhui gongzuo jihua, sheng renwei de pifu [Proposals and reports of South Jiangxi Administrative Office, Special Office, Lushan Administration Bureau, counties, and cities on health work, and regulation of urban restroom and feces management in Nanchang, and Provincial People's Committee's reply to Nanchang Sports Committee's work proposal].

JXA: X035-05-398, 1963. Sheng weishengting (dangwei) guanyu weisheng gongzuo de baogao, zongjie (baokuo 1951–1962 nian fangzhi shuyi gongzuo zongjie) jihua he shuyi fangzhi gongzuo shinian guihua [Reports and summaries of Provincial Department of Health (Party Committee) on health work, summary report (including report on 1951–1962 plague prevention and treatment].

JXA: X035-05-539, 1966. Weishengbu, guojia tiwei, caizheng, jiaoyubu guanyu weisheng, tiyu gongzuo de guiding, tongzhi [Regulations and announcements of Ministry of Health, State Sports Commission, Ministry of Finance, and Ministry of Education on health and sports].

JXA: X035-06-514, 1958. Jiangxi sheng nongye shehuizhuyi jianshe xianjin danwei daibiao huiyi wenjian [Documents of the Assembly of Jiangxi Outstanding Work Units in Agricultural Socialist Development].

JXA: X035-06-689, 1959. Jiangxi sheng chuhai miebing jiang weisheng gongzuo huiyi wenjian [Documents of Jiangxi Eliminating Pests and Diseases and Promoting Health Conference].

JXA: X039-01-421, 1–12/1957. Caiting yu sheng geji danwei guanyu wenhua jiaoyu weisheng minzheng dangqun shiye deng de lianhe tongzhi zhishi [Joint announcements and directives of Provincial Department of Finance and different levels of provincial agencies on culture, education, health, and civil administration and relationship between the Party and people].

JXA: X039–01–571, 1959. Wenjiao xingzheng caiwu gongzuo shouce (shehui wen-jiao caiwu bufen digao) [Work manual on culture, education, administration, and finance work (draft on society, culture, education, and finance sections)].

JXA: X039–03–432, 1/1957–12/1957. Sheng renwei guanyu weisheng shiye caiwu guanli zhishi pifu tongzhi guiding [Replies and regulations of Provincial People's Committee on health work and finance management].

JXA: X039–04–421, 11/27/1965–12/26/1966. Zhongyang youguan buwei sheng renwei caizheng wenjiao weisheng minzheng deng ting ju guanyu wenjiao weisheng minzheng deng biaozhun zhidu guiding de tongzhi [Announcements of related agencies of Central Committee of CCP, Provincial People's Committee, Department of Finance, Department of Culture and Education, and Department of Health and Department of Civil Administration on standard regulations on culture, education, health, and civil administration].

JXA: X045–01–017, 1956. Jiaoyuting, weishengting guanyu zuzhi bianzhi gongzuo de qingshi baogao he sheng bianwei pifu, tongzhi, fuhan [Proposals of Provincial Department of Education and Department of Health on organizational establishment and replies from Provincial Organizational Establishment Committee].

JXA: X045–01–044, 1957. Sheng weishengting, honghui, xuefang wurenzu guanyu fazhan Hongshizihui he fanyi, xuefang, yaocai gongsi jigou bianzhi de baogao he sheng bianwei de tongzhi [Reports of Provincial Department of Health, Red Cross, and Schistosomiasis Prevention Five-Person Small Group on developing Red Cross and organizational establishment of epidemic prevention, schistosomiasis prevention, and medicine supply agencies, and announcement of Provincial Organizational Establishment Committee].

JXA: X111–01–030, 3/2/1955–12/27/1955. Jiangxi sheng weishengting, dangwei, weishengting dangzu guanyu gaijin zhongyi gongzuo he Yushan xian xuexichongbing zhongdian qu fangzhi wenti de baogao ji shengwei wenjiao dangzu de pishi [Reports of Jiangxi Provincial Department of Health and Party unit on improving Chinese medical services and issues of schistosomiasis-affected areas in Yushan County, and replies from provincial Party unit of Culture and Education Department].

JXA: X111–01–078, 3/19/1957–11/30/1957. Jiangxi sheng weishengting, dangzu, shengwei, weishengting dangzu guanyu weisheng jigou xiajiao he renyuan xiafang ji lingdao guanxi wenti de baogao, pifu [Reports and replies of Jiangxi Provincial Department of Health, Party units, Party Committee, and Party unit of Department of Health on delegating health agencies and sending health service personnel to the countryside and the issues of leadership].

JXA: X111–02–087, 1954. Weishengting sheng xuefangsuo ji dui zu xuefang gongzuo zongjie tongzhi [Work summaries and announcements of the Schistosomiasis Prevention Center of Provincial Department of Health and related groups on the prevention of schistosomiasis].

JXA: X111–02–140, 1955. Shangrao zhuanqu yi er xuefangzhan xuefang gongzuo zongjie [Work summary of No. 12 Schistosomiasis Prevention Station in Shangrao Special Administrative Area on the prevention of schistosomiasis].

JXA: X111–02–200, 1956. Sheng guanyu xuefang zhishi jigou bianzhi zongjie jihua [Summary proposal of Jiangxi Province on the establishment of directive organizationas of schistosomiasis prevention].

JXA: X111–02–201, 2/1957. Jiangxi sheng weishengting, 1956 nian fangzhi xuexichongbing gongzuo ziliao huibian [Collected materials on the prevention of schistosomiasis, 1956, by Jiangxi Provincial Department of Health].

JXA: X111–02–266, 1957. Sheng xuefang wuren xiaozu ji bangongshi de zhishi zongjie deng wenjian [Directives and related documents of Provincial Schistosomiasis Prevention Five-Person Small Group and Office].

JXA: X111–02–268, 1957. Gedi shixian niandu xuefang gongzuo zongjie [Summary reports of different cities and counties on schistosomiasis prevention].

JXA: X111–02–269, 12/1957. Jiangxisheng weishengting, Jiangxi shengwei chuhai miebing lingdao xiaozu bangongshi, 1957 nian xuexichongbing fangzhi gongzuo ziliao huibian [1957 collected materials on the prevention and treatment of schistosomiasis by Jiangxi Provincial Department of Health and Leadership Small Group Office of Jiangxi Eliminating Pests and Diseases].

JXA: X111–03–089, 1959. Zhongyang xuefang jiuren xiaozu bangongshi bianyin de chuhai mie bing gongzuo jianbao (1–24 hao) [Work bulletins on eliminating pests and diseases by Schistosomiasis Prevention Nine-Person Small Group Office of the Central Committee of CCP (numbers 1–24)].

JXA: X111–04–052, 1951. Jiangxi weishengting, yaozhengju, yadanzi kang nueji liaoxiao de yanjiu [Study of treating malaria with java brucea fruit, by Jiangxi Provincial Department of Health and Bureau of Drug Administration].

JXA: X111–04–423, 1956. Shangrao zhuanqu gexian xuefang gongzuo jihua zongjie ji jiancha baoga [Proposals of counties of Shangrao Special Administrative Area on the prevention of schistosomiasis and study reports].

JXA: X111–04–604, 1958. Quanguo bensheng xueyanhui guanyu keyan de zongjie jihua fangzhi xuexichongbing ziliao huibian [Collected materials of the summary proposals of state and provincial schistosomiasis study institues on scientific study of the prevention and treatment of schistosomiasis].

JXA: X111–05–128, 1961. 1961 nian quanguo xue xi chongbing yanjiu weiyuanhui changwei kuoda huiyi ziliao [Materials of 1961 extended session of National Schistosomiasis Research Standing Committee].

JXA: X111–05–345, 1963. Ji'an zhuanqu sheng zhi qita shichang xuefang zongjie ji diaocha wenjian [Reports and study materials of Ji'an Special Administrative Area and other agencies on the prevention of schistosomiasis].

Qingpu Area Archive

QPA: 95-1-1, 3/1951. Qingpu xian, xuexichongbing fangzhizhan, benzhan xuefang gongzuo zongjie [Report on the work of the schistosomiasis prevention station, by Qingpu County Schistosomiasis Prevention and Treatment Station].

QPA: 95-1-2, 1–10/1952. Qingpu xian renmin zhengfu, xuexichongbing fangzhi zhan, benzhan xuefang gongzuo qingkuang baogao [Report on the work of the schistosomiasis prevention station, by Schistosomiasis Prevention and Treatment Station of Qingpu County Government].

QPA: 95–1-4, 1953. Qingpu xian weishengju, xuexichongbing fangzhi zhan, benzhan kaizhan weisheng fangyi gongzuo jihua zongjie [Proposal and summary of the station on launching the work of epidemic prevention, by Schistosomiasis Prevention and Treatment Station, Qingpu County Health Bureau].

QPA: 95–1-6, 1954. Qingpu xian, xuexichongbing fangzhi zhan, benzhan xuefang gongzuo jihua, zongjie [Proposal and summary of the station on schistosomiasis prevention, by Qingpu County Schistosomiasis Prevention and Treatment Station].

QPA: 95–1-8, 3/1955. Qingpu xian, xuexichongbing fangzhi zhan, chengbei shidian zu fangzhi gongzuo jihua zongjie baogao [Proposal and summary of schistosomiasis prevention and treatment at Chengbei experimental unit, by Qingpu County Schistosomiasis Prevention and Treatment Station].

QPA: 95–1-10, 1956–1958. Qingpu xian, xuexichongbing fangzhi zhan, chengbei shidian zu fangzhi gongzuo jihua zongjie baogao [Report of Qingpu County Health Bureau, Schistosomiasis Prevention and Treatment Station, County Party Committee on the prevention and treatment of schistosomiasis].

QPA: 95–1-11, 1–12/1956. Qingpu xian renmin zhengfu, Qingpu xianwei xuexichongbing fangzhi zhan, zhonggong Qingpu xianwei xuefang bangongshi, guanyu fangzhi gongzuo qingkuang baogao [Report of Qingpu County Government, County Schistosomiasis Prevention and Treatment Station, and Schistosomiasis Prevention and Treatment Office of Qingpu County Party Committee on the prevention and treatment of schistosomiasis].

QPA: 95–1-12, 1956. Qingpu xian, xuexichongbing fangzhi zhan, Chengbeixiang fangzhi gongzuo jihua qingkuang baogao zongjie [Proposal and summary of schistosomiasis prevention and treatment at Chengbei experimental unit, by Qingpu County Schistosomiasis Prevention and Treatment Station].

QPA: 95–1-15, 1957. Qingpu xian, xuexichongbing fangzhi zhan, benzhan xuefang gongzuo jihua qingkuang baogao zongjie [Proposal and summary of the station on schistosomiasis prevention, by Qingpu County Schistosomiasis Prevention and Treatment Station].

QPA: 95–1-28, 1962. Qingpu xian weishengju, xuexichongbing fangzhi zhan, yijiuliuer nian sanyue guanyu xuefang tizhi gaige huiyi cailiao [Conference materials on the reform of schistosomiasis prevention system, by Schistosomiasis Prevention and Treatment Station, Qingpu County Health Bureau, March 1962].

QPA: 95–1-29, 1/3/1962. Qingpu xian weishengju, xuexichongbing fangzhi zhan, benzhan xuefang gongzuo jihua zongjie huibao [Proposal and summary of the station on schistosomiasis prevention, by Schistosomiasis Prevention and Treatment Station, Qingpu County Health Bureau].

QPA: 95–2-2, 10/25/1952. Qingpu xian weishengju, xuexichongbing fangzhi zhan, weisheng zhi yi gongzuo qingkuang [Report on health and epidemic prevention, by Schistosomiasis Prevention and Treatment Station, Qingpu County Health Bureau].

QPA: 95-2-4, 1952. Qingpu xian weishengju, xuexichongbing fangzhi zhan, weisheng fangyi gongzuo kaizhan qingkuang, aiguo weisheng, yufang zhushe xiaozu [On the development of health and epidemic prevention work, Patriotic Public Health Campaign, and preventive shots small group, by Schistosomiasis Prevention and Treatment Station, Qingpu County Health Bureau].

QPA: 95-2-5, 10/1953–9/1955. Qingpu xian weishengju, xuexichongbing fangzhi zhan, baogao, tongzhi, han [Reports, announcements, and letters of Schistosomiasis Prevention and Treatment Station, Qingpu County Health Bureau].

QPA: 95-2-6, 12/1953. Qingpu xian, xuexichongbing fangzhi zhan, benzhan ge xuefang zu jihua qingkuang huibao, zongjie [Proposal and summary of the station's schistosomiasis prevention group, by Qingpu County Schistosomiasis Prevention and Treatment Station].

QPA: 95-2-7, 1953. Qingpu xian weishengju, xuexichongbing fangzhi zhan, benzhan kaizhan weisheng fangyi gongzuo qingkuang [On the development of health and epidemic prevention work in the station, by Schistosomiasis Prevention and Treatment Station, Qingpu County Health Bureau].

QPA: 95-2-9, 1953. Archive title unknown.

QPA: 95-2-11, 1954–1955. Qingpu xian weishengju, xuexichongbing fangzhi zhan, weisheng fangyi gongzuo kaizhan qingkuang [On the development of health and epidemic prevention work, by Schistosomiasis Prevention and Treatment Station, Qingpu County Health Bureau].

QPA: 95-2-12, 12/1954. Qingpu xian, xuexichongbing fangzhi zhan, ge xuefang zu fangzhi gongzuo jihua, zongjie huibao [Work proposals and summaries of different schistosomiasis prevention groups, by Qingpu County Schistosomiasis Prevention and Treatment Station].

QPA: 95-2-13, 12/1954. Qingpu xian weishengju, xuexichongbing fangzhi zhan, zhong yi, baihou, kajiemiao, jihua zongjie [Proposal on vaccination, diphtheria, and BCG vaccination, by Schistosomiasis Prevention and Treatment Station, Qingpu County Health Bureau].

QPA: 95-2-18, 1–12/1954. Qingpu xian renmin zhengfu, Qingpu xian xuexichongbing fangzhi zhan, benzhan baogao, tongzhi [Reports and announcements of the station, by Qingpu County Schistosomiasis Prevention and Treatment Station, Qingpu County Government].

QPA: 95-2-19, 1955. Qingpu xian weishengju, xuexichongbing fangzhi zhan, weisheng fangyi gongzuo kaizhan qingkuang (jihua, zongjie, huibao deng) [Proposals, summaries, reports on the development of health and epidemic work, by Schistosomiasis Prevention and Treatment Station, Qingpu County Health Bureau].

QPA: 95-2-20, 1/29/1955. Qingpu xian weishengju, xuexichongbing fangzhi zhan, guanyu xuefang gongzuo jihua, zongjie [Proposals and summaries on schistosomiasis prevention, by Schistosomiasis Prevention and Treatment Station, Qingpu County Health Bureau].

QPA: 95-2-21, 12/1955. Qingpu xian weishengju, xuexichongbing fangzhi zhan, benzhan ge xuefang zu fangzhi gongzuo jihua qingkuang baogao [Work proposals and summaries of different schistosomiasis prevention groups, by Schistosomiasis Prevention and Treatment Station, Qingpu County Health Bureau].

QPA: 95-2-23, 1956. Qingpu xian weishengju, xuexichongbing fangzhi zhan, xuefang ziliao, weisheng fangyi ziliao [Materials on schistosomiasis prevention, health and epidemic prevention, by Schistosomiasis Prevention and Treatment Station, Qingpu County Health Bureau].

QPA: 95-2-26, 1956. Archive title unknown.

QPA: 95-2-27, 1956. Qingpu xian weishengju, xuexichongbing fangzhi zhan, benzhan lianhe zhensuo zhongyi zhongyao zhiliao xuexichongbing qingkuang baogao zongjie [Report on joint station's treatment of schistosomiasis with Chinese medicine, by Schistosomiasis Prevention and Treatment Station, Qingpu County Health Bureau].

QPA: 95-2-32, 1–12/1957. Qingpu xian weishengju, xuexichongbing fangzhi zhan, ben xian weixie ge fanghui guanyu xuefang gongzuo jihua, huibao, zongjie ji weixiegongzuo qingkuang baogao [Proposals, reports, summaries of branches of County Health Association on schistosomiasis prevention, by Schistosomiasis Prevention and Treatment Station, Qingpu County Health Bureau].

QPA: 95–2-44, 1958. Qingpu xian, xuexichongbing fangzhi zhan, Qingpu xian ge lianhe zhensuo xuexichongbing fangzhi zu huibao zongjie [Reports of Qingpu County joint stations on schistosomiasis prevention and treatment groups, by Qingpu County Schistosomiasis Prevention and Treatment Station].

QPA: 95–2-45, 1958. Qingpu xian, xuexichongbing fangzhi zhan, Qingpu xian weisheng jianchazu, ge fangzhi zu jihua huibao [Proposals and reports of various prevention and treatment groups, by Qingpu County Schistosomiasis Prevention and Treatment Station and Qingpu County Health Check Group].

QPA: 95-2-75, 1961. Qingpu xian weishengju, xue xi chongbing fangzhi zhan, guanyu xuefang gongzuo zhuanti qingkuang baogao [Special reports on schistosomiasis prevention, by Schistosomiasis Prevention and Treatment Station, Qingpu County Health Bureau].

QPA: 95-2-76, 1961. Qingpu xian weishengju, xuexichongbing fangzhi zhan, benzhan ge xuefang zu liu luo gongzuo jihua zongjie [Report of Schistosomiasis Prevention Group of the station's Six-Snail Project, by Schistosomiasis Prevention and Treatment Station, Qingpu County Health Bureau].

QPA: 95-2-85, 1/19/1962. Benzhan, xian chu ban, weisheng ke deng, xuefang gongzuo ziliao [Materials on schistosomiasis prevention, by Schistosomiasis Prevention and Treatment Station, County Eliminating Pests and Diseases Office, and Health Department, etc.].

QPA: 95-2-108, 1965. Qingpu xian weishengju, xuexichongbing fangzhi zhan, guanyu xuefang gongzuo de jihua, yijian, baogao, zongjie deng [Proposals, reports, and summaries on schistosomiasis prevention, by Schistosomiasis Prevention and Treatment Station, Qingpu County Health Bureau].

QPA: 95-2-117, 1965–1966. Benzhan, xian chu ban shi xue yan suo xuefang gongzuo ziliao [Materials on schistosomiasis prevention, by Schistosomiasis Prevention and Treatment Station, County Eliminating Pests and Diseases Office, and Municipal Schistosomiasis Research Institute].

Yujiang County Archive at the Commemorative Museum

YJA: 1, 1953. Sheng xuefang suo: Diaocha baogao, gongzuo zongjie, #1 [Study and work reports of Provincial Schistosomiasis Prevention Institute, #1].

YJA: 2, 4–11/1953. Sheng fangyizhan, xuefang suo, guanyu diaodong renyuan, jigou bianzhi, fafang gongzi guiding de tongzhi, #3 [Announcements of Provincial Epidemic Prevention Station and Schistosomiasis Prevention Institute on transferring personnel, organizational establishment, and wage regulation, #3].

YJA: 3, 1954. Sheng zhuan xuefang suo zhan: 1954 nian quannian he fenyue gongzuo zongjie, #1 [Provincial Special Schistosomiasis Prevention Station: 1954 annual and monthly work reports, #1].

YJA: 4, 1954. Zhuanqu diyi xuefang zhan: 1954 nian diaocha, fenbian shidian, liaoxiao fucha deng zongjie, #2 [Special Administrative Area's No. 1 Schistosomiasis Prevention Station: Reports on 1954 study, feces control experimental unit, and recovery checkup, #2].

YJA: 5, 1–12/1954. Sheng weishengting, fangyizhan, xuefang suo: Guanyu peibei huandengpian, zhizuo biaoben, shou jianmian yaofei, bingyuan biaoyang jianding deng [Provincial Department of Health, Epidemic Prevention Station, Schistosomiasis Prevention Center: On equipping slides, making specimens, medical fee exemptions, and patient commendation evaluation].

YJA: 6, 1954. Yujiang xuefang zhan: Zonghe [General report of Yujiang Schistosomiasis Prevention Station].

YJA: 7, 1955. Zhuanqu diyi xuefang zhan: 1955 nian diaocha, wan xue zhiliao, mie luo deng zongjie, #2 [Special Administrative Area's No. 1 Schistosomiasis Prevention Station: Summaries on 1955 study, treatment of advanced schistosomiasis, eliminating snails, #2].

YJA: 8, 1–12/1955. Zhuanqu diyi xuefang zhan: 1955 nian quannian he fenyue gongzuo zongjie, #3 [Special Administrative Area's No. 1 Schistosomiasis Prevention Station: 1955 annual and monthly work reports, #3].

YJA: 9, 1–12/1956. Xianwei xuefang wuren xiaozu jici xuefang huiyi zongjie tongzhi, dianxing cailiao, #2 [Summaries and materials of several schistosomiasis prevention conferences of Five-Person Small Group, County Party Committee, #2].

YJA: 10, 1–12/1956. Xian xuefang wuren xiaozu, fangzhi weiyuanhui xuefang gongzuo diaocha, mie luo zhibing, guan fen de baogao zongjie, #3 [Summary report of County Schistosomiasis Prevention Five-Person Small Group, Prevention Committee, on schistosomiasis prevention, eliminating snails, treatment, and feces management, #3].

YJA: 11, 1–12/1956. Xian xuefangban, xuefang gongzuo huibao, jianbao, #4 [Reports and bulletins of County Schistosomiasis Prevention Office on schistosomiasis prevention, #4].

YJA: 12, 1956. Yujiang xuefang zhan zonghe [General report of Yujiang Schistosomiasis Prevention Station].

YJA: 13, 1–12/1957. Xian xuefang wuren xiaozu, xuefang zhan, 1957 nian xuefang
jihua, huibao, huiyi, zongjie, #1 [Proposals, reports, conference summaries of
County Schistosomiasis Prevention Five-Person Small Group and Schistosomiasis Prevention Station on 1957 schistosomiasis prevention, #1].

YJA: 14, 1–12/1957. Xianwei, xian renwei, xianwei xuefangban: Guanyu mie luo
huiyi, mie luo shiyan de tongzhi baogao, #2 [County Party Committee, County
People's Committee, Schistosomiasis Prevention Office of County Party Committee: Announcement on snail elimination conference and snail elimination
test, #2].

YJA: 15, 1957. Yujiang xuefang zhan: Zonghe [General report of Yujiang Schistosomiasis Prevention Station].

YJA: 16, 1958. Yujiang xuefang zhan: Fang Zhichun zai genchu xuexichongbing qing-
gong huiyi jianghua [Yujiang Schistosomiasis Prevention Station: Fang Zhichun's
speech at the conference of celebrating total elimination of schistosomiasis].

YJA: 17, 1–12/1959. Guanyu jinian genchu xuexichongbing yi zhounian de wen-
zhang zongjie diaocha baogao, #1 [Report on commemorating the first anniversary of total elimination of schistosomiasis, #1].

YJA: 18, 1–12/1961. Xian xuefang zhan, 1961 nian xuefang gonggu gongzuo jihua
anpai diaocha yanjiu gongzuo zongjie, #2 [1961 report of County Schistosomiasis
Prevention Station on strengthening the work of schistosomiasis prevention and
study, #2].

YJA: 19, 1–12/1961. Xianwei: Chuhai mie bing, xuefang gonggu gongzuo huiyi wenjian, #3 [County Party Committee: Conference documents on eliminating diseases in the sea and strengthening the work of schistosomiasis prevention, #3].

YJA: 20, 1–12/1962. Xian xuefang zhan, zhonggong Yujiang xianwei pizhuan xuefang gonggu zhuanye huiyi wenjian, #1 [Transmitted conference documents of
County Schistosomiasis Prevention Station and Yujiang County Party Committee of CCP on strengthening the work of schistosomiasis prevention, #1].

YJA: 21, 1–12/1962. Xian xuefang zhan, xuefang zhuanjia shicha jishi, #2 [Field study
of schistosomiasis prevention experts, by County Schistosomiasis Prevention Station, #2].

YJA: 22, 1–12/1962. Xian xuefang zhan, xuefang gonggu gongzuo jihua zongjie shiyan yanjiu fangan baogao, #3 [Summaries and reports of County Schistosomiasis
Prevention Station on strengthening the work of schistosomiasis prevention, testing, and research, #3].

YJA: 23, 1–12/1962. Xian xuefang zhan, cun shi, jiashi, xue xi chongbing liuxing shi,
#8 [Village history, family history, and the epidemic history of schistosomiasis, by
County Schistosomiasis Prevention Station, #8].

YJA: 24, 1–12/1962. Xian xuefang zhan, guanxin he reai xuefang gongzuo de dan-
gzhengqun xianjin renwu de shiji, #9 [The good deeds of outstanding party members and people who care and devote themselves to the work of schistosomiasis
prevention, by County Schistosomiasis Prevention Station, #9].

YJA: 25, 1962. Yujiang xuefang zhan: Znghe [General report of Yujiang Schisto-somiasis Prevention Station].

YJA: 26, 1–12/1963. Yujiangxian xuefang quan zong, zhonggong Yujiang xianwei, guanyu xuefang gonggu gongzuo huiyi wenjian de pishi, #1 [Directives of Yujiang County Schistosomiasis Prevention Station and Yujiang County Party Commit-tee of CCP on the conference of strengthening the work of schistosomiasis pre-vention, #1].

YJA: 27, 1–12/1963. Xianwei: Xuefang gonggu gongzuo jixiang guiding, xian, she, chang jingyan jieshao, #2 [County Party Committee: Directives on strengthen-ing the work of schistosomiasis prevention and introductions to the experiences of county, communes, and farms, #2].

YJA: 28, 1963. Yujiang xuefang zhan: Zonghe [General report of Yujiang Schisto-somiasis Prevention Station].

YJA: 29, 1–12/1964. Xianwei, chu ban, minzhengju: Xuefang gonggu ruogan zhidu zongjie huibao; xuefang zhan xianjin shiji wufan zhenggai fangan; dangyuan dengji, ganbu diaodong, laoruocan zhigong bianwai baopi biao gei shi ming wan xue bingren jiujikuan, #1 [County Party Committee, Schistosomiasis Prevention Office, Bureau of Civil Administration: Summary report on strengthening the work of schistosomiasis prevention and certain systems; proposal on good deeds in the Schistosomiasis Prevention Station and Five-Antis reform; party member registration, shifting cadres, staff status of old, weak and disabled workers, and relief fund for ten patients with advanced schistosomiasis, #1].

YJA: 30, 1964. Xuefang zhan: Zonghe [General report of Schistosomiasis Preven-tion Station].

YJA: 31, 1965. Xuefang zhan: Zonghe [General report of Schistosomiasis Prevention Station].

YJA: 32, 2–10/1967. Xian lin weihui, wei san zhan: Guanyu jinian "Song wenshen" fabiao jiu zhounian, zhaokai xuefang hui, xiugai chenlieguan, deng tongzhi, baogao, #1 [County Interim Committee, three health stations: Announcements and reports on commemorating the ninth anniversary of the publication of "Fare-well to the god of plague," holding schistosomiasis prevention conferences and remodeling exhibition hall, #1].

YJA: 33, 1–12/1968. Shinian daqing deng weihui, yi zhi qi qi "Song wenshen" jianbao, #1 [Ten Years Celebration Committee, nos. 1–7 bulletins of "Farewell to the god of plague," #1].

YJA: 34, 1–12/1968. Shinian daqing deng wei bangongshi "Song wenshen" chenlie-guan wenzi dagang, #3 [Ten Years Celebration Committee Office outline for the description of the "Farewell to the god of plague" exhibition hall, #3].

YJA: 35, 1–12/1970. Xian xuefang lingdao xiaozu xuefang gonggu gongzuo de jin-gyan jieshao, #1 [Introduction to County Schistosomiasis Prevention Leadership Small Group's experience of strengthening the work of schistosomiasis preven-tion, #1].

YJA: 36, 1–12/1971. Xian xuefang lingdao xiaozu xianjin shiji, chenlieguan wenzi dagang, xuefang huibao tigang gaojian, #1 [Outstanding deeds of County Schistosomiasis Prevention Leadership Small Group, outline for description of exhibition hall and report outline of schistosomiasis prevention, #1].

YJA: 37, 1–12/1972. Xian ge wei baodao zu xuefang yiliao dui xuefang yiliao duiwu shiji fu bo zhiyuan xiaojie, #1 [Summary report of County Medical Report Group on the deeds of schistosomiasis prevention medical group assisting Boyang, #1].

YJA: 38, 1–12/1972. Xian gewei, shuiliju: Weisheng gongzuo huibao tigang, nongtian shuili jianshe jingyan, #2 [County Revolution Committee, Bureau of Water Resources: Outline report on health work and experience of farmland irrigation constructions, #2].

YJA: 39, 12/1972. Xianwei xuefang bangongshi: Ma gang dadui shang Huangcun wuzhong jiancha fangfa cha bing shidian gongzuo zongjie, #3 [County Schistosomiasis Prevention Office: Summary report on five ways of disease detection in Shanghuang Village, Magang Brigade, #3].

YJA: 40, 1–12/1973. Zhonggong Yujiang xianwei: Guanyu xuefang gonggu gongzuo huiyi de tongzhi, baogao, zongjie, jilu, #1 [Yujiang County Committee of CCP: Announcements, reports, summaries, and records on the conferences of strengthening the work of schistosomiasis prevention, #1].

YJA: 41, 1–12/1973. Xianwei, xian xuefangban: Iinian "Song wenshen" fabiao shiwu zhounian tongzhi, gongzuo zongjie he jihua, jiedai canguan, wan xue diaocha huibao, #2 [County Party Committee, County Schistosomiasis Prevention Office: Commemorating the fifteenth-anniversary of the publication of "Farewell to the god of plague" work proposals, receptions and visits, and study of advanced schistosomiasis, #2].

YJA: 42, 1–12/1979. 1979 nian xuefang gonggu gongzuo jidu, niandu zongjie, cha luo cha bing, keyan zongjie, huibao 1979, #1 [1979 annual report on strengthening the work of schistosomiasis prevention, year-end summary, detecting snails and diseases, and scientific study, #1].

YJA: 43, 12/1976. Zhonggong Yujiang xianwei xuefang lingdao xiaozu bangongshi [Schistosomiasis Prevention Leadership Small Group Office of Yujiang Party Committee of CCP]. "Jiangxi sheng Yujiangxian xuefang gongzuo ziliao huibian (1949–1975)" [Collected materials of schistosomiasis prevention in Jiangxi Yujiang County (1949–1975)]. Neibu ziliao [Unpublished in-house book of statistics].

YJA: 44. Yu Laixi, Zhonggong Yujiang xianwei xuefang lingdao xiaozu bangongshi [Yu Laixi, Schistosomiasis Prevention Leadership Small Group Office of Yujiang Party Committee]. "Jiangxi sheng Yujiang xian xuefang zhi: 1953–1980" [Yujiang County, Jiangxi Schistosomiasis Prevention Gazetteer: 1953–1980]. Unpublished, handwritten copy.

INTERVIEWS

Interview on November 13, 2008, with proctors of the Yujiang County schistosomiasis commemorative museum.

Interview on September 13, 2007, with personnel of the Shanghai Institute of Parasitic Diseases.

FILMS AND PICTURES

The Barefoot Doctors of Rural China, 1975. National Archives and Records Administration, Washington, D.C. ARC: 46549.
Pictorial sources from the collection of Fan Ka Wai, Hong Kong.
Pictorial sources from the Yujiang County Schistosomiasis Commemorative Museum, Dengfuzhen.
Zheng Junli, dir. *Kumu feng chun.* [Spring comes to the withered tree]. Shanghai: Haiyan Film, 1961.

CHINESE NEWSPAPER ARTICLES

Boerdeliefu, Zhonghua renmin gongheguo weishengbu sulian zhuanjia zuzhang [Boerdeliefu (Tikhon E. Boldyrev, 1900–1984), Soviet Union Expert Group Chief at the Ministry of Health, PRC]. "Guanyu xiaomie xuexichong bing cuoshi de jidian yijian" [Several suggestions on schistosomiasis elimination]. *Jiankang bao,* no. 425, February 17, 1956.
"Boyang xuefang zhan yijia dang san jia: Jiejue xianweijing buzu de kunnan" [Boyang Schistosomiasis Prevention using one as three: Solving the problem of lacking microscopes]. *Jiangxi ribao,* no. 3221, May 15, 1958.
"Bu qiu shenxian zhi qiu yi" [Seeking help not from gods, but only from doctors]. *Qingpu bao,* no. 9, August 11, 1956.
Cui Yitian. "Dali zhankai huadong nongcun xuexichongbing fangzhi gongzuo" [Vigorously develop the work of prevention and treatment of schistosomiasis in east China]. *Jiefang ribao,* no. 885, November 9, 1951.
Dai Chun. "Pengze xian fangzhi xuexibing gongzuo weishenme mei gaoqilai?" [Why didn't Pengzi County's prevention and treatment of Schistosomiasis work?]. *Jiangxi ribao,* December 15, 1956.
"Ge xiang xuexichongbing pujian zhiliao jinbubiao" [Chart of each township's schistosomiasis survey treatment progress]. *Qingpu bao,* no. 205, August 2, 1958.
Huang Lanyan. "Sunan xuexichongbing yufang gongzuo" [Prevention and treatment of schistosomiasis in south Jiangsu]. *Jiankang bao,* no. 202, November 8, 1951.
Lü Qizuo. "Ganzou wenshen" [Expel the god of plague]. *Jiankang bao,* no. 695, November 26, 1958.
"Nong mu relie huanying Mao zhuxi pailai de yiliaodui" [Peasants and herders warmly welcome medical teams sent by Chairman Mao]. *Renmin ribao,* October 6, 1965.

"Qingpu xian xiaomie xuexichongbing jiangli banfa (caoan)" [Reward guidelines on elimination of schistosomiasis in Qingpu County]. *Qingpu bao,* no. 207 August 7, 1958.

"Quanguo gedi honghong lielie daban kexue shiye" [Vigorously develop the cause of science in the nation]. *Qingpu bao,* no. 188, June 26, 1958.

Wang Lun. "Xuefang zhanzhang" [Head of a prevention station]. *Jiangxi ribao,* October 5, 1957.

Wang Qingyuan. "Shi xuexichongbing fangzhi gongzuo yu aiguo weisheng yundong jiehe qilai" [Unite the work of schistosomiasis prevention and treatment and Patriotic Health Campaign]. *Jiankang bao,* no. 412, November 25, 1955.

"Weishengbu mianli xinnian qu nongcun de yiyao weisheng renyuan nuli zuodao" [On New Year's the Ministry of Public Health urges medical workers going to the countryside to make great accomplishments]. *Renmin ribao,* December 31, 1965.

"Wuchengzhen de xuexichongbing fangzhi xiaozu" [Wucheng Town Schistosomiasis Prevention and Treatment Group]. *Jiangxi ribao,* no. 2341, December 3, 1955.

"Yishi dapo mixin, xiaxiang shuxue qiangjiu bingren" [Doctors smash superstitions, rushing to the countryside to save sick people]. *Qingpu bao,* no. 193 July 8, 1958.

"Zunzhao Mao zhuxi guanyu 'yingdang jiji de yufang he yiliao renmin de jibing' de jiaodao" [Obey Chairman Mao's guidance to "actively prevent and treat the people's diseases"]. *Renmin ribao,* June 26, 1973.

OTHER PUBLISHED SOURCES

Allen, Edwin Joseph, Jr. "Disease Control in China: An Investigation into the Ways In Which Public Health Propaganda Effects Changes in Medicine and Hygiene, with Emphasis on Schistosomiasis Control." Master's thesis, Columbia University, 1965.

Andreano, R. L. *"Farewell to the God of Plague": The Economic Impact of Parasitic Disease (Schistosomiasis) in Mainland China.* Report No. 3. Madison, WI: Health Economics Research Center, 1971.

———. *More on the God of Plague: Schistosomiasis in Mainland China.* Report No. 7. Madison, WI: Health Economics Research Center, 1971.

Andreas, Joel. *Rise of the Red Engineers: The Cultural Revolution and the Origins of China's New Class.* Stanford, CA: Stanford University Press, 2009.

Anting People's Commune, Jiading County, Shanghai. "Drive Away the God of Plague with Gleaming Mattocks and Mighty Arms." *Chinese Medical Journal* 87.11 (1968): 662–68.

Arrow, Kenneth J., Claire Panosian, and Hellen Gelband, eds. *Saving Lives, Buying Time: Economics of Malaria Drugs in an Age of Resistance.* Washington, D.C.: National Academies Press, 2004.

Ashford, Bailey K., and Pedro Gutiérrez Igaravidez. *Uncinariasis (Hookworm Disease) in Porto Rico: A Medical and Economic Problem.* Washington, D.C.: Government Printing Office, 1911.

"Association News." *Chinese Medical Journal* 76.1 (January 1958): 101–2.

"Association News: Visit of Japanese Schistosomiasis Specialists." *Chinese Medical Journal* 75.1 (January 1957): 84.

Balasegaram, Mangai, and Alan Schnur. "China: From Denial to Mass Mobilization." In *SARS: How a Global Epidemic Was Stopped*. Geneva: World Health Organization, Western Pacific Region, 2006.

Banister, Judith. "Population, Public Health and the Environment in China." *China Quarterly* 156 (December 1998): 986–1015.

Barnett, A. Doak. *Cadres, Bureaucracy, and Political Power in Communist China.* New York: Columbia University Press, 1967.

Bennett, Gordon. *Yundong: Mass Campaigns in Chinese Communist Leadership.* China Research Monograph No. 12. Berkeley: Center for Chinese Studies, University of California, 1976.

Blumenthal, David, and William Hsiao. "Privatization and Its Discontents—the Evolving Chinese Health Care System." *New England Journal of Medicine* 353.11 (September 15, 2005): 1165–70.

Bonner, J. "Medicine and Public Health." *China Science Notes* 3.1 (January 1972): 6–8.

Borthwick, Sally. *Education and Social Change in China: The Beginnings of the Modern Era.* Stanford, CA: Hoover Institution Press, 1983.

Bowers, J. Z. "Medicine in Mainland China: Red and Rural." *Current Scene: Developments in Mainland China* 8.12 (June 15, 1970): 1–11.

Brookes, Tim. *Behind the Mask: How the World Survived SARS, the First Epidemic of the 21st Century.* Washington, D.C.: American Public Health Association, 2005.

Brown, Peter J. "Malaria, Miseria, and Underpopulation in Sardinia: The 'Malaria Blocks Development' Cultural Model." *Medical Anthropology* 17.3 (1997): 239–54.

Bruun, Ole. "The Fengshui Resurgence in China: Conflicting Cosmologies between State and Peasantry." *China Journal* 36 (July 1996): 47–65.

Buhs, Joshua Blu. *The Fire Ant Wars: Nature, Science, and Public Policy in Twentieth-Century America.* Chicago: University of Chicago Press, 2004.

Cao Xueqin. *Honglou meng* [Dream of the Red Chamber]. 1791. Beijing: Renmin wenxue chubanshe, Xinhua shudian faxing, 1996.

Cell, Charles P. *Revolution at Work: Mobilization Campaigns in China.* New York: Academic Press, 1977.

Chan, Anita, Richard Madsen, and Jonathan Unger. *Chen Village: The Recent History of a Peasant Community in Mao's China.* Berkeley: University of California Press, 1984.

Chekiang, Chia-shan Hsien, Anti-epidemic Station Revolutionary Leading Group. "As Chairman Mao Directs, We Follow: How Schistosomiasis in Jiashan County Was Wiped Out by 'People's War.'" *China's Medicine* 10 (October 1968): 603–9.

Chen, C. C. *Medicine in Rural China: A Personal Account.* Berkeley: University of California Press, 1989.

Chen, Honggen, and Dandan Lin. "The Prevalence and Control of Schistosomiasis in Poyang Lake Region, China." *Parasitology International* 53.2 (2004): 115–25.

Chen, Pi-chao. *Population and Health Policy in the People's Republic of China.* Occasional Monograph Series No. 9. Washington, D.C.: Interdisciplinary Communications Program, Smithsonian Institution, December 1976.

Chen, William Y. "Medicine and Public Health." In *Sciences in Communist China: A Symposium Presented at the New York Meeting of the American Association for the Advancement of Science, December 26–27, 1960,* edited by Sidney H. Gamble. Washington, D.C.: American Association for the Advancement of Science, 1961.

Chen Qilin. "Dengfuzhen chujian fenguan de huiyi" [Recollection of the start of shit management in Dengfuzhen]. In *Song wenshen jishi* [Record of farewell to the god of plague campaign], vol. 43, edited by Liu Yurui and Wan Guohe. Nanchang: Jiangxi sheng zhengxie wenshi ziliao yanjiu weiyuanhui, 1992.

Chen Xianyi et al. "Schistosomiasis Control in China: The Impact of a 10-year World Bank Loan Project (1992–2001)." *Bulletin of the World Health Organization* 83 (2005): 43–48.

Chen Zhengyan. "Wo shi dangnian de chijiaoyisheng" [At that time, I was a barefoot doctor]. *Wenshi bolan* 4 (2014): 46–48.

Cheng Tien-hsi. "Schistosomiasis in Mainland China: A Review of Research and Control Programs since 1949." *American Journal of Tropical Medicine and Hygiene* 20.1 (January 1971): 26–53.

Ch'ien Hsin-chung. "Summing Up of Mass Technical Experiences with a View to Expediting Eradication of the Five Major Parasitic Diseases." *Chinese Medical Journal* 77.6 (January 1958): 521–32.

China Health Care Study Group. *Health Care in China, an Introduction: The Report of a Study Group in Hong Kong.* Geneva: Christian Medical Commission, 1974.

"China Produces First Documentary on Disasters." www.china.org.cn/english/culture/96762.htm. Accessed March 10, 2006.

Chung, Arthur W. *Of Rats, Sparrows and Flies . . . : A Lifetime in China.* Stockton, CA: Heritage West Books, 1995.

Coale, Ansley J. *Rapid Population Change in China, 1952–1982.* Committee on Population and Demography Report No. 27. Washington, D.C.: National Academy Press, 1984.

Croizier, Ralph C. "Medicine and Modernization in China: An Historical Overview." In *Medicine in Chinese Cultures,* edited by Arthur M. Kleinman et al. Washington, D.C.: U.S. Department of Health, Education and Welfare, National Institutes of Health, 1975.

———. *Traditional Medicine in Modern China: Science, Nationalism, and the Tensions of Cultural Change.* Cambridge, MA: Harvard University Press, 1968.

Davis, A. "Schistosomiasis." Chapter 80 in *Manson's Tropical Diseases,* 21st ed., edited by Gordon C. Cook and Alimuddin I. Zumla. Philadelphia: Saunders, Elsevier Science, 2003.

Deng Shilin, oral history compiled by Shu Mingliang. "Bingfang she zai wode jia" [Establishing a ward in my house]. In *Song wenshen jishi* [Record of farewell to the god of plague campaign], vol. 43, edited by Liu Yurui and Wan Guohe. Nanchang: Jiangxi sheng zhengxie wenshi ziliao yanjiu weiyuanhui, 1992.

"Di yici quanguo renkou pucha" [The first national census]. Posted at the National Bureau of Statistics, June 25, 2002. www.stats.gov.cn. Accessed May 6, 2008.

Dobson, M. J., M. Malowany, and R. W. Snow. "Malaria Control in East Africa: The Kampala Conference and the Pare-Taveta Scheme; A Meeting of Common and High Ground." *Parassitologia* 42 (2000): 149–66.

Editor. "The Mao-Liu Controversy over Rural Public Health." *Current Scene* 7.12 (June 15, 1969): 1–18.

Endicott, Stephen, and Edward Hagerman. *The United States and Biological Warfare: Secrets from the Early Cold War and Korea.* Bloomington: Indiana University Press, 1998.

Engels, Friedrich. *Ludwig Feuerbach and the Outcome of Classical German Philosophy.* London: M. Lawrence, 1934.

———. "The Part Played by Labour in the Transition from Ape to Man." *Dialectics of Nature.* Translated and edited by Clemens Dutt. New York: International Publishers, 1940.

Engle, H. N., and P. Engle. *Poems of Mao Tse-tung.* New York: Simon and Schuster, 1973.

Fan, Ka wai, and Honkei Lai. "Mao Zedong's Fight against Schistosomiasis." *Perspectives in Biology and Medicine* 51.2 (Spring 2008): 176–87.

Fan Xingzhun. "You guan riben zhuxuexichongbing de zhongyi wenxian de chubu tantao" [A preliminary investigation of the Chinese medical literature relating to schistosomiasis]. *Zhonghua yixue zazhi* 11 (1954): 862–64.

Fang Xiaoping. *Barefoot Doctors and Western Medicine.* Rochester, NY: University of Rochester Press, 2012.

Farley, John. *Bilharzia: A History of Imperial Tropical Medicine.* New York: Cambridge University Press, 2003.

Faust, Ernest, and Henry Meleney. *Studies on Schistosomiasis Japonica.* Monograph Series No. 3. Baltimore: American Journal of Hygiene, 1924.

Fee, Elizabeth. *Disease and Discovery: A History of the Johns Hopkins School of Hygiene and Public Health, 1916–1939.* Baltimore: Johns Hopkins University Press, 1987.

Fee, Elizabeth, and Liping Bu. "Models of Public Health Education: Choices for the Future?" *Bulletin of the World Health Organization* 85.12 (December 2007): 901–80.

Feurtado, Gardel MacArthur. "Mao Tse-tung and the Politics of Science in Communist China, 1949–1965." Ph.D. dissertation, Stanford University, 1986.

"First County to Wipe Out Schistosomiasis." *China Reconstructs* (July 17, 1968): 12–16.

Fluehr-Lobban, Carolyn. "Frederick Engels and Leslie White: The Symbol versus the Role of Labor in the Origin of Humanity." *Dialectical Anthropology* 11.1 (1986): 119–26.

Foucault, Michel. *Discipline and Punish: The Birth of the Prison.* New York: Vintage, 1979.

———. *The History of Sexuality.* Vol. 1. New York: Vintage, 1990.

Friedman, Edward, Paul G. Pickowicz, and Mark Selden. *Chinese Village, Socialist State.* New Haven, CT: Yale University Press, 1991.

———. *Revolution, Resistance, and Reform in Village China.* New Haven, CT: Yale University Press, 2005.

Frolic, Michael B. *Mao's People: Sixteen Portraits of Life in Revolutionary China.* Cambridge, MA: Harvard University Press, 1980.

Fu Lien-Chang. "An Address to the Members of the Medical Profession among the Delegates to the Peace Conference of the Asian and Pacific Regions." *Chinese Medical Journal* 71 (January–February 1953): 1–6.

———. "Summing-Up of the Ninth General Conference of the Chinese Medical Association Held in Peking on December Fourteenth to Seventeenth, 1952." *Chinese Medical Journal* 71 (March–April 1953): 159–62.

Gao, Mobo. *Gao Village: Rural Life in Modern China.* Honolulu: University of Hawai'i Press, 1999.

Garrett, Laurie. *The Coming Plague: Newly Emerging Diseases in a World Out of Balance.* New York: Penguin, 1994.

Gettleman, Jeffrey. "Meant to Keep Malaria Out, Mosquito Nets Are Used to Haul Fish In." *New York Times,* January 24, 2015.

Greenhalgh, Susan. *Just One Child: Science and Policy in Deng's China.* Berkeley: University of California Press, 2008.

Guo Jiagang. "Schistosomiasis Control in China: Strategy of Control and Rapid Assessment of Schistosomiasis Risk by Remote Sensing (RS) and Geographic Information System (GIS)." Ph.D. dissertation, University of Basel, 2003. http://edoc.unibas.ch/245/1/DissB_7169.pdf. Accessed July 26, 2015.

Hackett, L. W. *Malaria in Europe: An Ecological Study.* London: Oxford University Press, 1937.

Hanson, Marta. "The Art of Medicine: Maoist Public-Health Campaigns, Chinese Medicine, and SARS." *Lancet* 372 (October 25, 2008): 1457–58.

Harding, Harry. *Organizing China: The Problem of Bureaucracy, 1949–1976.* Stanford, CA: Stanford University Press, 1981.

Harrison, Gordon. *Mosquitoes, Malaria and Man: A History of the Hostilities since 1880.* New York: E. P. Dutton, 1978.

He Lianyin. "Policy Making and Organization in Managing Tropical Diseases in China." *Chinese Medical Journal* 114.7 (2001): 769–71.

"Health Work Serving the Peasants." *Chinese Medical Journal* 85.3 (March 1966): 143–49.

Heggenhougen, H. Kristian, Veronica Hackethal, and Pramila Vivek. *The Behavioral and Social Aspects of Malaria and Its Control: An Introduction and Annotated Bibliography.* Geneva: World Health Organization, 2003.

Helitzer-Allen, Deborah L., Carl Kendall, and Jack J. Wirima. "The Role of Ethnographic Research in Malaria Control: An Example from Malaŵi." *Research in the Sociology of Health Care* 10 (1993): 269–86.

"The Henry Lester Institute and Hospital." *Science* 69.1785 (March 15, 1929): 290–91.

Hillier, S. M., and J. A. Jewell. *Health Care and Traditional Medicine in China, 1800–1982.* London: Routledge & Kegan Paul, 1983.

Horn, Joshua. *Away With All Pests: An English Surgeon in People's China, 1954–1969.* New York: Monthly Review Press, 1969.

———. "Building a Rural Health Service in the People's Republic of China." *International Journal of Health Services* 2.3 (August 1972): 377–83.

Hou Tsung-Ch'ang, Chung Huei-Lan, Ho Lien-Yin, and Weng Hsin-Chih. "Achievements in the Fight against Parasitic Diseases in New China." *Chinese Medical Journal* 79 (December 1959): 493–515.

Hsiao, William C. L. "The Chinese Health Care System: Lessons for Other Nations." *Social Science and Medicine* 41.8 (October 1995): 1047–55.

Hsu, H. F., and Li S. Y. Hsu. "Schistosomiasis in the Shanghai Area." In *China Medicine as We Saw It,* edited by Joseph R. Quinn and John E. Fogarty International Center, DHEW Publication No. (NIH) 75–684. Washington, D.C.: U.S. Department of Health, Education, and Welfare, 1974.

Huang, Yanzhong. "The SARS Epidemic and Its Aftermath in China: A Political Perspective." In *Learning from SARS: Preparing for the Next Disease Outbreak; Workshop Summary,* edited by Stacey Knobler, Adel Mahmoud, Stanley Lemon, Alison Mack, Laura Sivitz, and Katherine Oberholtzer. Washington, D.C.: National Academies Press, 2004.

Huang Qijing and Luo Zhuliu. "Tongxin xieli song wenshen—qing puxiang xue xi chongbing yiqing ji fangzhi chengguo" [Unite together to say farewell to the god of plague—achievements of prevention and treatment of epidemic of schistosomiasis in Qingpu County]. In *Qingpu wenshi, di si qi* [Qingpu culture and history, vol. 4]. Qingpu [Shanghai]: Zhongguo renmin zhengzhi xieshang huiyi Qingpu xian weiyuanhui wenshi ziliao weiyuanhui, 1989.

Hubei sheng weishengting [Hubei Provincial Department of Health]. *Xuexichongbing fangzhi zhishi jianghua* [Speech on schistosomiasis prevention and treatment knowledge]. Wuhan: Hubei sheng weishengting, 1966.

Hughes, Thomas Parke. *American Genesis: A Century of Invention and Technological Enthusiasm, 1870–1970.* Chicago: University of Chicago Press, 2004.

Hvistendahl, Mara. "The Numbers Game." *Science* 340 (May 31, 2013): 1037–38.

Iijima Wataru. "'Farewell to the God of Plague': Anti–*Schistosoma japonicum* Campaign in China and Japanese Colonial Medicine." *Memoirs of the Toyo Bunko* 66 (2008): 45–79.

Issii, Akira, Miyasu Tsuji, and Isao Tada. "History of Katayama Disease: Schistosomiasis Japonica in Katayama district, Hiroshima, Japan." *Parasitology International* 52.4 (December 2003): 313–19.

Jiangsu sheng nongcun jingji 50 nian [50 years of Jiangsu's rural economy]. Beijing: Zhongguo tongji chubanshe, 2000.

Jiangsu sheng xuexichongbing fangzhi yanjiusuo [Jiangsu Schistosomiasis Prevention and Treatment Research Institute]. *Youguan zhiliao xuexichongbing de ziliao* [Materials on treatment of schistosomiasis]. Nanjing: Jiangsu sheng xuexichongbing fangzhi yanjiusuo, 1965.

"Jiangxi sheng xuexichongbing ji fangzhi dashiji, 1909–1991" [Great event of Jiangxi Province's schistosomiasis prevention and treatment, 1909–1991]. In *Song wenshen jishi* [Record of farewell to the god of plague campaign], vol. 43, edited by Liu Yurui and Wan Guohe. Nanchang: Jiangxi sheng zhengxie wenshi ziliao yanjiu weiyuanhui, 1992.

Jiangxi sheng xuexichongbing yanjiu weiyuanhui [Jiangxi Provincial Schistosomiasis Research Committee]. *Xuexichongbing yanjiu, 1956–1985* [Study of schistosomiasis, 1956–1985]. Nanchang: Jiangxi sheng xuexichongbing yanjiu weiyuanhui, [198?].

Jin Jiqing, ed. *Qingpu xian fangzhi xuexichongbing sanshiwu nian: Tubiao ji* [Thirty-five years of treating and prevention schistosomiasis in Qingpu County: Chart collection]. Shanghai: Shanghai kexue jishu chubanshe, 1986.

Jin Yimin and Qingpu xian shuiliju [Jin Yimin and Qingpu County Bureau of Water Resources]. "Shuili xing ze wenming cun—Qingpu xian shuilishi qiantan" [Great water resources preserve civilization—brief introduction to the history of water resources in Qingpu County]. In *Qingpu wenshi, di yi qi* [Qingpu culture and history, vol. 1]. Qingpu [Shanghai]: Zhongguo renmin zhengzhi xieshang huiyi Qingpu xian weiyuanhui wenshi ziliao weiyuanhui, 1989.

Johnson, Chalmers. "Chinese Communist Leadership and Mass Response: The Yenan Period and the Socialist Education Period." In *China in Crisis: China's Heritage and the Communist Political System,* edited by Ping-ti Ho and Tang Tsou. Chicago: University of Chicago Press, 1968.

Kan Huai-chieh and Yao Yung-tsung. "Some Notes on the Anti–Schistosomiasis Japonica Campaign in Chih-huai-pan, Kaihua, Chekiang." *Chinese Medical Journal* 48.4 (April 1934): 323–36.

Kau, Michael, and John Leung, eds. *The Writings of Mao Zedong, 1949–1976.* Vol. 1. Armonk, NY: M. E. Sharpe, 1986.

———. "Circular Requesting Opinions on 17 Articles on Agricultural Work" (December 21, 1955).

———. "Comment on Department of Public Health" (1953).

———. "Conversation with Security Guards" (mid-July, 1955).

———. "Criticism of the Ministry of Public Health" (October 1953).

———. "Directive on Work in Traditional Chinese Medicine" (July 30, 1954).

———. Editors' notes on *Upsurge of Socialism in China's Countryside* (December 27, 1955).

———. "Implementing Correct Policy in Dealing with Doctors of Traditional Chinese Medicine" (October 20, 1954).

———. "Instruction on Leadership Work of Health Department of Military Commissions" (April 3, 1953).

———. "Resolving the Problem of the 'Five Excesses'" (March 19, 1953).

———. "Second Preface to *Upsurge of Socialism in China's Countryside*" (December 27, 1955).

Kau, Michael, and John Leung, eds. *The Writings of Mao Zedong, 1949–1976.* Vol. 2. Armonk, NY: M. E. Sharpe, 1992.

———. "Instructions on Report on Schistosomiasis Prevention Conference" (March 7, 1956).

———. "On the Ten Great Relationships" (April 25, 1956).

———. "RMRB Editorial on Cultivating Traditional Chinese Medicine" (May 27, 1956).

———. "Talk with Music Workers" (August 24, 1956).

Kaufman, Joan. "SARS and China's Health-Care Response: Better to Be Both Red and Expert!" In *SARS in China: Prelude to Pandemic?,* edited by Arthur Kleinman and James L. Watson. Stanford, CA: Stanford University Press, 2006.

Kerr, Richard A., and Richard Stone. "A Human Trigger for the Great Quake of Sichuan?" *Science* 323.5912 (January 16, 2009): 322.

Kiangxi, Yü-chiang Hsien, Revolutionary Committee, Culture, Education, Health, and Antischistosomiasis Section, with Yü-chiang Antischistosomiasis Station. "A Great Victory of Mao Zedong's Thought in the Battle against Schistosomiasis: The 10 Years Since the Eradication of Schistosomiasis in Yukiang County in 1958." *China's Medicine* 10 (October 1968): 588–602.

Kleinman, Arthur. "Traditional Doctors." In *Rural Health in the People's Republic of China: Report of a Visit by the Rural Health Systems Delegation, June 1978,* by Committee on Scholarly Communication with the People's Republic of China, NIH Publication No. 81–2124. Washington, D.C.: U.S. Department of Health and Human Services, Public Health Service, National Institutes of Health, November 1980.

Komiya, Y. "Recommendatory Note for the Control Problem of Schistosomiasis in China." *Japanese Journal of Medical Science and Biology* 10.6 (1957): 461–71.

Kwok, D. W. Y. *Scientism in Chinese Thought, 1900–1950.* New Haven, CT: Yale University Press, 1965.

Lai Hongyi. "Local Management of SARS in China: Guangdong and Beijing." In *The SARS Epidemic: Challenges to China's Crisis Management,* edited by John Wong and Zheng Yongnian. Singapore: World Scientific Publishing Company, 2004.

Lampton, David M. *Health, Conflict, and the Chinese Political System.* Michigan Papers in Chinese Studies No. 18. Ann Arbor: University of Michigan, 1974.

———. *The Politics of Medicine in China: The Policy Process, 1949–1977.* Boulder, CO: Westview Press, 1977.

Lee, Vincent. "Snail Scare." *Shanghai Star,* June 24, 2004.

Leiper, R. T., and E. L. Atkinson. "Observations on the Spread of Aseatic Schisto-somiasis." *Chinese Medical Journal* 29.3 (May 1915): 143–49.

Lenin, V. I. "The Taylor System—Man's Enslavement by the Machine" (1914). In *Collected Works,* vol. 20. Moscow: Foreign Languages Publishing House, 1964.

Li Guohua. "Chabing, zhibing, de jijian wangshi" [A few past incidents regarding the inspection and curing of the disease]. In *Song wenshen jishi* [Record of fare-well to the god of plague campaign], vol. 43, edited by Liu Yurui and Wan Guohe. Nanchang: Jiangxi sheng zhengxie wenshi ziliao yanjiu weiyuanhui, 1992.

Li Junjiu. "Diyi mian hongqi shi zenyang chashang de" [How the first red flag was put in place]. In *Song wenshen jishi* [Record of farewell to the god of plague cam-paign], vol. 43, edited by Liu Yurui and Wan Guohe. Nanchang: Jiangxi sheng zhengxie wenshi ziliao yanjiu weiyuanhui, 1992.

Li Keqiang. "National Schistosomiasis Treatment and Prevention Working Confer-ence—Li Keqiang's Attendance and Speech," September 6, 2010. www.gov.cn /ldhd/2010–09/06/content_1697124.htm. Accessed October 15, 2010.

Li Zhenglan, compiled by Ning Haisheng. "Wo canjia xuefang kepu gongzuo" [I participated in the work to popularize the science of prevention]. In *Song wenshen jishi* [Record of farewell to the god of plague campaign], vol. 43, edited by Liu Yurui and Wan Guohe. Nanchang: Jiangxi sheng zhengxie wenshi ziliao yanjiu weiyuanhui, 1992.

Li Zhisui. *The Private Life of Chairman Mao.* New York: Random House, 1994.

Liansheng People's Commune, Qingpu County, Shanghai. "Struggle against Schis-tosomiasis." *Chinese Medical Journal* 87.11 (1968): 669–72.

Lieberthal, Kenneth. *Governing China: From Revolution through Reform.* New York: W. W. Norton & Company, 1995.

Liu Wei. "Hunan Province Takes Measures to Prevent Spread of SARS." *China Radio International,* April 22, 2003. http://english.cri.cn/144/2003-4-23 /14@10764.htm. Accessed January 31, 2015.

Logan, O. T. "A Case of Dysentery in Hunan Province Caused by the Trematode *Schistosoma japonicum.*" *Chinese Medical Journal* 19 (1905): 243–45.

Lü Liang. "Xu" [Preface]. In *Song wenshen jishi* [Record of farewell to the god of plague campaign], vol. 43, edited by Liu Yurui and Wan Guohe. Nanchang: Jiangxi sheng zhengxie wenshi ziliao yanjiu weiyuanhui, 1992.

Luo Chengqing. "Songzou wenshen zhanhongtu—wei min zaofu shi qianqiu—ji Fang Zhichun tongzhi lingdao xiaomie xuexichongbing gongzuo pianduan" [See-ing off the god of plague developing a great plan to bring benefits for the people for one thousand generations—fragmentary remembrances of comrade Fang Zhichun's leadership in schistosomiasis elimination work]. In *Song wenshen jishi* [Record of farewell to the god of plague campaign], vol. 43, edited by Liu Yurui and Wan Guohe. Nanchang: Jiangxi sheng zhengxie wenshi ziliao yanjiu weiy-uanhui, 1992.

Ma Xuewen. *Qingpu xian zhi* [Qingpu County gazeteer]. Shanghai: Shanghai ren-min chubanshe, 1990.

MacFarquhar, Roderick. *The Origins of the Cultural Revolution.* Vol. 1, *Contradictions among the People, 1956–1957.* New York: Columbia University Press, 1974.

———. *The Origins of the Cultural Revolution.* Vol. 2, *The Great Leap Forward, 1958–1960.* New York: Columbia University Press, 1983.

———. *The Origins of the Cultural Revolution.* Vol. 3, *The Coming of the Cataclysm, 1961–1966.* New York: Columbia University Press, 1997.

MacFarquhar, Roderick, and Michael Schoenhals. *Mao's Last Revolution.* Cambridge, MA: Belknap Press of Harvard University Press, 2006.

Mao Huiren, Li Guifa, and Jiangxi sheng Yujiang xian xianzhi bianzuan weiyuanhui bianji [Mao Huiren, Li Guifa, and Jiangxi Yujiang County Gazetteer Compilation Committee]. *Yujiang xianzhi* [Yujiang County gazetteer]. Nanchang: Jiangxi renmin chubanshe, 1993.

Mao Shou-Pai. "Parasitological Research in Institutes in China." Chapter 10 in *Parasitology: A Global Perspective,* edited by Kenneth S. Warren and John Z. Bowers. New York: Springer-Verlag, 1983.

Mao Zhixiao. "Wo canjia song wenshen de licheng (Guangfeng)" [The process of my participation in bidding farewell to the god of plague (Guangfeng County)]. In *Song wenshen jishi* [Record of farewell to the god of plague campaign], vol. 43, edited by Liu Yurui and Wan Guohe. Nanchang: Jiangxi sheng zhengxie wenshi ziliao yanjiu weiyuanhui, 1992.

———. "Xuefang Jishi" [Record of prevention]. In *Guangfeng xian wenshi ziliao,* vol. 3 [Guangfeng county culture and history, vol. 3]. Guangfeng xian: Zhongguo renmin zhengzhi xieshang huiyi Jiangxi sheng Guangfeng xian wenshi ziliao yanjiu weiyuanhui, 1989.

Marks, Robert B. *Tigers, Rice, Silk, and Silt: Environment and Economy in Late Imperial South China.* New York: Cambridge University Press, 1998.

McNally, Christopher A. "Baptism by Storm: The SARS Crisis' Imprint on China's New Leadership." In *The New Global Threat: SARS and Its Impacts,* edited by Tommy Koh, Aileen Plant, and Eng Hin Lee. Singapore: World Scientific Publishing Company, 2003.

McNeil, Donald G., Jr. "Gate Foundation's Influence Criticized." *New York Times,* February 16, 2008.

Mechanic, David, and Arthur Kleinman. "Ambulatory Care." In *Rural Health in the People's Republic of China: Report of a Visit by the Rural Health Systems Delegation, June 1978,* by Committee on Scholarly Communication with the People's Republic of China, NIH Publication No. 81–2124. Washington, D.C.: U.S. Department of Health and Human Services, Public Health Service, National Institutes of Health, November 1980.

"Medical Activities in New China." *Chinese Medical Journal* 76.5 (1958): 105–6.

Meisner, Maurice. *Mao's China and After: A History of the People's Republic.* Revised and expanded 1st ed. New York: Free Press, 1986.

———. *Marxism Maoism and Utopianism: Eight Essays.* Madison: University of Wisconsin Press, 1982.

Morris, Andrew. "'Fight for Fertilizer!': Excrement, Public Health, and Mobilization in New China." *Journal of Unconventional History* 6.3 (Spring 1995): 51–76.

Munson, E. L. "Cholera Carriers in Relation to Cholera Control." *Philippine Journal of Science* 10B (January 1915): 1–9.

Najera, J. A. "Malaria and the Work of WHO." *Bulletin of the World Health Organization* 67.3 (1989): 229–43.

National Schistosomiasis Research Committee. "Studies on Schistosomiasis Japonica in New China." *Chinese Medical Journal* 78.4 (1959): 368–79.

"News and Notes." *Chinese Medical Journal* 85.4 (1966): 274–76.

"News and Notes." *Chinese Medical Journal* 85.9 (1966): 633–34.

"News and Notes." *Chinese Medical Journal* 87.11 (1968): 683–84.

Oldham, C. H. G. "Science and Technology Policies." *Proceedings of the Academy of Political Science* 31.1 (March 1973): 80–94.

"The Orientation of the Revolution in Medical Education as seen in the Growth of 'Barefoot Doctors': Report of an Investigation from Shanghai." Reprinted from *Hongqi*, no. 3 (1968), *Chinese Medical Journal* 87.10 (1968): 574–81.

Ou Risheng and Li Baojia, eds. *Zhongguo jindai guanchang xiaoshuo xuan*. Vol. 2, *Guanchang xianxing jixia* [Selected short stories of China's recent officials, vol. 2, notes on officials' real selves]. Hohhat: Neimenggu renmin chubanshe, 2003.

Packard, Randall M. "Malaria Dreams: Postwar Visions of Health and Development in the Third World." *Medical Anthropology* 17.3 (1997): 279–96.

Pan, Phillip P. "Village by Village, China Fights Virus; SARS Battle Shows Party Can Still Mobilize the Masses." *New York Times,* June 8, 2003.

"Parasites—Schistosomiasis." Centers for Disease Control and Prevention. www.cdc.gov/parasites/schistosomiasis. Accessed July 26, 2015.

Parish, William L., and Martin King Whyte. *Village and Family in Contemporary China*. Chicago: University of Chicago Press, 1978.

Qian Xinzhong. *Zhonghua renmin gongheguo xuexichongbing dituji, shangce, zhongce* [Atlas of schistosomiasis in the People's Republic of China, vols. 1 and 2]. Shanghai: Zhonghua dituxue she chuban, 1987.

Qianjunwanma song wenshen [Farewell to the god of plague: An account of the mass movement to prevent and cure schistosomiasis]. Guangzhou: Zhongguo chukou shangpin jiaoyihui, 1973.

Qingpu xian fangzhi xuexichongbing sanshiwu nian weiyuanhui [Qingpu County Thirty-Five Years of Schistosomiasis Prevention and Treatment Committee]. *Qingpu xian fangzhi xuexichongbing sanshiwu nian: Dashiji ji* [Thirty-five years of schistosomiasis prevention and treatment in Qingpu County: Collected chronical of events]. Shanghai: Shanghai kexue jishu chubanshe, 1988.

———. *Qingpu xian fangzhi xuexichongbing sanshiwu nian: Zonglunji* [Thirty-five years of prevention and treatment of schistosomiasis in Qingpu County: General introduction]. Shanghai: Shanghai kexue jishu chubanshe, 1987.

Quanguo fangzhi wu da jishengchongbing jingyan jiaoliu huiyi [National exchange meeting for experience treating and preventing the five key parasitic diseases].

Renmin shouce 1959 nian [The people's 1959 handbook]. Beijing: Renmin ribao chubanshe, 1960.

Reed, John Harland. "Brass Butterflies of the Thoughts of Mao Tsetung: The Sociology of Schistosomiasis Control in China." Ph.D. dissertation, Cornell University, 1979.

"Report of the American Schistosomiasis Delegation to the People's Republic of China." *American Journal of Tropical Medicine and Hygiene* 26.3 (1977): 427–62.

Reynolds, Richard C. "Hospital Care." In *Rural Health in the People's Republic of China: Report of a Visit by the Rural Health Systems Delegation, June 1978*, by Committee on Scholarly Communication with the People's Republic of China, NIH Publication No. 81–2124. Washington, D.C.: U.S. Department of Health and Human Services, Public Health Service, National Institutes of Health, November 1980.

Rogaski, Ruth. "Nature, Annihilation, and Modernity: China's Korean War Germ-Warfare Experience Reconsidered." *Journal of Asian Studies* 61.2 (May 2002): 381–415.

Rogers, Everett M. "Barefoot Doctors." In *Rural Health in the People's Republic of China: Report of a Visit by the Rural Health Systems Delegation, June 1978*, by Committee on Scholarly Communication with the People's Republic of China, NIH Publication No. 81–2124. Washington, D.C.: U.S. Department of Health and Human Services, Public Health Service, National Institutes of Health, November 1980.

Rosenthal, Marilyn M., and Jay R. Greiner. "The Barefoot Doctors of China: From Political Creation to Professionalization." *Human Organization* 4.4 (1982): 330–41.

Ross, A. G., et al. "Schistosomiasis in the People's Republic of China: Prospects and Challenges for the 21st Century." *Clinical Microbiology Reviews* 14.2 (2001): 270–90.

Russell, Edmund P., III. "'Speaking of Annihilation': Mobilizing for War against Human and Insect Enemies, 1914–1945." *Journal of American History* 82.4 (March 1996): 1505–29.

Saich, Tony. "Is SARS China's Chernobyl or Much Ado about Nothing?" In *SARS in China: Prelude to Pandemic?*, edited by Arthur Kleinman and James L. Watson. Stanford, CA: Stanford University Press, 2006.

Sandbach, F. R. "Farewell to the God of Plague—the Control of Schistosomiasis in China." *Social Science and Medicine* 11 (1977): 27–33.

———. "The History of Schistosomiasis Research and Policy for Its Control." *Medical History* 20.3 (July 1976): 259–75.

SARS: Clinical Trials on Treatment Using a Combination of Traditional Chinese Medicine and Western Medicine. Geneva: World Health Organization, 2004.

Scheid, Volker. *Chinese Medicine in Contemporary China: Plurality and Synthesis.* Durham, NC: Duke University Press, 2002.

"Schistosomiasis." World Health Organization. www.who.int/schistosomiasis/en. Accessed October 17, 2013.

"Schistosomiasis." World Health Organization, Fact Sheet No. 115, February 2010. www.who.int/mediacentre/factsheets/fs115/en/index.html. Accessed October 17, 2013.

Schmalzer, Sigrid. "On the Appropriate Use of Rose-Colored Glasses: Reflections on Science in Socialist China." *Isis* 98.3 (2007): 571–83.

———. *The People's Peking Man: Popular Science and Human Identity in Twentieth-Century China.* Chicago: University of Chicago Press, 2008.

Schram, Stuart R., ed. *Mao's Road to Power: Revolutionary Writings, 1912–1949.* Vol. 1, *The Pre-Marxist Period, 1912–1920.* Armonk, NY: M. E. Sharpe, 1992.

———. "The Founding and Progress of the 'Strengthen Learning Society'" (July 21, 1919).

———. "Letter to Li Jinxi" (June 7, 1920).

Schram, Stuart R., ed. *Mao's Road to Power: Revolutionary Writings, 1912–1949.* Vol. 3, *From the Jinggangshan to Establishment of the Jiangxi Soviet, July 1927–December 1930.* Armonk, NY: M. E. Sharpe, 1995.

———. "Oppose Bookism" (May 1930).

Schurmann, Franz. *Ideology and Organization in Communist China.* Berkeley: University of California Press, 1968.

Selected Works of Mao Tse-tung: Vols. 1–9, Poems, and *Red Book.* Vols. 1–5 originally published by Foreign Language Press, Peking. Vols. 6–9 originally published by Kranti Publications, Hyderabad. www.marxists.org/reference/archive/mao/selected-works/index.htm. Accessed April 22, 2010.

———. "Basic Tactics" (1937), vol. 6.

———. "Be Concerned with the Well-Being of the Masses, Pay Attention to Methods of Work" (January 27, 1934), vol. 1.

———. "Directive on Public Health" (June 26, 1965), from *Long Live Mao Tse-tung Thought,* a Red Guard publication, vol. 9.

———. "Methods of Work of Party Committees" (March 13, 1949), vol. 4.

———. "On Practice" (July 1937), vol. 1.

———. "Sixty Points on Working Methods—a Draft Resolution from the Office of the Centre of the CPC" (February 2, 1958), vol. 8.

———. "Strengthen Party Unity and Carry forward Party Traditions" (August 30, 1956), vol. 5.

———. "A Study of Physical Education" (April 1917), vol. 6.

———. "Talk on Health Services" (January 24, 1964), from *Long Live Mao Tse-tung Thought,* a Red Guard publication, vol. 9.

———. "Twenty Manifestations of Bureaucracy" (February 1970), vol. 9.

———. "22. Methods of Thinking and Methods of Work" (February, 5, 1940; originally from "On Practice," July 1937), *Red Book.*

———. "The United Front in Cultural Work" (October 20, 1944), vol. 3.

———. "We Must Learn to Do Economic Work" (January 10, 1945), vol. 3.

Shah, Sonia. *The Fever: How Malaria Has Ruled Humankind for 500,000 Years.* New York: Sarah Crichton Books, 2010.

Shanghai kexue daxue liuxingbingxue jiaoyanshi [Shanghai Science University Epidemiology Teaching and Research Section]. *Su Delong jiaoshou lunwen xuanji* [Selected papers from Professor Su Delong]. Tianjin: Tianjin kexue jishu chubanshe, 1985.

Shanghai shi aiguo weisheng yundong weiyuanhui bangongshi [Shanghai Patriotic Health Campaign Committee Office]. *Chu qi hai* [Eliminating seven-pests]. Shanghai: Shaonian ertong chubanshe, 1958.

Shanghai shi difangzhi bangongshi [Shanghai Gazetteer Office]. "Diba pian zhuan bing fangzhi, diyi zhang xuexichongbing, disan jie jigou" [Chapter 8: Treatment and prevention of special diseases; section 1: schistosomiasis; part 3: organizations]. *Shanghai weishengzhi* [Shanghai health gazetteer]. www.shtong.gov.cn/node2 /node2245/node67643/node67655/node67719/node67847/userobject1ai65180 .html. Accessed September 29, 2013.

Shanghai Zhongyi xueyuan deng bian [Shanghai College of Traditional Chinese Medicine et al., eds.]. *"Chijiao yisheng" shouce* ["Barefoot doctor" handbook]. Shanghai: Shanghai shi chuban geming zu, 1970.

Shangrao Prevention Station. "Xiaomie weihai renmen jiankang de xuexichongbing" [Eliminating schistosomiasis that endangers the people's health]. In *Shangrao shi wenshi ziliao,* vol. 9. Jiangxi: Zhengxie Shangrao Shi weiyuanhui wenshi ziliao bangongshi, 1989.

Shankman, David, and Qiaoli Liang. "Landscape Changes and Increasing Flood Frequency in China's Poyang Lake Region." *Professional Geographer* 55.4 (2003): 434–45.

Shapiro, Judith. *Mao's War against Nature: Politics and the Environment in Revolutionary China.* Cambridge: Cambridge University Press, 2001.

Shen Ch'i-chen. "Report on Prevention of Schistosomiasis." In *Speeches Given at the Second Session of the Second National People's Congress, Communist China.* Washington, D.C.: U.S. Joint Publications Research Service, 1961.

Shirly, Aaron. "Community Health." In *Rural Health in the People's Republic of China: Report of a Visit by the Rural Health Systems Delegation, June 1978*, by Committee on Scholarly Communication with the People's Republic of China, NIH Publication No. 81–2124. Washington, D.C.: U.S. Department of Health and Human Services, Public Health Service, National Institutes of Health, November 1980.

Shu Xiangmao, oral history compiled by Lei Yu. "Shouzhan Magang" [First battle at Magang]. In *Song wenshen jishi* [Record of farewell to the god of plague campaign], vol. 43, edited by Liu Yurui and Wan Guohe. Nanchang: Jiangxi sheng zhengxie wenshi ziliao yanjiu weiyuanhui, 1992.

Shue, Vivienne. *The Reach of the State: Sketches of the Chinese Body Politic.* Stanford, CA: Stanford University Press, 1988.

Sidel, Victor W., and Ruth Sidel. *Serve the People: Observations on Medicine in the People's Republic of China.* Boston: Beacon Press, 1974.

Skinner, G. William, and Edwin A. Winckler. "Compliance Succession in Rural Communist China: A Cyclical Theory." In *A Sociological Reader on Complex Organizations,* 2nd ed., edited by Amitai Etzioni. New York: Holt, Rinehart and Winston, 1969.

Snow, Edgar. *Red Star over China.* New York: Grove Press, 1994.

"Some Aspects of Research in the Prevention and Treatment of Schistosomiasis Japonica in New China." *Chinese Medical Journal* 72 (March–April 1955): 100–106.

"Southern China Launches Antischistosomiasis Campaign." *Chinese Medical Journal* 3.4 (July 1977): 286–87.

Spence, Jonathan D. *The Search for Modern China.* 2nd ed. New York: W. W. Norton & Company, 1999.

Su De-long and Carl E. Taylor. "The Community Health Teaching Center in China." *American Journal of Public Health* 72.9, suppl. (September 1982): 89–91.

Sun Yongjiu. "Gonggu chengguo ying nan er shang; ba xuefang hongqi ju de genggao" [Solidifying the achievements, facing the difficulties and going ahead; raising the red flag of prevention even higher]. In *Song wenshen jishi* [Record of farewell to the god of plague campaign], vol. 43, edited by Liu Yurui and Wan Guohe. Nanchang: Jiangxi sheng zhengxie wenshi ziliao yanjiu weiyuanhui, 1992.

Suttmeier, Richard P. *Science, Technology and China's Drive for Modernization.* Stanford, CA: Hoover Institute Press, 1980.

Sze, Szeming. *China's Health Problems.* Washington, D.C.: Chinese Medical Association, 1943.

Tanner, Marcel, and Don de Savigny. "Malaria Eradication Back on the Table." *Bulletin of the World Health Organization* 86.2 (February 2008): 82.

Taylor, Frederick Winslow. *The Principles of Scientific Management.* 1911. New York: W. W. Norton & Company, 1967.

Taylor, Kim. *Chinese Medicine in Early Communist China, 1945–1963: A Medicine of Revolution.* New York: RoutledgeCurzon, 2005.

Thompson, Roger R., trans. *Mao Zedong: Report from Xunwu.* Stanford, CA: Stanford University Press, 1990.

Timberg, Craig, and Daniel Halperin. *Tinderbox: How the West Sparked the AIDS Epidemic and How the World Can Finally Overcome It.* New York: Penguin, 2013.

Tong Xianghan. "Shiziyan" [The lion cliff]. In *Song wenshen jishi* [Record of farewell to the god of plague campaign], vol. 43, edited by Liu Yurui and Wan Guohe. Nanchang: Jiangxi sheng zhengxie wenshi ziliao yanjiu weiyuanhui, 1992.

Tootell, George T. "Tartar Emetic in Schistosomiasis Japonica." *Chinese Medical Journal* 38.4 (April 1924): 276–77.

Utzinger, Jürg, et al. "Conquering Schistosomiasis in China: The Long March." *Acta Tropica* 96 (2005): 69–96.

Wang, Jessica Ching-Sze. *John Dewey in China: To Teach and to Learn.* New York: SUNY Press, 2008.

Wang, L. D., H. G. Chen, et al. "A Strategy to Control Transmission of *Schistosoma japonicum* in China." *New England Journal of Medicine* 360.2 (January 8, 2009): 121–28.

Wang, L. D., J. G. Guo, et al. "China's New Strategy to Block *Schistosoma japonicum* Transmission: Experience and Impact beyond Schistosomiasis." *Tropical Medicine and International Health* 14.12 (December 2009): 1475–83.

Wang, L. D., J. Utzinger, and X. N. Zhou. "Schistosomiasis Control: Experiences and Lessons." *Lancet* 372.9652 (November 2008): 1793–95.

Wang Jingui. "Song zou wenshen, renshou nianfeng: De'an xian xuexichongbing fangzhi gongzuo de huigu" [Saying farewell to the god of plague, longevity, and plenty: Review of De'an County's work preventing and treating schistosomiasis]. In *De'an xian wenshi ziliao,* vol. 3. Jiangxi: De'an xian xuexichongbing fangzhi lingdao xiaozu bangongshi, 1989.

Wang Ximeng. *Shanghai xiaomie xuexichongbing de huigu* [Review of elimination of schistosomiasis in Shanghai]. Shanghai: Shanghai kexue jishu chubanshe, 1988.

Wang Zude, Chen Zhengxuan, Wang Bosheng, and Bianzhuan weiyuanhui bian [the Compilation Committee]. *Shanghai nongye zhi* [Shanghai agriculture gazeteer]. Shanghai: Shanghai Shehui kexueyuan, 1996.

Warren, Kenneth S. "'Farewell the Plague Spirit': Chairman Mao's Crusade against Schistosomiasis." In *Science and Medicine in Twentieth-Century China: Research and Education,* edited by John Z. Bowers, J. William Hess, and Nathan Sivin. Ann Arbor: Center for Chinese Studies, University of Michigan, 1988.

Watt, John R. *Saving Lives in Wartime China: How Medical Reformers Built Modern Healthcare Systems amid War and Epidemics, 1928–1945.* Leiden: Brill, 2014.

Wei, Chunjuan Nancy, and Darryl E. Brock, eds. *Mr. Science and Chairman Mao's Cultural Revolution: Science and Technology in Modern China.* Lanham, MD: Lexington Books, 2013.

Wei Wenbo. "Farewell the 'God of Plague.'" In *Mao Zedong: Biography-Assessment-Reminiscences,* compiled by Zhong Wenxian. Beijing: Foreign Language Press, 1986.

Wei Wen-po [Wei Wenbo]. "Battle against Schistosomiasis." Translated and reprinted from *Hongqi,* no. 2 (1960), *Chinese Medical Journal* 80.4 (1960): 299–305.

———. "The People's Boundless Energy during the Current Leap Forward: New Victories on the Anti-schistosomiasis Front." *Chinese Medical Journal* 77 (1958): 107–11.

Weller, Robert. *Discovering Nature: Globalization and Environmental Culture in China and Taiwan.* New York: Cambridge University Press, 2006.

White, Lynn T., III. "SARS, Anti-populism, and Elite Lies: Temporary Disorders in China." In *The New Global Threat: SARS and its Impacts,* edited by Tommy Koh, Aileen Plant, and Eng Hin Lee. Singapore: World Scientific Publishing Company, 2003.

Whorton, James. *Before Silent Spring: Pesticides and Public Health in Pre-DDT America.* Princeton, NJ: Princeton University Press, 1974.

Wu Ningkun. *A Single Tear: A Family's Persecution, Love, and Endurance in Communist China.* New York: Atlantic Monthly Press, 1993.

Wu Zaocun. "Feng zheng jin zu qu wenshen" [With righteous manners we will have enough strength to expel the god of plague]. In *Song wenshen jishi* [Record of farewell to the god of plague campaign], vol. 43, edited by Liu Yurui and Wan Guohe. Nanchang: Jiangxi sheng zhengxie wenshi ziliao yanjiu weiyuanhui, 1992.

"Xin Zhongguo zai fangzhi xuexichongbing wentishang suo kaizhan de yi xie yanjiu gongzuo" [New China's launch of research work on problems with treating and preventing schistosomiasis]. *Zhonghua yixue zazhi* [Chinese medical journal], no. 7 (1955): 394.

Xiong Peikang. "Zhenma qiepi, Zhansheng wenshen (Boyang xian)" [Acupuncture anesthesia on the spleen, overcome the god of plague (Boyang County)]. In *Song wenshen jishi* [Record of farewell to the god of plague campaign], vol. 43, edited by Liu Yurui and Wan Guohe. Nanchang: Jiangxi sheng zhengxie wenshi ziliao yanjiu weiyuanhui, 1992.

Xu Fuzhou. "Fangbing zhibing zaofu renmin—Qingpu weisheng gongzuo si shin-ian" [Prevention and treatment of diseases, bringing benefits to people—Forty years of health work in Qingpu]. In *Qingpu wenshi, di si qi* [Qingpu culture and history, vol. 4]. Qingpu [Shanghai]: Zhongguo renmin zhengzhi xieshang huiyi Qingpu xian weiyuanhui wenshi ziliao weiyuanhui, 1989.

Xue xianjin gan xianjin xianjin geng xianjin chu sihai, xiaomie xuexichongbing jin-gyan [Learning advances, pursuing advances, advances even more advances, experience eliminating the four-pests, schistosomiasis, and parasitic diseases]. Nanchang: Jiangxi renmin chubanshe, 1958.

Yang Daozheng. "Qumo you dang yizhi jian yin chu pikai xin tiandi (Fengxin)" [The Party has unwavering determination to expel demons, a silver hoe can cleave open a new universe (Fengxing County)]. In *Song wenshen jishi* [Record of fare-well to the god of plague campaign], vol. 43, edited by Liu Yurui and Wan Guohe. Nanchang: Jiangxi sheng zhengxie wenshi ziliao yanjiu weiyuanhui, 1992.

Yang Hsiao. *The Making of a Peasant Doctor.* Peking: Foreign Language Press, 1976.

Yang Nianqun. "Disease Prevention, Social Mobilization and Spatial Politics: The Anti Germ-Warfare Incident of 1952 and the 'Patriotic Health Campaign.'" *Chinese Historical Review* 11.2 (Fall 2004): 155.

———. "Memories of the Barefoot Doctor System." In *Governance of Life in Chinese Moral Experience,* edited by Everett Zhang, Arthur Kleinman, and Tu Weiming. New York: Routledge, 2011.

Yang Ruidong. "Wo canjia xuefang gongzuo de pianduan huiyi" [Partial recollec-tion of my participation in prevention work]. In *Jingjiang wenshi ziliao,* vol. 7. Jingjiang xian: Zhongguo renmin zhengzhi xieshang huiyi Jiangsu sheng Jin-gjiang xian weiyuanhui wenshi ziliao yanjiu weiyuanhui, 1987.

Yao Yuanxiang. *Zhonggong Qingpu dangshi dashiji* [Chronicle of Qingpu Party history]. Shanghai: Shanghai shehui kexueyuan chubanshe, 1994.

Ye Songling. "Xuexichongbing fangzhi gongzuo de huigu (De'an)" [Recollection of the work to prevent and cure schistosomiasis (De'an County)]. In *Song wenshen jishi* [Record of farewell to the god of plague campaign], vol. 43, edited by Liu

Yurui and Wan Guohe. Nanchang: Jiangxi sheng zhengxie wenshi ziliao yanjiu weiyuanhui, 1992.

Yeh Wen-hsin. *Shanghai Splendor: Economic Sentiments and the Making of Modern China, 1843–1949*. Berkeley: University of California Press, 2007.

Yip, Ka-Che. *Health and National Reconstruction in Nationalist China: The Development of Modern Health Services, 1928–1937*. Ann Arbor, MI: Association for Asian Studies, 1995.

Yu, Dongbao, et al. "Cost-Effectiveness Analysis of the Impact on Infection and Morbidity Attributable to Three Chemotherapy Schemes against *Schistosoma japonicum* in Hyperendemic Areas of the Dongting Lake Region, China." *Southeast Asian Journal of Tropical Medicine Public Health* 33.3 (September 2002): 441–57.

Yu Laixi. "Yi fenguan laoren Wan Fengxin" [Recollecting the feces management of the elder Wan Fengxin]. In *Song wenshen jishi* [Record of farewell to the god of plague campaign], vol. 43, edited by Liu Yurui and Wan Guohe. Nanchang: Jiangxi sheng zhengxie wenshi ziliao yanjiu weiyuanhui, 1992.

———. "Yujiang renmin fangzhi xuexichongbing de weida douzheng" [The people of Yujiang's mighty battle to treat and prevent schistosomiasis]. In *Song wenshen jishi* [Record of farewell to the god of plague campaign], vol. 43, edited by Liu Yurui and Wan Guohe. Nanchang: Jiangxi sheng zhengxie wenshi ziliao yanjiu weiyuanhui, 1992.

Yu Laixi and Zhonggong Yujiang xianwei xuefang lingdao xiaozu bangongshi [Yu Laixi and Schistosomiasis Prevention Leadership Small Group Office of Yujiang Party Committee of CCP]. *Jiangxi sheng Yujiang xian xuefang zhi: 1953–1980* [Jiangxi Yujiang County gazetteer of schistosomiasis prevention: 1953–1980]. Yujiang: Zhonggong Yujiang xianwei xuefang lingdao xiaozu bangongshi, 1984.

Yudkin, J. "Medicine and Medical Education in the New China." *Journal of Medical Education* 33.7 (July 1958): 517–22.

Zhang Jiwan, oral history compiled by Xiong Yangsheng. "Jianmiao baifo xinqiancheng wanminan miao bu anmin—wanminan jiangcun duanrenyan zao huimie qinjian qinli ji" [Establishing temples and bowing to the Buddha with sincere heart, Wanminan temple does not give the people peace—personally experienced record of Wanminan Jiang villagers' meeting with disaster and being eliminated]. In *Song wenshen jishi* [Record of farewell to the god of plague campaign], vol. 43, edited by Liu Yurui and Wan Guohe. Nanchang: Jiangxi sheng zhengxie wenshi ziliao yanjiu weiyuanhui, 1992.

Zhang Yi. "Chen Yun hui guxiang, diaocha xuexichongbing fangzhi qingkuang" [Chen Yun returning to hometown, study of the prevention and treatment of schistosomiasis]. In *Qingpu wenshi, di san qi* [Qingpu culture and history, vol. 3]. Qingpu [Shanghai]: Zhongguo renmin zhengzhi xieshang huiyi Qingpu xian weiyuanhui wenshi ziliao weiyuanhui, 1989.

Zhang Yufeng, Bai Gengsheng, and Qiao Mingxian, eds. *Zhongguo minjian gushi quanshu: Henan, nanzhao juan* [A comprehensive volume of Chinese folktales: Henan, book of southern stories]. Beijing: Zhishi chanquan chubanshe, 2011.

Zhejiang kexue jishu puji xiehui and Zhejiang weisheng shiyanyuan [Zhejiang Science and Technology Dissemination Society and Zhejiang Health Laboratory]. *Xiaomie xuexichongbing guatu* [Eliminating schistosomiasis charts]. Beijing: Renmin weisheng chubanshe, 1956.

Zheng Yongnian and Lye Liang Fook. "SARS and China's Political System." In *The SARS Epidemic: Challenges to China's Crisis Management,* edited by John Wong and Zheng Yongnian. Singapore: World Scientific Publishing Company, 2004.

Zhong Zubiao and Jiangxi sheng jiachu xuexichongbing fangzhi zhan [Zhong Zubiao and Jiangxi Schistosomiasis Prevention of Domestic Animals Station]. *Jiangxi sheng jiachu xuefang zhi: 1956–1996* [Jiangxi gazetteer of schistosomiasis prevention of domestic animals: 1956–1996]. Nanchang: Jiangxi sheng jiachu xuexichongbing fangzhi zhan, 1989.

Zhonggeng Jiangxi sheng weifangzhi xuexichongbing wuxiaozu banggongshi bianxie [Compilation of the People's Republic, Jiangxi Province Office of the Five-Person Small Group for Prevention and Treatment of Schistosomiasis]. *Yujiang xian shi zenyang genzhi xuexichongbing de* [How Yujiang County is fundamentally curing schistosomiasis]. Nanchang: Jiangxi renmin chubanshe, 1958.

Zhonggong zhongyang fangzhi xuexichongbing jiuren xiaozu bangongshi [Schistosomiasis Prevention and Treatment Nine-Person Small Group Office of Central Party Committee of CCP]. *Song wenshen* [Farewell to the god of plague]. Shanghai: Shanghai wenyi chubanshe, 1961.

Zhonggong zhongyang nanfang shisan sheng, shi, qu xuefang lingdao xiaozu bangongshi [Thirteen Provincial, City, and District Party Schistosomiasis Prevention Leadership Small Group Offices in South China]. *Song wenshen: Huace* [Farewell to the god of plague: Pictorial work]. Beijing: Zhonggong zhongyang nanfang shisan sheng, shi, qu xuefang lingdao xiaozu bangongshi, 1978.

Zhou Fukai, oral history compiled by Xiong Xiangsheng. "Yongyi mocai, jifu sangming" [Quacks cheat them, and the stepfather loses his life]. In *Song wenshen jishi* [Record of farewell to the god of plague campaign], vol. 43, edited by Liu Yurui and Wan Guohe. Nanchang: Jiangxi sheng zhengxie wenshi ziliao yanjiu weiyuanhui, 1992.

Zhou Xiaonong et al. "Application of Geographic Information Systems and Remote Sensing to Schistosomiasis Control in China." *Acta Tropica* 79.1 (2001): 97–106.

Zhu, Qin. "SARS in Beijing: An Urban Response." In *SARS from East to West,* edited by Eva Karin Olsson and Lan Xue. Lanham, MD: Lexington Books, 2012.

Zou Huayi. *Kuayue siwang didai* [Leaping over the dead zone]. Nanchang: Baihuazhou wenyi chubanshe, 1993.

Zou Keyuan. "SARS and the Rule of Law in China." In *The SARS Epidemic: Challenges to China's Crisis Management,* edited by John Wong and Zheng Yongnian. Singapore: World Scientific Publishing Company, 2004.

INDEX

bureaucratic organization *(continued)* 204, 207; scientific management and, 208–9

burial, snail suffocation by, 131–32. *See also* snail elimination campaigns; effectiveness of, 64, 133, 134–35, 141, 219; labor demands of, 133–34, 138; as method of choice, 131–32, 138–39, 221; origin of method, 33, 90

campaign personnel. *See also* educated youth; local cadres; medical personnel: grassroots activists and, 189–94; ineptness and, 147–48; morale of, 46, 71, 74, 135–36, 139, 150; pyramidal structure for, 225–26; recordkeeping and, 215; relationships between villagers and, 82, 146, 149–50, 155–60; salaries of, 57, 66–67; traditional celebrations and, 188–89; transfers among, 56–57

campaign structure: attacks on leadership and, 38; compliance and, 108–13; LSG system in, 38, 47–51, 238–39; research organization and, 32–33; restructuring and, 58–59

caretaking needs: campaign personnel and, 65–66, 73; communes and, 161–62; family relationships and, 58, 161, 191; patient costs and, 69; support for Party and, 45, 191–94, *192*

cattle treatment, 168–69, 299n77. *See also* water buffalo

CCP. *See* Chinese Communist Party

cercariae, 3, 92, 94, 95–96, 98

cesspools, 119, 120, 125, 149, 218

Chen, C. C., 98

Chengbei Township, Qingpu County (national test site), 8, 82, 111, 137–38, 288n91; leadership and, 53, 57; scientific tools and, 105, 217, 218–19, 226

Chen Hongting, 147

Chen Qiguo, 97

Chen Yun (Chinese Vice Premier), 19

Chinese Academy of Medical Science, 171

Chinese Communist Party (CCP). *See also* ideology; propaganda strategies; scientific consolidation; scientific socialist

society: commitment of top leadership in, 19; control over MPH and, 30; educational strategies and, 88–97; global scientific leadership and, 18–19; government structure and, 47–48; grassroots activists and, 189–94; leadership challenges for, 43–44; planning process and, 208–9; popular support for, 192–200; scientific legitimation and, 181–202; snail fever as priority and, 16–19, 247–48

Chinese Medical Journal, 157–58

Chinese medicine. *See also* herbal medicine; medical personnel; united clinics: compensation of doctors and, 71–73, 82; Mao's unity goals and, 27–29, 157, 159, 171, 183; practitioner skill level and, 153–54; role in health campaigns, 28, 225; rural appeal of, 157; villager attitudes toward, 82, 152–53, 157–58

Chiyonosuke Yokote, 31

chopsticks, as eradication tool, 106

chronic disease, 3–4, 152

Chung, Dr. (medical expert), 172

coercive strategies. *See also* advanced producers' cooperatives; communes: local participation and, 238–40, 248, 252; medical treatment and, 195; SARS campaign and, 249; science education and, 92

commode-washing, 117, 118, 124, 125, 127, 275n7. *See also* feces management; feces vats; public toilets; stool sampling; as job, 125, 139, 199–200, 276n40

commune-level hospital system, 23

communes, 27. *See also* advanced producers' cooperatives; cooperatives, early forms of; model test sites; campaign resources and, 52, 59, 63–64, 66, 67, 70, 73, 146; compliance and, 108, 122, 195; education and, 92; famine period and, 286n71, 288n92; feng shui and, 122; medical facilities and, 8, 23, 37, 172, 173, 297n39; prevention work and, 135; production efforts and, 142–43; propaganda and, 115; sanitation campaigns and, 125, 128; scientific consolidation and, 203–4, 215, 221; snail killing and, 33; statistics and,

eradication, as goal. *See also* burial, snail suffocation by; snail elimination campaigns: funding and, 61, 245; impossibility of, 10, 243–44; logic of prevention activities and, 101–2; malaria campaign and, 243–46; political nature of, 20; popular engagement and, 103, 135–36; technical advances and, 247

evaluation, 217, 218, 220, 297n41

experimentation. *See also* scientific performances: drug treatments and, 167; grassroots science and, 106–8, 207, 209, 218–20; model test sites and, 218, 219–21

family relationships: barriers to treatment and, 163–64, 177; caretaking and, 191–92; hygiene campaign and, 111–12; treatment compliance and, 108–10

famine period. *See also* Great Leap Forward (1958-61): collapse of campaign in, 135–37; resurgence of disease in, 166–67; treatment compensation and, 73

Fang Zhichun, 38, 54–55, 58, 61, 80, 139

Fan Ka wai, 25–26

Faust, Ernest, 6, 33

feces management, 123–27. *See also* cesspools; commode-washing; feces vats; private land rights; public toilets; cooperatives and, 194–200; economic sabotage and, 67; fermentation and, 107, 117, 125, 142, 218, 280n120; fertilizer control and, 117, 125, 126, 195–200; grassroots creativity and, 107; personnel and, 124, 125, 139, 280n118; as prevention strategy, 33, 117; village cleanup days and, 189

feces vats: commode concept and, 126; feng shui and, 120, 121; fertilizer control and, 198; funding and, 118; management of, 117, 119, 123, 218; personnel and, 119, 124

Fenghuang Mountains (Hubei), 6

feng shui. *See also* traditional culture and beliefs: campaign work and, 115, 116, 120–23, 143, 185; disease causality and, 152; grassroots science and, 241

fermentation, and feces management, 107, 117, 125, 142, 218, 280n120

festivals and celebrations: educational entertainment at, 89, *90*; health campaign co-opting of, 188–89

fever paranoia, 250–51

financing of campaign. *See also* unfunded mandate, health campaign as: campaign as unfunded mandate and, 35, 50, 61–82; Cultural Revolution treatment subsidies and, 68, 73–74, 169–70, 268n75; eradication as goal and, 245; famine and recovery period and, 34–35; fee collection and, 69–70; outside support in Yujiang and, *83–84*; in recovery period (1961-65), 35; in Reform era, 247–48; in rural vs. urban areas, 36, 37; SARS campaign and, 251; study site diversity and, 8

fishing community, 8, 126–27, 195, 277n58

Five-Anti Campaign (1952), 197

flamethrowers, 131, 176

forms and records: CCP planning and, 208–9, 228; grassroots reports and, 222; introduction of, 214–17; patient information and, 297n32, 297n39; scientific consolidation and, 214–17; stool testing and, 147–48

Foucault, Michel, 289n112

Four Harms campaign *(sihai yundong),* 101–2, 106

"Fourteen Articles on Science" (government directive), 35–36

Fulian (Women's Federation), 165, 190

Gao Mobo, 153

Gates Foundation, 245

gender differences, 124, 190. *See also* women

germ warfare, 19, 99, 110

Gilbreth, Frank, 206

Gilbreth, Lillian, 206

global malaria campaign: public resistance and, 99, 146–47, 282n22; snail fever campaign and, 242–46; technical problems and, 296n24, 296n26

global scientific leadership, 18–19, 287. *See also* Maoist primary health care model

global warming, 247

government intrusiveness: Party framing of, 166, 181–82; popular resistance and, 117, 143–44, 145–49, 177 grassroots science. *See also* scientific consolidation; scientific tools: experimentation and, 207, 209; expert snubbing of, 243; ideological value of, 204–6, 240–42; impacts of scientific tools in, 223–28; innovative prevention activities and, 106–8; local leadership and, 10, 11; local medical practitioners and, 22–23; Mao's view of science and, 207; role of, 9–12; rural empowerment and, 241 (*see also* feng shui)

Great Leap Forward (1958-61). *See also* famine period: campaign effectiveness and, 10, 116, 224; claims of disease elimination during, 116; disease rebound during, 34–35, 166–67; focus on science in, 87 (*see also* scientific knowledge); grassroots creativity in, 107; participation in treatment and, 160–61, 165; patterns of labor in, 295n16; professional physicians and, 34; scientific tool use and, 210, 215–16, 218; treatment efficacy and, 159

Greenhalgh, Susan, 187, 298n59

Gutiérrez Igaravidez, Pedro, 186

Hangzhou, November 1955 meeting at, 25

Han Songling, Dr., 173

Harding, Harry, 52–53, 210

health, villager vision of, 152–53. *See also* disease causality

health campaigns. *See also* grassroots science; scientific consolidation: collectivization and, 27; colonial subjects and, 148–49; concepts of disease causality and, 96–97; denunciation strategies and, 111–12; eradication of superstition and, 186, 187–89, 241; as mass science campaigns, 240–42; pedagogical agenda of, 88–97; political legitimation and, 181–202, 240–42; role of Chinese medicine in, 27–29; scientific mind-set and, 102–8, 241; as unfunded mandates, 61–82

He Cheng, 25, 30, 249

herbal medicine. *See also* Chinese medicine: availability of, 158; experimental use of, 159; late-stage patients and, 90, 158–59; practitioner knowledge and, 23,

153, 156, 172, 243; rural beliefs and, 152; treatment costs and, 71, 72, 153; treatment efforts using, 28, 37, 90, 158–59

holidays. *See* festivals and celebrations

Horn, Joshua, 2, 108–9, 153, 189, 227–28

household responsibility system, 239, 250–51

Hughes, Thomas P., 207–8

Hundred Flowers Campaign (1957), 33, 184

Hu Shi, 207

hygiene practices. *See* commode-washing; public toilets; sanitation campaign

ideology, 16–19. *See also* propaganda strategies; scientific consolidation; scientific socialist society; malaria campaign and, 242–43; Maoist health campaigns and, 240–42; prevention work and, 139–40; sanitation activities and, 117–18; SARS campaign and, 249–50; science-based change and, 181–202; scientific knowledge and, 87–88; scientific tools and, 222–23, 235–36

Iijima Wataru, 31

"integrated strategy," 248

irrigation system. *See also* environmental reconstruction: feng shui and, 121; as snail habitat, 29–30, 129, 134–35, 137

Japanese snail fever experts, 19, 26, 30–32. *See also* Komiya, Yoshitaka

Jiangsu Province, 5, 7, 9. *See also* Qingpu County, Jiangsu Province; accomplishments of campaign in, *175, 176*; Dantu County in, *132*; funding and, 67–73; impediments to campaign in, 47, 49, 54–55, 56, 57, 64; incidence of disease in, 16, 19; Jiangdu County in, 193–94, 195, 231; Kunshan County in, 54, 97; medical personnel in, 57, 172–73; model test sites and, 231; Nanhui County and, 64; Party loyalty in, 193–94; prevention efforts in, 128, 131, *132*, 134, 135, 136, 138; recordkeeping and, 215; research efforts in, 219, 221; science and superstition in, 184; scientific mindset and, 87, 97, 103, 105; Songjiang Prefecture in, 16; treatment in, 67–73, 149, 152, 158, 169, 173

local knowledge base, 172, 243. *See also* Chinese medicine; grassroots science; traditional culture and beliefs

Logan, O. T., 6

LSG system. *See* leadership small group system

Lu Guang, *80*

L Liang, 65, 138

Ma Jincai, 194

malaria campaign. *See* global malaria campaign

manure vendors, 197

Maoist primary health care model: assessments of, 1–3, 237–38; key components of, 237–38, 248–49; long-term government commitment and, 238, 240–42; popularity of, 1, 252; role of grassroots science in, 11–12; rural effectiveness of, 238–40; SARS campaign and, 242, 248–52

Mao Shou-Pai, 7

Mao Zedong, 18, *21. See also* speeches and writings of Chairman Mao; campaign takeover by, 20–21, 25–34, 48, 123–28; Chinese and Western treatment unity and, 27–29, 72, 73–74, 157, 159, 183; crusade against bureaucracy and, 44, 140, 204, 207; deleterious effects and, 39–40; focus on elimination and, 10, 32–33, 102; legacy of, 39–40; persistence of, 240–42

Mao Zedong Thought, 37, 38, 83, 205

Mao Zhixiao (barefoot doctor), 161, 172–73, 227

mass mobilization: as coercive strategy, 238; concept of prevention and, 97–102; educational strategies and, 88–97; good leadership and, 46–47; grassroots activists and, 189–94; long-term success and, 112–13, 114; militaristic approach to campaign and, 110–13; producers' cooperatives and, 32–33, 92, 105, 106, 110–11, 114; SARS campaign and, 249–50; scientific mindset and, 102–8; scientific tools and, 204–6

Mawangdui tombs (Hunan), 6

medical classics, 6

medical experts. *See also* professional physicians; urban medical establishment; Western medicine: campaign diversity and, 8, 9; in Japan, 6; MPH and, 22; in Nationalist era, 7; sidelining of, 22, 244

medical personnel. *See also* barefoot doctors; campaign personnel; Chinese medicine; professional physicians: antipathy toward testing and, 149–50; competence of, 167–68; Cultural Revolution and, 171–74; fee collection and, 69–70; lack of, 38–39, 55–56, 174; morale of, 46, 71, 74, 135–36, 139, 150; MPH efforts and, 22–23; in 1970s, 38–39; regional diversity and, 8–9; salary dynamics and, 70–74, 268n64; villager attitudes toward, 69, 72, 153–56, 158, 177

medicines. *See* antimony treatment; drug treatment; herbal medicine; shots

Meisner, Maurice, 185

Meleney, Henry, 6, 33

microscopes: as educational tools, 92–95, 96–97, 113, 271n32; as testing method, 281n7

military fitness, 15, 16, 24–25, 110

military imagery, *46, 132*–33, 244–45

military medical teams, 171

Ministry of Public Health (MPH), 21–25; campaign takeover by Mao and, 20–21, 25–26, 36, 48; critiques of, 20, 24–25, 26, 27–30, 171; Department of Parasitology, 6; establishment of, 6; impact of prevention work by, 119–20; personal sanitation efforts by, 116–20; snail fever campaign under, 21–25, 32; urban focus of, 27–28, 29–30, 36

miracidia, 3, 92, 96–97

mobile units, 34, 48, 58, 171, 172, 288n98

mock battles, 111

model test sites. *See also* Qingpu County, Jiangsu Province; Yujiang County, Jiangxi Province: application of results from, 61, 137–38; campaign funding and, 74–81; data collection practices and, 213, 214, 216, 218; evaluation and, 217, 218, 220, 297n41; experimentation

Taiwan, 15
Taylor, Frederick Winslow, 206, 208
teacake (molluscicide), 221
technical advances. *See also* scientific tools:
    grassroots creativity and, 106–7;
    Reform era campaign and, 246–47;
    skin test and, 150, 151; urban vs. rural
    access to, 150–51
technical bureaucracy, 203, 205
temples, as wards, 187–88. *See also* tradi-
    tional culture and beliefs
testing, 45, 168, 170–71. *See also* skin test;
    stool sampling
theatrical productions, 89, *90*
Three-Anti Campaign (1951-52), 23–24, 52
Three Gorges Dam basin, 247
tiao/kuai system, 47
toilets. *See* commode-washing; public
    toilets; pit toilets
Tomb-Sweeping Day *(qingmingjie),* 188
top leadership. *See* Chinese Communist
    Party; Ministry of Public Health; urban
    medical establishment
tracking systems. *See* forms and records
traditional culture and beliefs. *See also* feng
    shui; festivals and celebrations; science-
    superstition dyad: educational strategies
    and, 94, 98, 99–100; health campaigns
    in eradication of, 187–89; neophilia and,
    103–4; Party agenda and, 182–87,
    291n22; Party reinforcement of, 89,
    99–*100*; sanitation efforts and, 117;
    scientific mindset and, 102–8; treatment
    efforts and, 104, 152–53, 156–57
training methods. *See also* scientific knowl-
    edge: barefoot doctors and, 172–73, 227,
    289n108; for educators, 92; scientific
    tools and, 222, 223, 224–25
transparency. *See also* forms and records;
    model test sites; public presentations:
    local cadres and, 11, 209, 229, 241, 251;
    SARS campaign and, 251; scientific
    tools and, 209, 229, 241
treatment campaign, 246–47. *See also*
    barriers to treatment; caretaking needs;
    stool sampling; testing; wards; accom-
    plishments of, 167–76, *175*, 246–47, 252;
    coercive tactics and, 160, 195; Cultural

Revolution successes and, 167–76; cure
    rates and, 159–60; early incidences of
    snail fever and, 6; economic barriers
    and, 37, 61, 65, 67–70, 82, 104, 169, 170;
    evaluation in, 166–67; during famine
    period, 166–67; Mao's support of,
    33–34, 70, 73–74, 169–70; negative
    reactions and, 158–59; peer support for,
    108–10; priority populations and,
    169–70, 173; production activities and,
    66, 67–70; recordkeeping and, 214–15,
    216–17; sex bias and, 164–65; short-
    course regimens and, 159–60, 167, 170;
    treatment fees and, 69–70, 71–74
treatment facilities. *See* wards
Trotsky, Leon, 207–8

unfunded mandate, health campaign as.
    See also financing of campaign: eco-
    nomic sabotage tactics and, 65–67;
    villager problems with, 67–70
united clinics, 8, 23, 71, 267n52
universal testing, 171
urban medical establishment, 2, 27, 29–30,
    31, 37, 60, 71, 72, 171, 264n31, 288n98.
    See also professional physicians
urban study site. *See* Shanghai

vaccination campaigns, 97–98
villager participation. *See also* barriers to
    treatment; financing of campaign; mass
    mobilization; popular resistance; tradi-
    tional culture and beliefs: advanced
    producers' cooperatives and, 194–200;
    coercive strategies and, 111–12, 238–40;
    collectivization and, 32–33, 92, 105, 106,
    110–11, 194–200; famine period and,
    135–36; prevention activities and, 33,
    97–102, 110–11, 115 *(see also* popular
    resistance); role of activists in, 189–94;
    scientific mindsets and, 107–8; snail
    killing and, 128–35; success of campaign
    and, 10, 237–39

Wan Fengxin, 107
Wang, Jessica Ching-Sze, 206
wards: behavior in, 45, 155; campaign diver-
    sity and, 8; conditions in, 63, 71, 145,

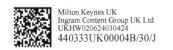

Milton Keynes UK
Ingram Content Group UK Ltd.
UKHW020624030424
440333UK00004B/30/J